Ecological Medicine

Herbal Antibiotics, revised and expanded second edition

Healing Lyme

*Healing Lyme Disease Coinfections: Complementary and
   Holistic Treatments for Bartonella and Mycoplasma*

Pine Pollen: Ancient Medicine for a New Millennium

Herbs for Hepatitis C and the Liver

The Natural Testosterone Plan

The Fasting Path

The Transformational Power of Fasting

Vital Man

Nonfiction

Ensouling Language

Gaia's Mind (in press)

The Secret Teachings of Plants

The Lost Language of Plants

Sacred Plant Medicine

One Spirit, Many Peoples

Sacred and Herbal Healing Beers

Poetry

*The Taste of Wild Water: Poems and Stories Found While
   Walking in Woods*

HERBAL ANTIVIRALS

NATURAL REMEDIES
FOR EMERGING RESISTANT AND EPIDEMIC VIRAL INFECTIONS

STEPHEN HARROD BUHNER

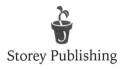

Storey Publishing

For Our Children

The mission of Storey Publishing is to serve our customers by publishing practical information that encourages personal independence in harmony with the environment.

Edited by Nancy Ringer
Art direction by Cynthia N. McFarland, based on a book design
    by Mary Winkelman Velgos
Text production by Tina Henderson, LLC
Front cover photography by © Arco Images GmbH/Alamy, top left; © luisapuccini/
    iStockphoto.com, top right; and © FrancoDeriu/iStockphoto.com, bottom
Indexed by Nancy D. Wood

This publication is intended to provide educational information for the reader on the covered subject. It is not intended to take the place of personalized medical counseling, diagnosis, and treatment from a trained health professional.

Storey Publishing
210 MASS MoCA Way
North Adams, MA 01247
www.storey.com

Printed in the United States by McNaughton & Gunn
10 9 8 7 6 5 4 3 2 1

Storey Publishing is committed to making environmentally responsible manufacturing decisions. This book was printed on paper made from sustainably harvested fiber.

Library of Congress Cataloging-in-Publication Data

Buhner, Stephen Harrod, author.
  Herbal antivirals / Stephen Harrod Buhner.
    p. ; cm.
  Includes bibliographical references and index.
  ISBN 978-1-61212-160-4 (pbk. : alk. paper)
  ISBN 978-1-61212-385-1 (ebook)
  I. Title.
  [DNLM: 1. Antiviral Agents. 2. Phytotherapy. 3. Plant Preparations—
    therapeutic use. 4. Virus Diseases—drug therapy. WB 925]
RM411
615.7'924—dc23
                    2013009932

CONTENTS

WHY THIS BOOK EXISTS

It serves little purpose merely to be scared by viruses. But it serves a good deal of purpose to understand them.
— **Frank Ryan, MD, *Virus X: Tracking the New Killer Plagues***

If you aren't skeptical about your skepticism, you aren't a skeptic.

For several decades now, I have been deeply interested in antibiotic resistance, the intelligence of bacteria, and the use of treatment approaches that are, ultimately, more elegant than pharmaceuticals. Plant-based medicines, unlike pharmaceuticals, don't cause resistance problems, they are much safer, *and* they are ecologically sound — they are biodegradable *and* renewable, which most pharmaceuticals are not.

My long-term interest in herbal antibacterials resulted, after a considerable time (and an early initial look at the topic), in a very deep exploration of systemic herbal antibacterials for resistant infections (*Herbal Antibiotics*, second edition, Storey Publishing, 2012). And during that exploration, many aspects of plant medicine not hitherto developed in the West began to reveal themselves (such as the importance of plant synergists).

This book is the beginning, for me, of a similar exploration into the world of viruses, emerging and resistant viral diseases, and more ecologically responsible (and often more effective) forms of treatment. In this book you will find information on some of the best broad-spectrum, systemic, antiviral herbs on Earth. As with herbal antibiotics, they are easy to use, easy to grow, and easy to make into medicines for yourself, your family, your patients. And they are very, very effective for emerging and resistant viral infections. For the plants themselves learned long ago, just as they did with bacteria, how to stop viruses from killing them. Plants can't run but they sure can do chemistry.

The concept of herbal antibiotics as primary interventives has, over the past several decades, become common in cultures outside the Western industrialized nations. Medical systems in Africa, Asia, and South and Central America are turning away from pharmaceuticals as a first-line treatment for bacterial infections because of resistance problems and, most especially, because pharmaceutical corporations make a great deal too much money off the suffering of their populations. Cultures other than those in the West have realized that they just can't afford corporate greed any longer — *and* they are unwilling to let the poorer members of their populations die because of it. Researchers in cultures across the globe have found that plant antibacterials are often *more* effective than pharmaceuticals. So they are exploring which ones are most potent, which forms of preparation are most effective, and how best to grow them. Then they are traveling throughout their regions (especially in Africa), giving seeds to local villages, teaching them all they have learned, and letting them get on with their healing. There is no middleman raking off profits in the process. A new model of health care is coming into being — and it's about time.

It is my hope that this same kind of movement will begin in the treatment of viral diseases. (And in China, they are already years ahead of us; they *see* the writing on the wall.) We need a new paradigm of healing. We need new ways of thinking about viruses, their emergence, and their treatment — just as we have needed them about bacteria. (Even in the herbal communities in the West, our approaches to viral infections and viruses have been extremely shallow.) There is a lot we can do to create a more effective healing paradigm in our world, one that is ecologically sustainable while at the same time being more human friendly ... if we step outside the box that our thinking has been trapped by.

I hope that you find the material in this book stimulating to your thinking. I hope that you begin, yourself, to add to this emerging paradigm of healing, one that is slowly extricating itself from the outmoded thinking of the past. We have a great opportunity to create something new, something that reflects more accurately the world around us, something that truly addresses the healing needs of the people who come to us.

I think the viruses are going to be pretty insistent that we do so. And soon.

1

EMERGING VIRUSES: WHAT WE ARE FACING

It is naive to think we can win.

— David Livermore, MD

Viral diseases, caused by pathogenic virus infections which have high morbidity and mortality rates, are still the leading cause of death in humans worldwide. . . . Moreover, the emergence of viral resistance to drugs, as well as the serious adverse effects induced by antiviral drugs, has caused serious medical problems, particularly when [the drugs are] administered in combination over prolonged treatment periods. . . . And these drugs are quite costly, thus limiting their use in developing countries, where infection is most prevalent.

— Kaio Kitazato et al., "Viral Infectious Disease and Natural Products with Antiviral Activity"

For much of the twentieth century, infectious diseases in human populations of Western countries have been in retreat, as we learnt to sanitize our cities, cleanse our water supplies, improve domestic hygiene, use antibiotics, control vector organisms and vaccinate. As a result the developed world became rather complacent, naively welcoming the false dawn of a life mostly free of infectious disease. Since the 1980s things have looked much less secure, however, with the emergence of many previously unrecognized infectious diseases, and the re-emergence of known infectious diseases that were thought to be under control. This trend has continued until the present time and many infectious pathogens, predominantly viruses, have been newly identified.

— Thijs Kuiken et al., "Emerging Viral Infections in a Rapidly Changing World"

During the summer of 2006 a hitherto little-known viral disease
swept across a large and diverse range of islands in the Indian Ocean.
On the island of Réunion 265,000 people became critically ill — out of
a population of 770,000. Very few of those infected were asymptomatic; the illness was, in nearly every case, severe. Health-care workers
and the island's hospital system were overwhelmed. Even if they had
not been, there was little they could do. So, they offered "supportive"
care. In other words, they watched. They waited. Either the person's
immune and bodily systems would fight it off, or they wouldn't. For
many, they didn't.

The virus soon jumped to India, where an estimated 1.3 million
people became ill. The culprit? A relatively little-known viral disease,
chikungunya fever.[1] The virus is known to medical science but not
well; it's not a common disease. But it had mutated. Later analysis
showed that the mutation had occurred sometime between the
spring and fall of 2005. Within 6 months it had become pandemic in
the region. By the end of 2006 over two million people had become
infected.

The disease is attended by severe joint pain (somewhat like dengue
fever). The ankles and wrists are the most impacted; conjunctivitis
and a rash often occur. The pain in the joints can last for weeks … or
months, and it is debilitating. There is no treatment and there is no
cure. The physicians recommended the use of acetominophen for the
pain. The cause of death for many of those who died? Liver damage …
from the acetominophen.

People visiting the region who traveled back to their homes in the
United States and Europe brought the disease with them. Over 1,000
in the United States were diagnosed with it; person-to-person trans-
mission occurred in a number of instances, infecting new hosts. Then,
luckily for most of us, the epidemic just … faded away.

The disease is primarily spread by mosquitoes (similarly to most of
the diseases discussed in this book), specifically *Aedes albopictus*. This
is a mosquito that was once limited in its geographical range but has,
in the past 50 years, spread to every continent on Earth.

This is an example of just how fast a new viral pathogen can spread in the global village. It began with an African virus entering an Asian mosquito that traveled with people by plane and boat to the Indian Ocean and India. And from there, it went everywhere. This same dynamic is now playing out everyplace on Earth. The chikungunya outbreak is not an uncommon event. West Nile encephalitis virus emerged in the United States in a large outbreak in 1999. It soon spread throughout the world and is now endemic in Europe and Asia. In the fall of 2002, SARS emerged in China and quickly spread throughout the pan-Asian region. The epidemiologists who studied the SARS outbreak discovered that it had initially emerged in a small region in China. The physician who attended the ill then visited Hong Kong, where he infected 16 people. Some of them traveled and in doing so spread the disease worldwide in a matter of weeks.

Then came swine flu and headlines like these:

Doctors shocked by spread of swine flu — and its severity

— Jeremy Lawrence, *The Independent*, December 22, 2010

460 flu victims fighting for life as experts admit 24 deaths from swine strain may be only a fraction of the true number

— Sophie Borland, *Mail Online*, December 24, 2010

Flu crisis hits cancer surgery: Hospitals struggle to cope as deaths rise and Britain teeters on the brink of an epidemic

— Sophie Borland, *Mail Online*, December 27, 2010

And only a year later, in the fall of 2011, a worldwide epidemic of dengue fever began in northern Africa. It soon spread to the Philippines and Puerto Rico, crossing the ocean in both directions. Finally it hit Brazil. By April of 2012 over 50,000 people had been admitted to hospitals in Brazil. Five hundred newly infected people were being admitted each week.

Viral diseases such as these are emerging in new and potent forms everyplace on Earth. There are few medical treatments for them if a reliable vaccine does not exist. And for most of them it does not.

Welcome to the twenty-first century.

But We Won . . . Didn't We?

When the first antibiotic, penicillin, came into common use in 1946 it was heralded as the beginning of the end for infectious diseases. And as each new antibiotic was discovered, and ever more diseases conquered, the voices proclaiming the end of infectious diseases grew louder. The success of antibiotics stimulated concerted medical assaults on epidemic viral diseases, primarily through the development and use of vaccines. The first widespread success was the polio vaccine.

Though it is not widely known, nearly everyone in a given region, when the polio virus spread to that area, became infected. It was, in fact, a very common virus with very few symptoms for most people. For over 90 percent there were no symptoms at all. Only about 8 percent or so had mild to moderate symptoms, generally a self-limited flu-like condition (which nearly every virus causes). But for about 1 percent of the population, the virus entered the nervous system and those people developed what most people think of as polio. It caused shrunken limbs or paralysis or even, for some, the loss of the capacity to breathe on their own. For those, the rest of life was lived encased in a shell that raised and lowered the chest mechanically.

Oddly enough, given the memories that some people still have of the disease — and the fear it engendered prior to the late twentieth century — it was relatively uncommon. Polio epidemics, as such, were unknown throughout most of human history. But by 1910 major epidemics of the disease began to sweep the world. It became the scourge of the industrialized nations.

The success of antibiotics after World War II combined with the deep public fear of the disease drove a powerful medical movement in the search for a cure. And as with most viral diseases, the focus was on a vaccine. It didn't take long. The Salk vaccine was discovered in 1955 and, after trials, in 1962 it was licensed for widespread use. Worldwide epidemics soon faded from memory, and infections declined from the millions to the hundreds of thousands, and by 2007 to a mere 1,652, almost all in Asia and Africa. It was a powerful success story and the belief that medical science could defeat all infectious diseases spread.

A 1963 comment by the Australian physician Sir F. Macfarlane Burnet, a Nobel laureate, is typical. By the end of the twentieth century, he said, humanity would see the "virtual elimination of infectious disease as a significant factor in societal life."[2] Seven years later, Surgeon General William Stewart testified to Congress that "it was time to close the book on infectious diseases."[3] And for a while, it seemed they might be right, for the next viral disease they attacked was smallpox.

Though they rarely get credit for it, it was Russian physicians in 1958 who began to press for a worldwide program to permanently eradicate smallpox. By 1967 the program was in full swing with some 250 million vaccinations occurring throughout the world each year. Within a decade, mostly due to the efforts of an American physician and epidemiologist, Donald Henderson, the last regions still endemic for the disease were cleared. And the world celebrated. For the first time a major human disease pathogen had been eradicated from the planet. (Though to be fair to the virus, both the Russians and the Americans kept just a little around, in case they needed it later — you know, for the kids.)

The triumph over smallpox was the apex of the success of the medical assault on microbial disease pathogens — though few knew it at the time. It was thought to be the beginning of the end for every disease pathogen on Earth. The hubris level, already immense by 1963, grew larger. If humans could defeat smallpox, they could defeat every virus on Earth. The word spread; the newspapers were filled with optimistic scenarios of a future without disease. Researchers were quoted extensively (as they still are) as saying that, soon, in just a few years, none of us would die from infectious diseases. Most people in the industrialized world accepted this at face value . . . as they still do. It is, regrettably, part of the utopian future-myth of science (especially medical science) that many people take for granted. But it never has, and never has had, much to do with reality. As physician and researcher Frank Ryan comments, "Perhaps it reflected, in part, a regrettable separation of clinicians from basic scientists."

> In fact those people whose living depended upon a study of microbes, of their potential and durability, were never deluded. A prescient few, such as René' Dubos, warned us openly that the optimism was unjustified. But on the whole people were not inclined to listen. Most doctors, never mind members of the public, were infected with the prevailing overconfidence, hardly perceiving the growing threat of social changes to the "global village." They seemed unable to grasp the new potential afforded to a very ancient peril arising from world travel.... Today, as one after another of the dismissed plagues returns to haunt us, as new plagues every bit as deadly as anything seen in previous history threatens our species, it is obvious that the postwar years were an age of delusion. It was comforting, a very understandable delusion, but a delusion nonetheless.[4]

As it happens, the scientific and medical beliefs about the Earth and its interrelated life forms, including bacteria and viruses, that have been widely spread are not very accurate. Lynn Margulis and Dorion Sagan, in their book *What Is Life?*, note that once "the germ theory of contagion finally caught on, it did so with a vengeance. Different types of bacteria were implicated in anthrax, gonorrhea, typhoid, and leprosy. Microbes, once amusing little anomalies, became demonized.... [They] became a virulent 'other' to be destroyed."[5] But there are many problems with this belief about microbes. Two stand out for me. The first comes from the particular medical paradigm in use in the West and the second from a very inaccurate, outmoded nineteenth-/early-twentieth-century view of nature.

The medical paradigm problem is simple enough, though it's rarely recognized for the problem it is. Specifically: Most physicians and medical researchers commonly speak of the "cause of death" when speaking of mortality. The assumption, deeply embedded within that communication, is that the bacteria or virus (or heart disease or stroke) caused the death. Even deeper is the communication that if all "causes" of death were defeated, then there would be no more death. As Harvard researcher and zoologist Richard Lewontin puts it, "The claims made by medicine imply this possibility without explicitly stating it. Medical scientists speak of 'preventing' deaths by curing disease, but the evidence is that death cannot be prevented, only post-poned at best. Moreover, the postponement has not been as effective as is sometimes claimed during the last fifty years of great progress in physiology, cell biology, and medicine.... [The truth is] that although the proximate causes of death can be dealt with, death itself cannot. So, there must be a cause of death as a *phenomenon*, as distinct from the individual cases."[6] In other words, if *every* "cause" of death were removed, in spite of what physicians (and news reports) say, there would still be death. Death is inherent in this place. The unstated and deeply buried assertion that microbes "cause" death is not only false, it stimulates people to view microbes as enemies, as participants in a war against us — and this is very far from the truth.

Bacteria and viruses are not a "virulent other." They are, instead, intimately interwoven into the underpinnings of life on this planet. They cannot be killed off without killing off every form of life on Earth. This is the great error of the nineteenth-/early-twentieth-century view of nature that continues to plague us. Or, as Lynn Margulis once put it, "The more balanced view of microbe as colleague and ancestor remains almost unexpressed. Our culture ignores the hard-won fact that these disease 'agents,' these 'germs,' also germinated all life."[7] We are, counterintuitively and most upsettingly, only a form of bacteria ourselves — in extremely elegant, symbiogenic, innovative shapes. Bacteria are the foundation of every life form on this planet. Had bacteria not developed resistance to antibiotics all life on this planet would have already become extinct simply from the millions of tons of antibiotics now present in the environment.

With bacteria the paradigm problem is bad enough, but when viruses enter the picture, the complexity rises by orders of magnitude. Viruses are not and never have been parasites, though they may act as or seem to be parasites when we fall sick with one. They, in fact, perform highly elegant ecosystem functions — as everything on this planet does. Viruses, as Frank Ryan comments, "weave in and out of

11

the genomes of every form of life on earth. As a result, terrestrial life [has] become a dense web of genetic interactions."[8]

DNA is not, and never has been, a computer program (and neither is RNA). It is, as Nobel Prize winner Barbara McClintock once noted, a living organ of the cell. DNA and RNA are both similar structures and they are deeply interactive with the world around them. DNA is a double-stranded molecule, RNA is single-stranded, but both of them are intimately involved in the structural formation of life forms. DNA contains information about the genetic development of living organisms. RNA is a messenger molecule used to carry genetic information that directs, in part, the synthesis of proteins, proteins that are needed for the structural formation of organisms. But again, these nucleic acids are not fixed in form. They change. We live in the midst of constant genetic rearrangements. And these gene rearrangements occur not only in response to impulses within the organism but also, as Barbara McClintock observed, to communications from the environment around it.

There is, in fact, no discrete inside and outside, no "us" and "them," even though it seems (within our nineteenth-century paradigm) that there is. The life forms on this planet are living organisms and that means they possess soft boundaries, *very* soft boundaries. There is a constant exchange (of energy, for example) between the inside and outside in all living systems. But to be more direct there is a constant inflow and outflow of life through those soft boundaries. The nature of the ecological reality of this world demands it.

As Richard Lewontin observes,

> Even virus particles, which do not metabolize energy, can reproduce only when they become integrated into the metabolic apparatus of the cells they infect. At the time of viral replication, there is a complete abolition of the previously existing boundary between the virus and its cellular environment.... Organisms do not find already existent ecological niches to which they adapt, but are in the constant process of defining and remaking their environments. At every moment natural selection is operating to change the genetic composition of populations in response to the momentary environment, but as that composition changes it forces a concomitant change in the environment

itself. Thus organism and environment are both causes and effects in a coevo-
lutionary process. . . . Small changes in environment lead to small changes in
the organism which, in turn, lead to small changes in the environment. . . . In
general the organism and the environment must track each other continuously or life would long ago have become extinct.[9]

Specifically, viruses have the capacity to enter cells, snip off
sections of DNA (or RNA), and weave them into their own genetic
structure. They can then weave those sections, as well as sections
of their own genome, into other living organisms. One of their main
functions in fact is the genetic intermingling of all life forms on Earth.
Or as Frank Ryan puts it, "Viruses are vehicles for genetic exchange
between the disparate species that make up the matrix of life on
earth."[10] Our genome, as that of all life on this planet, contains snippets of the genetic codes of multiple other life forms. It also contains
snippets of viral genes. Our forms, our shapes, are an expression of a
communication that has been ongoing since life has been. We *are* the
enemy we have been fighting.

In short, the perspectives of most scientists at the beginning of the
antibiotic era were limited, more limited than even the most prescient
knew. And the view of the world that they disseminated was deeply
flawed. Viruses are deeply interwoven into the ecological matrix of
this planet and they serve functions that are essential. Further, they
are extremely adaptable. They can alter their structure very rapidly
and take on new forms seemingly at will. All based on their analysis
of the environment that surrounds them. They are highly intelligent.
They are not in fact stupid. But we certainly were (and are) when we
thought them so.

The paradigm of medicine that emerged in the twentieth century
was wrong and we are now paying the price for applying it so compre-
hensively. We now face the emergence of epidemics more devastating
than any known before. If *we* are to adapt, we have to see with different
eyes, understand through a different paradigm. We have to realize that
viruses are not what we thought them to be. We have to learn to see
them as they are.

Viruses

To begin with, if you have ever read much about viruses, or if you have looked closely at some of the words I have used while writing this, you might have noted that many people refer to viruses as "particles." There is a widely held belief among scientists that viruses are not alive. Many insist that they are merely organic structures that interact with living organisms. Some say they are "organisms at the edge of life" but really aren't organisms in any meaningful sense. This is, they say, because they lack a cellular structure, don't have their own metabolism, and can only reproduce *inside* cellular structures — and besides they don't use cellular division to do it either. If asked where the definition of life comes from, a definition that precludes viruses, biologists will admit, under duress, that people invented the definition but nevertheless, it's true anyway. (This explains why manufacturers put a warning label on those sun shields people occasionally place in the front windows of their cars to protect the interior from the sun: "Warning: do not drive with shield in place.")

Oddly enough some bacteria such as rickettsia and chlamydia are considered bacteria and thus living despite having similar limitations. (And the Earth is not alive, though it may "act" like a living system. Why? Because it consumes its own waste, which, as everyone knows, living organisms *never* do ... apparently they have not met my neighbor's dog.)

There are a lot of viruses on this planet. Estimates are that the Earth contains 10^{31} viruses, that is, a 10 with 31 zeros after it. Technically (for wonks) that is somewhere between a nonillion and a decillion (though if you just say bajillion you are close enough). Essentially — a whole lot. And there are multitudes of different kinds. In every 200 liters of water (about 50 gallons or the contents of a typical hot water tank) some 5,000 different viral genotypes are present. There are viruses in the coldest, most inhospitable parts of this planet and viruses inside boiling hot springs. There are viruses high in the atmosphere and in the deepest wells on Earth. They live on top of moun-

14

tains and in the furthest depths of the ocean. And, sometimes, they even travel into space. They are a part of life on this planet; there is no avoiding them.

Viruses, unlike bacteria, have no nucleus and no cell wall. They are the minimum of life honed to a structural simplicity. Though there are many kinds, in general, a virus is a strand of DNA or RNA surrounded by a mathematically elegant polyhedron, called a capsid, whose shape is virus specific. For what are called "enveloped" viruses, the capsid is surrounded by one or more protein envelopes. This simplified structure makes them different than bacteria, for example, but no less alive. They *are* a unique life form (but that is no reason to discriminate against them). They are very much like seeds (or spores): They only grow when they find the right soil in which to do so. And like seeds, even though in a suspended state, they constantly monitor the exterior world around them.

The surface of the viral protein envelope is studded with receptors, specific kinds of sensory organs that tell viruses about their surroundings. Viruses use these elegant sensory organs to analyze the environment in which they find themselves and to help them find the cells they are most suited for. As physician and researcher Frank Ryan comments,

> Viruses have a kind of sensation that could be classed as intermediate between a rudimentary smell or touch. . . . They have a way of detecting the chemical composition of cell surfaces. . . . This gives a virus the most exquisite ability to sense the right cell surfaces [allowing it to find its unique host cell]. It recognizes them through a perception in three-dimensional surface chemistry.[11]

Viruses have a highly sophisticated capacity to sense the environment around them, to determine its nature, to find the cellular organisms within which they can most easily reproduce, and to then stimulate the organisms in which those cells reside in order to spread the viruses to new hosts. And they are very good at surviving. They can analyze the nature of the immune response that occurs against them and they can alter themselves — or alter the host immune defense itself — in order to avoid it. They can *reason* by any useful definition of the term, that is: analyze inputs and create new behaviors based on what they have determined the meaning of those inputs to be.

Viruses are typed in a number of ways: by size or shape, presence or absence of an enclosing capsule (not all have one), whether DNA or RNA based (and from that whether single or double stranded, positive or negative sense), their type of protein structure, and their manner of replication. DNA viruses are fairly reliable as viruses go because they have a kind of "copy-check" mechanism that RNA viruses lack. This means that when a DNA virus is making more of itself within a host cell, it uses a biofeedback loop to make sure the copies of itself are reasonably accurate. In contrast an RNA virus can't. It tends to make a whole lot of copies that vary, sometimes a great deal, from the original. Some of these copy differences are initiated intentionally by RNA viruses to increase their genetic variation and, hence, survivability in the host. Because of this, while it is often possible to come up with a lasting vaccine for a DNA virus, it is very hard, if not impossible, to make one for an RNA virus. This also makes RNA viruses very hard to treat with pharmaceuticals; they, like bacteria, begin creating solutions to synthetic drugs the moment they encounter one. Evidence indicates that the mutation rate of the hepatitis C virus, for example, accelerates in response to interferon and ribavirin therapy in much the same way that bacterial alteration occurs in the presence of antibiotics. Infection with an RNA virus like West Nile or Japanese encephalitis is actually quite different than infection with a DNA virus.

> We live in an era of rapidly changing global landscapes and local environments. Viruses with RNA as their genetic material can quickly adapt to and exploit these varying conditions. . . . It comes as no surprise, then, that several prominent recent examples of emerging or re-emerging viruses are caused by RNA viruses.
>
> — *Stuart Nichol et al.,* "Emerging Viral Diseases"

While DNA viruses make billions more of themselves, RNA viruses make billions of similar but not identical viruses. It is something like a swarm of honeybees — all similar but all different. In fact it is much more accurate to think of an RNA infection as infection by a viral swarm. The ones most similar to each other are the ones that die off when the human immune system is first activated or a pharmaceutical drug that can recognize them is used. This leaves the others free to multiply unchecked and they multiply very fast indeed (some viruses producing a new generation every *minute*) while still making subtle changes in each new virus produced.

There is also evidence that both DNA and RNA viruses, like bacteria, share information among themselves in order to remain unaffected by medical treatments or immune systems. Similar viruses will actively share genetic structure to create very difficult-to-treat infections. Influenza viruses (for instance) specifically (and intentionally) both rearrange their genetic structures and insert entirely new genes within themselves on a regular basis in order to remain invisible to the human immune system. And they gather these new gene sequences from pigs and birds in Asia. This is why a new vaccine is needed every year for the flu.

Viruses, when not in a living cell, go into a state of hibernation much like plant seeds. In this state of dormancy they move with air currents, in water, or simply rest dormant on the ground until they come into contact with a life form that contains the cells they need to awaken from their long sleep. At that moment a virus's first task is to get inside the new host organism, bypass its protective mechanisms, and find the proper host cell. Viruses use highly elegant analysis to address these challenges; they actually begin experimenting with new combinations of genes to adapt to the environment they face. Most of them have also generated a genetic structure that facilitates their entry into other host organisms after an initial infection begins. The rabies virus, for instance, affects a part of the brain that then causes uncontrolled biting. At the same time, the virus swarms in its billions into the saliva of infected animals. Then, every time the animal bites something the virus is transmitted to a new host. Influenza, and other respiratory viruses, enter respiratory droplets and then stimulate coughing or sneezing. Those droplets are then breathed in by new hosts. And still other viruses, spread by mosquitoes, flood into the blood and there stimulate the release of chemicals through the host skin surface that calls mosquitoes to the infected host so that the virus can be picked up and spread to others. Viruses are very good at getting from *here* to *there*.

Viruses spread by ticks or mosquitoes take advantage of the compounds in the arthropod saliva to facilitate their entry into the new host. The salival compounds reduce certain immune responses in the host to allow the arthropod to feed and often anesthetize the bite location as well. The lowered immune responses at that location allow the viruses to enter the new host in a place where there will be little resistance. Once inside the viruses will make their way to the draining lymph node nearest the bite location and be carried to the spleen via the lymph. There they will begin altering the host's immune function, reducing the capacity of immune cells to recognize and kill invading microbes. Once that occurs, the viruses will catch a ride on immune cells, macrophages or monocytes usually, and begin spreading throughout the body. This is common for encephalitis viruses, for example. They will then travel in the lymph to the barrier between the brain and the rest of the body, release compounds that make the barrier more porous, enter the brain, and find the cells they really prefer: brain neurons.

Other viruses enter through being inhaled (influenza) or through sex (HIV) or through being eaten on food (enteroviruses). Once in the body, they hitch rides on whatever cells they have developed a taste for (usually immune cells, for those cells travel *everywhere*) and actively seek out their preferred location. Such is the case with HIV, which views T4 lymphocytes as the perfect host cells, or the Epstein-Barr virus, which has an affinity for human B cells, or the Japanese encephalitis virus, which loves monocytes.

To hitch rides, a virus uses chemotactic compounds that allow it to stick to its preferred "taxi" cell. The receptors on the surface of the virus fool the cell into thinking it is a compatible protein that has attached, and through a series of chemical communications, the virus gets the cell to let it inside. Basically, it gets the cell's confidence, then abuses it. From there the virus is carried everyplace it might need to go in the body. Once near its preferred location, it leaves its ride, attaches to the cell that is most specific for it, and once again fools the cell into taking it inside. Now it begins to replicate in its millions.

Once inside the primary habitat cell, the virus sheds its protein coat and begins taking over the cell. First it stops the cell from dying, which infected cells are programmed to do, and there it remains, protected from the rest of the immune system. It then breaks off pieces of itself and sends them into the nucleus of the cell, which is then tricked into making copies of the virus, using the viral proteins as a template. These new viral particles exit the nucleus, travel to the interior of the cell wall, and bubble out (viral budding, they call it). The cell dies during this process and bursts apart, and the viruses take up parts of the cell membrane and make themselves new viral protein coats with receptors for new host cells. And it all happens very quickly.

Thus the ancient struggle begins: finding out which is in better shape — the organism's immune system or the replicating virus. If the virus is particularly strong or if the immune system is compromised

> **The present period of unprecedented ecological change and the growing economic and social crises that are driving vast movements of hosts are together contributing to the resurgence of old pests and the appearance of new ones. Important components in this rapid evolution are the vulnerabilities of ecosystems and instabilities in climate.**
>
> — *Paul Epstein,*
> "Emerging Diseases and Ecosystem Instability: New Threats to Public Health"

in any way, the virus can really take hold and illness, sometimes severe illness, is inevitable.

Emerging Pathogenic Viruses

Similarly to antibiotic-resistant bacteria, many of the viruses long thought conquered are making comebacks. They are doing this through genetic rearrangements, through learned resistance to antivirals, and, most of all, because of changes in the world in which all of us live. And those changes are profound.

Here are some of the major alterations affecting the planet that researchers have identified as being behind the emergence of so many new (and old) pathogenic viruses. There is no place on the planet that has escaped them.

- **Demographic changes:** human population and refugee increases, accelerated mobility, worldwide urbanization, increasing population density in confined spaces such as inner cities and prisons
- **Medical care and technology:** medical-related infections in hospitals, concentrated microbial intermingling in hospitals and nursing homes, blood transfusions, organ transplantation, reuse of medical equipment, pharmaceutical contaminants, viral and antibiotic resistance
- **Economic and commercial trends:** overly extensive industrial agriculture with the resultant damage of ecosystem homeodynamis; worldwide disbursement of commercial food animals, food plants, and agricultural pharmaceuticals
- **Ecosystem disturbance:** deforestation, waterway disturbances, reduction in predator populations, destruction of wild plant populations
- **Climatic changes:** disruptions in climate homeodynamis by anthropogenic factors such as global warming, CO_2 increases, and pollutant gases

Viruses have lived for millions of years in balance with their host species (such as wild bee or buffalo populations). The disruption of healthy ecosystems by human incursions and the resultant loss of host species and their habitats stimulates viruses to jump species. And one of the species into which they jump is us (or the animals that survive well with us: pigeons, mice, pigs, and chickens — from whom they then easily move into us). After all, there are a lot more of *us* now (and our food animals) than any other large life form; we aren't that hard to find. As a matter of fact many of us live in the same places the viruses' former hosts did. And a home is a home. Our bodies are not all that different from the other animals on this planet. It is a simple adjustment for the viruses to make *us* their new hosts.

Some of the most common emerging, resistant, or newly virulent viruses are dengue virus (which infects millions worldwide every year), hepatitis C, enterovirus 71, HIV, and the eight members of the herpes family that affect humans, including cytomegalovirus and Epstein-Barr virus. But by far the ones that are causing the most worldwide concern (outside HIV) are the influenza and encephalitis viruses.

Influenza, which often seems a somewhat mild disease in many people's minds, just another "case of the flu," is actually a very potent viral pathogen. Epidemiologists have been warning, with increasing insistence, that a worldwide pandemic similar to the one that covered the globe in 1918, a pandemic that infected over 500 million people and caused some 100 million deaths, is due soon. Our factory farms (in whose pigs and chickens the viruses increase their virulence), our growing populations, the hubris and outdated nature of our medical system, and the intelligence of viruses make it certain that a pandemic strain will emerge again. It is only a matter of time. As Robert Heinlein once said, "Population problems have a horrible way of solving themselves."

The viruses are learning. We should, too.

2

VIRAL RESPIRATORY INFECTIONS AND THEIR TREATMENT

Persistent host-specific viral agents are the origin of emerging acute epidemic disease following adaptation of that virus to new host species. . . . These acute viruses have a high dependence on host population structure as described by the apparently accurate mathematical models that resemble predator-prey dynamics in which the viruses act as predators on their host prey. . . . Acute human influenza A represents a host species jump of a persisting viral agent of aquatic birds.

— **Luis Villarreal et al., "Acute and Persistent Viral Life Strategies and Their Relationship to Emerging Diseases"**

The major animal reservoirs of Influenza A are migratory birds and the majority of all the possible combinations of HA-NA subtypes have been isolated from them.

— **Andrew Pekosz and Gregory Glass, "Emerging Viral Diseases"**

Most of us think of the flu as a fairly minor disease, and for most of us it is. At worst we lie in bed for a week or so, feeling miserable. But for the old and the very young the flu can be deadly; it kills those with the weakest or least developed immune systems, some 30,000 people a year in the United States. But sometimes a real pandemic happens and the death rate rises. It has never risen more than it did in 1918.

The 1918 world influenza pandemic is the most deadly plague that human beings have *ever* experienced. It began in 1918, just as war was drawing to a close, and lasted until December of 1920. World War I (which ended in 1918) killed some 17 million people. In contrast, the influenza pandemic, spread around the world by returning soldiers, killed six times as many in half the time — perhaps as many as 130 million people. The first wave of the pandemic began in January of 1918 and it was fairly routine. People became ill but only the very old and very young died; it was, so far, a pretty typical flu. But the virus soon mutated. And the second wave? It was deadly. It killed those with the strongest immune systems. Half of those who died were between the ages of 20 and 40; nearly all were under age 65. And it killed them by the millions.

Instead of the usual respiratory infection, with death occurring as the lungs filled with fluid, massive hemorrhages took place. The infected lung cells, and those nearby, damaged by the virus-stimulated cytokine storm (see page 29 for more on cytokines), literally burst open from the inflammation. And unlike most viral influenzas this one did not stay confined to the respiratory system. It spread to the GI tract, the brain, and every mucous membrane system in the body. First it destroyed the infected mucosal epithelial cells, then the blood vessels that fed them inflamed and burst open. Bleeding was extensive from the nose, stomach, and intestines; hemorrhages from the skin and ears were common. The infected literally bled out. And nothing physicians tried would stop it.[1]

To understand the impact, consider the fact that, in a world reeling from war, *one-third* of the entire world's population contracted the disease — over 500 million people. In some places half the population was bedridden. As troops demobilized, the ships returning them home from war stopped at hundreds of ports along the way, and the infection spread across the globe. On the islands of Western Samoa 90 percent of the population fell ill — *simultaneously*. Thirty percent of the men, 22 percent of the women, and 10 percent of the children died.

In an attempt to stop the infection, port quarantines were put into effect around the world. Most were too late to do any good. One out of every three persons on Earth fell ill. One out of every five of those died. Five percent of the total world population — one out of every 20 people — did not survive the pandemic. Within the first 6 months 25 million people died, more than were killed in 5 years of war. Entire towns and cities were shut down.

There were few professionals to help the sick. Doctors and nurses were the first responders and they succumbed immediately. (The morticians followed soon after.) The infected filled the hospitals, school gymnasiums, auditoriums — every large building that could hold masses of people was pressed into service. The beds and the floors were awash in blood as the people died . . . and hemorrhaged by the hundreds and the thousands while doing it. And the bodies piled up. Steam shovels were brought in and mass graves dug — row after row after row of identically sized holes stretching across empty fields in a terrible mockery of industrial expediency. Then the trucks came, the bodies piled high on the wooden beds, and the masked workers dropped them in, hour by hour, day by day, month after month. And behind them, the steam shovels covered them over . . . one by one, day by day, for the 2 terrible years of the pandemic. There were few coffins and often no headstones. The system was completely overwhelmed. Not even a full century of the Black Plague had killed like this. In the history of human habitation of Earth, never had a disease spread so quickly around the world nor killed so many in so short a time. Only one place on Earth reported *no* infections: the tiny island of Marajó near Brazil in South America. And then, as inexplicably as it had begun, in a 1-month period of time, between November and December of 1920, the pandemic ended, simultaneously, around the globe.

Much effort has been expended in recent years in an attempt to understand what made that particular influenza strain so much more deadly than all the others people have known. It turns out that there were two interrelated events that came together in just the right way at just the right time in a terrible serendipity of the universe. From that intermingling came the worst pandemic the human species has ever experienced.

The first event was the emergence of a new strain of influenza at just the right time in human history. An analysis of the viral genome from 1918 has revealed that a new influenza strain had jumped species (from birds) just prior to 1913. By 1915 the virus had split into two types: one infecting pigs, the other humans. The second event was the war itself, which began with perfect timing in 1914.

Normally, when people fall ill with the flu, they go home and rest. The soldiers could not and the new influenza strain rapidly spread throughout the troops on both sides of the conflict. Constrained in cramped, unhealthy conditions, in hospital tents and in trenches, the soldiers were a perfect breeding ground for the virus. And sometime between 1915 and late 1917 the virus mutated again, this time into a form that could powerfully infect just that kind of population: the young. Then, the war over, the soldiers, millions of whom were infected, were crowded together in ships (there was no air travel then) that sailed from port to port to port, infecting as they went. Once home port was reached, the soldiers took trains, buses, and cars to their individual towns and cities. And the virus went with them, infecting everyone.

Re-created forms of the strain, patiently assembled in laboratories, when given to primates, have been found to generate the same symptoms as those described, in depth, by the physicians who treated the 1918 pandemic. An analysis of the physiological damage that occurs found that the reason the disease is so severe is that the virus creates a tremendously potent cytokine cascade in the body — a cytokine storm. A perfect storm. These cytokines are immunoregulatory proteins stimulated by the body's innate immune system in response to infection. The cytokine cascade is how the body attempts to kill off the invading pathogen. But this was much more than the usual immune response. The immune reaction was extreme, somewhere between 100 and 1,000 times what would be normal in those who were infected. And that overreaction, much more pronounced in those with strong immune systems, is what killed so many so quickly.

It is just this kind of influenza pandemic that epidemiologists and viral researchers fear will emerge once more. Given the current population density (and the crowding in prisons, nursing homes, hospitals, day care centers, and inner cities), the ecological disruptions that are occurring worldwide, the number of viruses that are jumping species, the rate of mutation, *and* the vast and very rapid movement of people via air travel, they say it is only a matter of time. And in spite of the many advances in medical technology, there is very little that modern medicine can do to treat a widespread pandemic of deadly influenza. Pharmaceutical antivirals are only partially effective for this kind of infection and the stocks of those antivirals are insufficient to deal with a true pandemic. And vaccines? Vaccines take time.

Flu vaccines have to be made for the specific virus that emerges *in that year*. This means that the disease will already be moving throughout the world before production even begins. And if it is a true pandemic of a deadly strain, by the time the vaccine is produced and shipped (normally a 3- to 6-month process), the infrastructure of the world will already be failing. The health-care workers, hospitals, and transportation workers will be the first to fall. Then the morticians and cemetery workers. The system will begin to shut down. Quarantines, forcing people to stay in their homes, will be put into effect to try and stop the spread. And people will survive as best they can, just as they always have.

The Influenza Virus

The influenza virus is a member of the Orthomyxoviridae family. It is an RNA virus and that means it alters its genetic structure very quickly. That is why a new flu shot is needed every year (for those in the Western world who have such things available). The old vaccine can only help prevent infection by the strain that has emerged in that particular year. The next year, it is not the same virus, merely a similar one. Influenza viruses spread around the world every year in seasonal epidemics; 250,000 to 500,000 people die from them each time.

About one-third of people who are infected remain asymptomatic; the rest get some degree of the "flu." The first symptoms are usually a feeling of being cold or achy and perhaps the beginnings of a fever. High fever alternating with severe chills sets in as the infection spreads. As the virus enters the lungs and sinus tissues mucous congestion begins. Coughing, body aches, fatigue, headache, and irritated eyes, nose, and throat are common. Some people will have diarrhea and abdominal pain. Vomiting. Sometimes. Yes.

The symptoms of the infection usually begin the third day after infection. But the virus is already well established by then. It starts replicating the second day, then begins "shedding" viral particles that are released in increasing numbers for the next 5 to 7 days. The higher the fever, the more viral organisms that are being released. Children are *extremely* infectious compared to adults, with very high viral loads. They also tend to have very high fevers.

As the virus invades the lungs it stimulates inflammation in the tissues. The lung cells, filled with viruses, soon bulge outward and explode — the essence of viral shedding. Then the virus stimulates coughing, spreading the virus to new hosts via respiratory droplets. Pneumonia, a severe inflammation of the lungs accompanied by massive fluid retention and an inability to breathe, is the main cause of death. People, in essence, drown.

There are three different groups of influenza viruses, denoted A, B, and C. Influenza A is the most virulent. Influenza B is a relatively stable virus and mutates much more slowly than A. Most people develop, in childhood, at least some immunity to it; it is much less dangerous. Influenza C is fairly rare. It does infect people, sometimes severely, but it usually causes only a mild illness, generally in children. When people talk about an influenza pandemic, what they are talking about is influenza A in one of its many genetically altered forms. The 1918 pandemic was caused by an influenza A strain.

There have been numerous pandemics of influenza over the years, each caused by a different strain of the virus. The one in 1918 was the beginning of the modern influenza pandemic era; such pandemics were much less common before then. There was a long rest after 1918. Since 1957, however, they have been occurring with greater frequency.

The most dangerous strains, currently, are H1N1, which caused the flu pandemic of 1918; H2N2, which caused the Asian flu pandemic in 1957; H3N2, which caused the Hong Kong flu pandemic in 1968; and a relatively new one, H5N1, known as avian or bird flu, which caused a pandemic in 2004. Then H1N1 came again. It was the source of the swine flu pandemic in 2009 and is a modified descendant of the 1918 H1N1 strain.

The influenza virus alters its genetic structure rather significantly every year by passing through both pigs and birds. And on that trip it exchanges genetic material with other viruses and reworks its own. Then it spreads around the world again by plane and boat, rail and car, infecting millions, causing what we call the yearly flu season. But every so often it develops a much more virulent strain, sometimes through unique genetic rearrangements, sometimes through species jumps, sometimes through both. The Asian flu pandemic in 2004 was a species jump. The swine flu epidemic of 2009 was a unique genetic rearrangement. It occurred when the virus took advantage of giant agribusiness animal crowding.

Viral geneticists have traced the lineage of the 2009 swine flu epidemic, a virulent H1N1 strain, to an H3N2 strain that emerged in 1998 in U.S. factory farms, specifically huge hog farms in which the animals are so tightly packed together that they literally cannot move. This H3N2 strain combined with another swine strain, a European H1N2 variant, rearranged genetic material into a new and very potent H1N1 form, and then emerged into the human population. The earliest infections occurred in La Gloria, Veracruz, Mexico, just adjacent to a huge hog farm. The workers became infected with the new strain, went home, infected others, many of whom traveled to other cities and towns, and the pandemic began. And it was particularly deadly for those who were infected. Among those hospitalized, depending on location, up to 31 percent were in intensive care units, and as many as 46 percent of those receiving intensive care died.

One of the main fears that epidemiologists and viral geneticists have is the possibility of a combined swine and avian flu strain. The crowding of human food animals, similar to the crowding of soldiers in trenches in World War I, continually allows for the emergence of potently virulent strains. Chicken farms, in which unique avian flu strains can emerge, and hog farms, in which unique swine strains can emerge, are perfectly positioned to allow the combination of the two into one potent, and very deadly, influenza strain. This kind of combined strain can then pass easily into farm workers and thence into the population at large.

Researchers have found that, indeed, the H3N2 swine flu virus easily combines with H5N1 strains of avian flu. When that occurs, a tremendously pathogenic form of the virus emerges. It is, they insist, only a matter of time until it occurs on its own. In fact, studies of pigs on large farms adjacent to poultry farms have found such viral combinations already infecting pigs. That combined viral strain has not infected people ... yet.

Infection Dynamics and the Cytokine Cascade

Cytokines are physiological signaling molecules produced by the body for a variety of reasons. They are produced in the largest numbers during infections. Cytokines (and their cousins, chemokines) are generally part of the innate (rather than the adapted) immune system. They are intended to respond to incursions into our bodies by viruses and bacteria. Another way to think of them is as inflammatory molecules. They cause various sorts of inflammation in the body — they are why, when you cut yourself, the wound gets red and tender and swells. The cytokines rushing to the area create conditions in which many bacteria and viruses find it difficult to survive. Unfortunately for us, bacteria and viruses have also learned how to use our own immune responses for their purposes. They subvert them, quite often, to facilitate their infection of the body *and* their destruction of certain areas of the body. This facilitates their reproduction and allows them to gather nutrients. Influenza viruses love the lungs and it is where they cause the greatest damage.

Unlike encephalitis viruses, which love brain neurons but have to find their way to the brain after being injected into people by mosquitoes, influenza viruses don't have to work nearly so hard. They are taken to the location they like best simply because we need to breathe.

Once inhaled, the viruses begin attaching to lung epithelial cells. They use a kind of agglutinin (a substance that glues things to itself — its name shares a root with the English word "glue"), a hemagglutinin, to bind to what are called sialic acid linkages on the surface of airway epithelial cells. (This is one mechanism by which plants such as Chinese skullcap and ginger stop influenza infections; they are hemagglutinin inhibitors.) All viruses do this in their own way; they have an affinity for a unique receptor on the surface of specific cells and in one way or another they get to that location and those particular cells. Once there, they attach to that part of the cells. In a sense they use that part of the host cells' membrane as a docking port.

As soon as it is attached to a cell, the virus begins to alter the permeability of the cell wall, inducing alterations in the cell's cytoskeleton and initiating endocytosis. In other words, it makes the cell surface more soft, causes the skeletal structure of the cell to bend apart, and tricks the cell into taking the virus inside it where it can't be found by the immune system. It does this by using a particular kind of enzyme, neuraminidase — which is sometimes also called a sialidase because such enzymes catalyze, or break apart, the sialic acid linkages on the host cell surface. This is why neuraminidase inhibitors (such as Tamiflu, i.e., oseltamivir) are effective in the treatment of influenza; they inhibit the ability of the virus to enter host cells. This stops the infection. (Chinese skullcap, elder, licorice, rhodiola, ginger, isatis, *Lespedeza bicolor*, *Angelica keiskei*, *Amorpha fruticosa*, quercetin, *Alpinia zerumbet*, *Erythrina addisoniae*, and *Cleistocalyx operculatus* are all neuraminidase inhibitors.) Neuraminidase inhibitors are effective against both influenza A and B strains.

During the process of endocytosis, the virus stimulates the cell to create what is called a vacuole, essentially a sealed bubble that will be held inside the cell. Cells do this to sequester substances that can damage them. Microbes have learned to use such vacuoles for their own purposes, usually to protect the virus or bacteria from intracellular antimicrobial actions.

The virus uses its hemagglutinin to bind itself to the inside of the vacuole membrane, where it opens a pore to the cell's cytoplasm, i.e., its interior spaces. To do this the virus uses what is called the M2 ion channel — ion channels are tiny pores in cells that allow charged molecules to enter and exit cells, bringing food in and allowing waste out. Using an M2 inhibitor blocks this process and literally stops the virus from replicating. (Lomatium is one of the most potent M2 inhibitors known, stronger than the pharmaceutical amantadine.) Use of the M2 channel is specific to the influenza A virus, which is why the development of blockers for it was considered crucial. Unfortunately, the extensive use of chemical M2 inhibitors such as amantadine in poultry farms has now created nearly complete resistance to them in all influenza A strains.

Once the pore is open, the virus disassembles itself and releases viral RNA and core proteins into the cytoplasm. (Chinese skullcap inhibits this kind of viral RNA release.) The core proteins and viral RNA form a complex that is taken into the nucleus of the cell, where the cell is stimulated to begin making copies of the viral RNA (each slightly different). The new viral RNA is combined with other newly manufactured virus components such as neuraminidase and hemagglutinin and assembled into new viruses. These attach to the inside of the host cell membrane, a bulge forms in the membrane, and the new viruses are expressed (viral budding or shedding) into the extracellular matrix surrounding the cell.

The cell is taken over by the virus in this process, its own components depleted during the creation of new viruses. Once its resources are gone, the cell dies and the newly created viruses move on to new host cells, beginning the process all over again.

The alveolar epithelial cells are specific sites for this process to occur. The alveoli are tiny sacs that are the terminal end of the respiratory tree. The air we breathe travels throughout the bronchial tree, eventually emerging into the alveoli, where the oxygen transfuses across very thin membranes into the blood. This is how our bodies remain oxygenated. In the cells lining those tiny sacs the viruses breed. They cause extreme inflammation, or swelling, of the cells in that location with resulting edema (fluid accumulation). All the infected cells burst open and die as new viruses are made. So, fewer alveoli are functional. Breathing is more difficult and the infected person has much less energy because oxygen is not making it into the blood in sufficient quantities. (This is why hospitals sometimes give the infected oxygen.) Pneumonia is when this process becomes severe, the sacs filling with increasing amounts of fluid while there are fewer and fewer functional alveoli.

Throughout the cellular infection and replication process, the virus is also stimulating the release of cytokines by the cell. These cytokines make the tight junctions between cells (and the cellular membranes) more porous and allow easier movement of viral particles through the extracellular matrix (and into the cells themselves). The cytokines are also stimulated in just such a way as to keep the parts of the immune system that can kill the viruses suppressed for as long as possible.

Toll-like receptors (TLRs) are pattern recognition receptors that can identify different types of microbes. The virus particles stimulate TLR3, which begins inducing the release of nuclear factor kappa-B (NF-κB) cytokines. NF-κB is an upstream cytokine, meaning that it is a powerful initiator of other inflammatory cytokines. NF-κB *begins* very specific types of cytokine cascades. Other types of initiators such as RIG-1, NOD2, and MDA5 are also released as part of the body's reaction to a viral infection. Normally, these would strongly stimulate type 1 interferon (IFN) production (IFN-α and IFN-ß). And influenza viruses are generally very susceptible to these interferons. However, the influenza virus uses a protein, the NS1 protein, which blocks the induction of type 1 IFNs long enough to get established in the body.

(Upregulating the production of type I interferons with herbs such as licorice will help reduce the severity of the infection.) The virus also inhibits dendritic cell maturation and activation, lowering the response levels of T and B cells. (Increasing T cell counts is particularly effective in reducing influenza severity. Licorice, elder, red root, and zinc are specific for this.) These cells are part of the adaptive immune response; suppressing them protects the virus from attack. The body response also stimulates the release of type III interferons, to which the virus is less susceptible and which it does nothing to suppress. These interferons have general, rather than specific, antiviral qualities and are upregulated within 3 to 6 hours of infection. This is what begins causing the general flu-like feelings that presage a full-blown flu episode. The virus itself does not make you feel "fluey."

During this same time period, the infected airway cells (tracheobronchial and alveolar epithelial cells) begin generating specific cytokines and chemokines: interleukin-1 beta (IL-1ß), IL-6, IL-18 (which causes spikes in IFN-γ production), C-C chemokine ligand 5 (CCL5, also known as RANTES, "regulated and normal T cell expressed and secreted"), C-X-C chemokine ligand 10 (CXCL10). Then, some 12 to 16 hours later, other cytokines are produced: tumor necrosis factor alpha (TNF-α), IL-8, and CCL2 (also known as monocyte chemoattractant protein-1 or MCP-1). The expressed cytokines make the epithelial structures more porous. This assists faster viral penetration of the cells. It also stimulates the migration of immune cells to the sites of infection.

Interferon-gamma (IFN-γ) is a type 2 interferon, sometimes called macrophage-activating factor. It is this IFN that is crucial in the cytokine overinflammation that occurs during severe influenza. By stimulating it, the virus initiates a positive feedback loop in the cytokine process that leads, in severe infections, to cytokine storms.

CCL2 causes the migration of blood-derived monocytes into the alveolar airspaces. TNF-α and IL-1ß upregulate adhesion molecules (which include intercellular adhesion molecule 1, a.k.a. ICAM-1, and E-selectin) on the surface of the endothelial cells that line blood vessels. This helps the endothelial lining become more porous and stimulates the transendothelial migration of neutrophils to those locations. TNF-α induces monocyte and neutrophil movement across the epithelium through ICAM-1 and VCAM-1 (vascular cell adhesion molecule-1) upregulation. The consequence of this is increasing amounts of white-blood-cell-filled mucus in the lungs. (This is what we cough up during a flu infection.)

The size of the drainage lymph nodes in the lungs begins to increase. This helps, during a healthy resolution of infection, to drain more of the fluids from the lungs, preventing suffocation. Within those lymph nodes, areas called the geminal centers increase their size and development. The germinal centers are the sites where B lymphocytes are produced and are differentiated in order to attack the specific infection that is occurring. This is part of the adaptive humoral immune response. These lymph node locations (as well as those in peripheral tissues) can become overfull during severe infections, slowing drainage and healthy adaptive immune responses. They can also, during severe influenza infections, be specifically attacked and damaged so that they do not function at all. This is a contributor to the mortality that sometimes occurs during cytokine storms. (This is why herbs such as red root, inmortal, and pleurisy root are useful; they all support the lymph structures in the lungs and periphery. Red root — *Ceanothus* spp. — is particular useful in the periphery for spleen and lymph enlargement and lymph drainage; inmortal — *Asclepias asperula* — is specific for optimizing lymph drainage from the lungs; pleurisy root — *Asclepias tuberosa* — is specific for reducing inflammation in the pleurae and lungs. They can be used interchangeably to some extent.) The lymph centers in the lungs are heavily affected during influenza, much more so than the periphery.

Similarly to many viruses, while influenza viruses reproduce most efficiently in the alveolar epithelial cells, they can also infect other cells, specifically dendritic cells, monocytes, macrophages, neutrophils, T cells, B cells, and natural killer (NK) cells. In response to being infected those cells also begin releasing cytokines and chemokines:

IFNs, IL-1α and IL-1ß, IL-6, TNF-α, CXCL8, CCL2 (MCP-1), CCL3 (a.k.a. macrophage inflammatory protein-1 alpha, or MIP-1α), CCL4, CXCL9, and CXCL10 through the ERK-1, ERK-2 (extracelluar-signal-regulated kinase 1 and 2), p38 MAPK (p38 mitogen-activated protein kinase), and JNK (c-Jun N-terminal kinase) pathways.

TNF-α, IL-1ß, IL-6, and IFN-γ are responsible for most of the negative effects of the cytokine cascade. Mice that are unable to produce TNF-α consistently show decreased mortality, a reduced symptom picture, and less severe course of the disease. This holds true even if they are infected with the reconstituted, and very virulent, 1918 virus. Inhibition of TNF-α (especially) and IL-1ß has been found to significantly reduce the cytokine-based inflammation that occurs during influenza, alleviating symptoms and inhibiting viral spread. (Herbs specific for inhibiting TNF-α are kudzu, Chinese senega root, Chinese skullcap, elder, ginger, houttuynia, licorice, boneset, and cordyceps. Herbs specific for inhibiting IL-1ß are Japanese knotweed, Chinese senega root, Chinese skullcap, cordyceps, kudzu, and boneset.)

The virus can also inhibit the production of macrophages over time. This occurs because, over time, macrophages will begin producing anti-inflammatory cytokines such as IL-4 and IL-10. Once the bodily system is macrophage-depleted a prolonged inflammatory process occurs, keeping the infection going. Lung levels of IL-1ß, IL-6, and TNF-α all increase considerably at that point. Stimulating monocyte and dendritic cell maturation (cordyceps) and inducing IL-4 and IL-10 (Chinese skullcap, elder, houttuynia, licorice, cordyceps) will help counteract this.

The virus is exceptionally sophisticated in its impacts. There are three stages of chemokine stimulation. The first, 2 to 4 hours postinfection, is attended by the production of CXCL16, CXCL1, CXCL2, and CXCL3. These chemokines are specific for attracting neutrophils, cytotoxic T cells, and NK cells. At 8 to 12 hours postinfection CXCL8, CCL3, CCL4, CCL5, CXCL9, CXCL10, and CXCL11 are being produced, which attract effector memory T cells. At 24 to 48 hours post infection, when dendritic cells are most present in the lymphoid tissues, the chemokine profile changes again in such a manner as to attract naive T and B cells. The effect of all this is the virus playing the immune system as a virtuoso plays a violin. Eventually the immune system catches up (usually) and the infection is stopped as influenza-specific antibodies are created.

Plants that reduce the other main cytokines that the virus stimulates will also help lessen disease severity and prevent lung damage. I think the most important are inhibitors of NF-κB (Chinese senega root, Chinese skullcap, ginger, houttuynia, kudzu, licorice, boneset, astragalus), IL-6 (kudzu, Chinese skullcap, isatis), IL-8 (cordyceps, isatis, Japanese knotweed), RANTES (licorice, isatis), MCP-1 (houttuynia), CXCL10 (boneset), CCL2 (boneset), the ERK pathway (kudzu, Chinese skullcap, cordyceps), the p38 pathway (Chinese skullcap, houttuynia, cordyceps), and the JNK pathway (Chinese skullcap, cordyceps, lion's mane). The reduction of these cytokines and pathways will reduce IFN-γ.

Each type of influenza has a slightly different cytokine profile with slightly different cytokines more strongly represented. However, the protocols herein, directed to this form of cytokine profile, will be specific enough for every strain, including the low pathogenic avian strain H9N2, which strongly upregulates transforming growth factor beta 2 (TGF-ß2), a different dynamic entirely. Medicinal plants already in use in the developed protocol are, however, specific for TGF-ß2, i.e., astragalus (the strongest) and Chinese skullcap. *Magnolia officinalis, Ginkgo biloba, Folium syringae, Nigella sativa, Paeonia lactiflora,* and *Lonicera japonica* are other plants specific for inhibiting TGF-ß2. (This is why lonicera, or Japanese honeysuckle, is commonly used in the treatment of respiratory infections in China — it alleviates wind heat and expels wind heat invasion. In other words, it reduces inflammation in the lungs and expels the virus or bacteria responsible.)

Normally, influenza viruses stay in the upper respiratory tract. However, during more severe infections they will infect the lower respiratory tract as well. Pneumonia is one serious complication from that. So are cytokine storms, should the disease really take hold.

Cytokine Storms

The more serious pandemic viruses (1918 H1N1, 2009 H1N1, and 2004 H5N1) cause severe pulmonary injury and inflammation. In these cases, the cytokine cascades become storms and the death rate correspondingly climbs. H5N1, for example, has around a 60 percent death rate in those who are infected, usually from acute respiratory distress and organ failure. The 1918 rate had a much lower mortality rate, around 20 percent, but the strain is much more infective, reaching about one-third of the population. (The emergence of a highly infective avian H5N1 strain is one of the things that keeps viral researchers up at night.)

While there is (usually) not a corresponding increase in viral replication during a viral storm, the cytokine increases in severe pandemic influenzas are significant and this is where the mortal damage comes from. Interferon-gamma (IFN-γ) production is usually increased, as is the expression of TNF-α, IL-1ß, CXCL10, RANTES, MIP-1α, MCP-1, MCP-3, and IL-6. The IFN-γ levels and the virus synergistically interact to significantly increase CXCL10 in airway epithelial cells. This causes a tremendous infiltration of immune cells into the airways. Blocking IFN-γ through the use of inhibitors has been found to significantly reduce airway infiltrates (houttuynia, cordyceps, Chinese skullcap, and licorice; note that licorice is an IFN-γ *modulator* — it inhibits its production when levels are high and stimulates its production, especially in T cells, when levels are low).

In particular, the inhibition of TNF-α, IFN-γ, IL-1ß, and IL-6 is crucial during infection with severe influenza pandemic strains. Those cytokines are found in exceptionally high levels in such instances and damage to the lungs is specific to them. If their levels rise high enough, the inflammation does not stay confined to the respiratory system but goes systemic. This kind of condition is called sepsis, essentially a whole-body inflammatory state. If severe enough it can lead to organ failure and cardiac arrest.

A particular cytokine-like protein has been implicated in sepsis-induced cytokine storms: high-mobility group box 1 protein (HMGB1).

This cytokine-like protein is highly elevated in all patients who die from sepsis, including sepsis generated by influenza. HMGB1 is also unique in that once stimulated, its secretion continues for a very long time. TNF-α, in comparison, lasts at peak levels for about 90 minutes once stimulated. HMGB1 peak levels last 18 hours before they begin to decline. Once HMGB1 is released it stimulates further cytokine releases *and* has the additional property of being synergistic with the other cytokines already present in the body, amplifying their effects. HMGB1 release is stimulated by macrophages and monocytes when a particularly potent cytokine cascade begins, specifically with high levels of NF-κB, TNF-α, RANTES, IL-6, and IFN-γ, in pretty much that order. The amount released is directly dose-dependent. In other words, the higher the cytokine levels, the more HMGB1 is released. And the more that is released, the higher the cytokine levels go. As examples, levels of IL-6 are nearly four times higher, IL-8 nearly three times higher, and IFN-γ more than two times higher during severe infections than in milder cases. Higher IL-6 concentrations are positively correlated with prolonged illness and hospitalization. As the storm progresses levels of IL-8, MCP-1, and H_2O_2-myeloperoxidase also significantly increase. Endothelial cells are strongly stimulated and begin to amplify the storm's cytokines. Hyperactivation of p38 MAPK with an accompanying inhibition of the adaptive immune system is a marker for these kinds of cytokine storms.

HMGB1 is also released when the nuclei of cells are damaged, as they are during influenza infections. HMG proteins are held in the nucleus to help in forming DNA complexes and regulating gene expression. When HMGB1 is expressed in lung tissue, as it is during severe influenza episodes, it causes massive neutrophil infiltration into the lungs and acute lung injury. As the storm progresses respiratory failure (requiring mechanical ventilation), acute renal failure, and systemic shock all occur. In severe cases such as these, antivirals (oseltamivir), antibiotics, and corticosteroids have all been found to be ineffective.

Common steroidal drugs (e.g., dexamethasone and cortisone) have consistently been found to have no effect on HMGB1 levels, and the

same can be said for NSAIDs such as aspirin, ibuprofen, and indomethacin — even at superpharmacological concentrations. However,
a number of herbs and herbal constituents do have direct suppressive
actions against the protein.

Direct inhibition of HMGB1 with herbs such as *Angelica sinensis*
and *Salvia miltiorrhiza* protects mice both before and 24 hours after
infection with normally lethal influenza viruses. The licorice constituent glycyrrhizin directly binds HMGB1, inactivating its actions in the
body. The green tea component epigallocatechin gallate (EGCG) also
inhibits HMGB1, as does quercetin. Counterintuitively, nicotine also
significantly lowers HMGB1 in the lungs. The pharmaceutical minocycline has also shown the ability to reduce HMGB1 levels; its use should
be explored in hospital and pharmaceutical settings.

During severe influenza infections reducing HMGB1 is essential.

Lung and Tissue Pathology during Severe Influenza Infections

Influenza viruses specifically invade lung tissues and cause both direct
and inflammatory-mediated damage. There are four primary pathological changes that occur: 1) diffuse alveolar damage; 2) necrotizing
bronchiolitis; 3) intense alveolar hemorrhage; and 4) severe fluid
accumulation.

The viruses infect specific cellular structures, in fact any that
possess linked sialic acids (alpha-2,6 and alpha-2,3) on their surface
membranes. But cells in the respiratory system express those acids
differently and different influenzal strains create different infection
profiles. The nonciliated cells of the lungs contain a higher proportion
of alpha-2,6-linked sialic acids while ciliated cells contain both alpha-
2,6- and alpha-2,3-linked sialic acid. H3N2 viruses prefer the non-
ciliated-cell sialic acids while the avian flu types (H5N1) exclusively
infect ciliated cells. This is part of the reason that the avian strains
tend to be more deadly. The cilia, when infected, are often killed and
their ability to move mucus up and out of the lungs destroyed. This

substantially increases mucous buildup in the lungs. The H5N1 strains prefer the alpha-2,3-linked sialic acids that are most strongly present on the ciliated cells but those acids exist on ciliated cells in higher quantities in the lower respiratory tract. So, the H5N1 strains infect not only the cilia but also the lower respiratory tract, causing a much deeper infection.

In severe cases, irrespective of strain, alveolar hemorrhage is often present, as is intra-alveolar edema and interstitial inflammation. The tissues surrounding blood vessels and lymph nodes and channels all inflame (perivasculitis). Microthrombi or tiny blood clots occur throughout the blood vessels in the lungs. IFN-γ levels are high in macrophages, alveolar epithelial cells, and vessels. TNF-α levels are high in alveolar macrophages and bronchial and vascular smooth muscle. There are massive infiltrates surrounding airways and in the alveolar walls. The spleen typically atrophies and presents with nonreactive white pulp. In the lymph nodes nonreactive follicles and sinusoidal erythrophagocytosis are common.

Protecting spleen and lymph structures and their function, cilial structures, and mucous membrane structures is essential.

Medical Interventions

If influenza is pharmaceutically treated, neuraminidase inhibitors such as oseltamivir (Tamiflu) or zanamivir (Relenza) are usually used. Sometimes adamantanes (amantadine and rimantadine) are as well; they inhibit the M2 ion channels. These pharmaceuticals are commonly referred to as antivirals but they are not, at least not in the same way that an antibiotic is an antibiotic, that is, something that specifically kills bacteria. They, more accurately, inhibit viral penetration of host cells (thus stopping or slowing the infection) or prevent the vacuole-enveloped virus from releasing viral proteins into the host cell interior (thus stopping or slowing the infection). They don't directly kill the virus. Ribavirin, a drug that interferes with RNA metabolism, is sometimes used but its effects are mixed and it has many serious side effects.

If there is significant inflammation, corticosteriods may be used to try and reduce it — but if HMGB1 levels are in play, corticosteroids will do nothing to reduce them. Hospitalization is common in severe cases, but other than passive care and the use of oxygen, little can be done. Intravenous liquids may be given but they may have serious side effects, since the main approach has been the use of a combination nutrient solution/glucose IV in an attempt to keep the patient's nutrient/energy levels high. Unfortunately, it turns out that the use of glucose during influenza infections significantly increases viral load and illness parameters. Insulin, on the other hand, reduces them considerably and also has the added benefit of lowering HMGB1 levels.

There is the bare beginnings within hospital settings of the use of cytokine inhibitors such as minocycline and HMGB1 inhibitors (e.g., anti-IFN-γ antibodies, intravenous immunoglobulin) but their use is not widespread. If microthrombi proliferate in the lungs then anti-coagulants may be used. Interestingly, both antithrombin III and thrombomodulin decrease HMGB1 in vitro. Very few of these HMGB1 interventions are commonly used, or known of, by practicing physicians.

To make matters worse, many influenza strains are developing resistance to the primary neuraminidase inhibitor used to treat them, oseltamivir, as well as to the primary adamantane M2 ion channel inhibitor, amantadine. Influenza virus samples from the 2007–2008 season showed 0.06 percent resistance, from the 2008–2009 season 1.5 percent resistance, and from the 2009–2010 season 28 percent resistance — a normal exponential learning curve for resistance. Research in late 2009 began finding strains resistant to the other major neuraminidase inhibitor, zanamivir. Resistance has become common as well to the other primary M2 ion channel inhibitor, rimantadine. Some areas report 100 percent resistance to amantadine and over 90 percent resistance to oseltamivir. Besides their overuse in agribusiness, there is another reason for resistance: human excretion.

Oseltamivir is immediately metabolized in the body to oseltamivir carboxylate. It is only active in this form. Unfortunately this form *is* the metabolized form and it is excreted out of the human body without any further alterations. It flows unaffected through wastewater treatment plants and ends up in waterways in low doses, where it comes into contact with waterfowl and thus is exposed to avian influenza strains. The avian strains develop resistance, and as the avian, human, and swine strains commingle the resistance is passed on into strains that can infect humans.

These drugs are also often used in large quantities during epidemic outbreaks. And the viruses quickly develop resistance to them. About 30 percent of those treated will develop resistant strains and will shed them for days afterward. The newly infected are then resistant to the drugs.

Less severe cases of the flu, if one sees a physician, are rarely treated (though, irresponsibly, some physicians will prescribe antibiotics, which are not active against viruses, for the flu). The usual medical advice is to "rest in bed, drink plenty of fluids, and take over-the-counter medications as needed." In other words, it is left up to the individual's immune system and some very limited self-care options to treat the infection. The Chinese don't have this kind of technological bias in place. Unlike those of us in the West, they have been developing both herb-alone and herb/pharmaceutical combination approaches in their treatment protocols. And their outcomes are very good when compared to Western approaches.

There are a great many interventions that are possible with plant medicines and unlike pharmaceuticals, viruses don't develop resistance to them.

Natural Treatment Protocols for Influenza

Again, just to emphasize this: *there are thousands of combinations of plant medicines that can be created to treat respiratory infections.* These are just the ones I have found useful. Please feel free to experiment, combine, innovate, and find your own unique combinations. There is no one right way to the truth.

An influenza infection can run the range from extremely mild to extremely severe. I break the disease down into four types, each needing a different approach: 1) early onset; 2) mild infection; 3) moderate infection; and 4) severe infection. I will go into some of the unique aspects of treating severe infections at the end of this section.

Early-Onset Treatment

I have found two approaches that can short-circuit a developing episode before it gets a good hold in the body: oscillococcinum and an herbal tincture combination.

OSCILLOCOCCINUM

I have found this homeopathic remedy to be extremely good for stopping the development of the flu *if you take it at the first signs of the flu*, that is, the *moment* you feel that first tingling sensation in your body that tells you that you are about to get sick.

Oscillococcinum comes as little sugar granules in tiny tubes. Take one tube every 6 hours, three per day, for 2 or 3 days in a row. This is often enough to stop the infection.

HERBAL TINCTURE COMBINATION

For many years I used a particular tincture combination: *Echinacea angustifolia* (now I use ginger juice — see page 44; and note: *E. purpurea* is useless for this; it won't work), red root, and licorice, in equal parts. The dosage is a full dropperful of the tincture (30 drops) *every hour*, every day, until the symptoms resolve themselves.

I have found this useful for stopping the development of a flu infection *if you take it at the first signs of tingling or soreness in your throat.* The tincture mix should be held in your mouth, liberally mixed with saliva, then swallowed, *slowly*, letting it dribble down the back of the throat.

For *Echinacea angustifolia* to work for a cold or flu *the herbal tincture must touch the affected membranes.* Echinacea *is* antiviral; it's been found active against HIV and influenza H5N1, H7N7, and H1N1 (swine origin). However, in order to inactivate the influenza strains, it needs *direct contact* with the affected cells just prior to or right at the moment of infection. Echinacea inhibits the receptor cell binding activity of the virus, interfering with its entry into the cells while at the same time strengthening the protective power of the mucous membranes through hyaluronidase inhibition. In essence, it strengthens the cellular bonds in the mucous membranes and makes it harder for a virus to penetrate. If the virus does penetrates deeper into the body, the herb just won't work because direct contact is not possible.

Goldenseal has some similar actions on mucous membranes, which is why the deplorable echinacea/goldenseal combinations are so common. They are only effective at the first signs of infection. (I reiterate: They are *only* effective at the first signs of infection. If the infection is full-blown, you are just wasting your money.) Again, *E. purpurea* (in the form in use in most of the West) will not work. The Germans use *only* the fresh, stabilized juice of the stalks, not the root, and it is the root that nearly every American herbalist and company use in their products. (Capsules, of any species, are completely useless for viral and bacterial infections.)

Mild Infection

If you do get sick but have a relatively mild case developing, then the following protocol, composed of two parts, will usually get rid of it.

FRESH GINGER JUICE TEA

Ginger is useful for the flu *only* if the juice of the fresh root is used. Dried ginger is useless.

At the first signs of an infection that is not going to stop, juice one to two pounds of ginger. (Squeeze the remaining pulp to get all the juice out of it, and keep any leftover juice refrigerated.) Pour 3 to 4 ounces of the juice into a mug, and add one-quarter of a lime (squozen), a large tablespoon of honey, $1/8$ teaspoon of cayenne, and 6 ounces of hot water. Stir well. Drink 2 to 6 cups daily.

This will usually end the infection within a few days. *If it does not* it is still tremendously useful as it will thin the mucus, slow the spread of the virus in the body, and help protect mucous membranes from damage.

Comment: Some people find that an elderberry syrup will provide the same effects.

Other Anti-Influenza Herbs and Supplements

A number of other plants have been found effective for influenza during in vitro, in vivo, or human studies:

Achillea millefolium (yarrow)

Aegle marmelos (bael)

Agathosma betulina

Agrimonia pilosa

Allium oreoprasum

Allium sativum (garlic)

Alpinia officinarum

Andrographis paniculata

Androsace strigilosa

Angelica keiskei

Aronia melanocarpa

Asparagus filicinus

Azadirachta indica (neem)

Bergenia ligulata

Camellia sinensis (green tea, EGCG)

Cephalotaxus harringtonia

Chaenomeles sinensis

Cistus incanus

Clinacanthus siamensis

Cocos nucifera (coconut oil, monolaurin)

Commelina communis

Eleutherococcus senticosus

Elsholtzia rugulosa

Geranium sanguineum

Ginkgo biloba

Holoptelea integrifolia

Hypericum japonicum

Justicia pectoralis

Myrica rubra

Narcissus tazetta

Nerium indicum

Ocimum sanctum (holy basil)

Olea europaea (olive)

Panax spp. (ginseng)

Pandanus amaryllifolius

Phyllanthus emblica

Propolis

Prunus mume

Punica granatum (pomegranate)

Rhinacanthus nasutus

Sanicula europaea

Saponaria officinalis

Schefflera heptaphylla

Terminalia chebula

Thalictrum simplex

Tinospora cordifolia

Toddalia asiatica

Trachyspermum ammi

Tussilago farfara (coltsfoot)

Uncaria rhynchophylla

Verbascum thapsus (mullein)

HERBAL TINCTURE COMBINATION

Tincture combination of 2 parts lomatium, 2 parts red root, 2 parts licorice, and 1 part isatis (e.g., 2 ounces of each of the first three, 1 ounce of the latter). Dosage: 30–60 drops each hour until the condition improves.

Moderate and Severe Infections

I treat moderate and severe influenza infections similarly, though with severe infections there needs to be a great deal of focus and persistence. The doses often need to be higher as well and additional formulations used as symptoms develop.

The primary interventions are:

- Direct antivirals that will inhibit viral penetration of host cells and replication. (The primary antiviral herbs for this are Chinese skullcap, isatis, licorice, houttuynia, lomatium, cordyceps, astragalus, rhodiola, boneset, elder, *Strobilanthes cusia*, *Forsythia suspensa*, and *Sophora flavescens*.)
- Reducing cytokine levels, thus inhibiting damage in tissues.
- Thinning the mucus and promoting fluid drainage from the lungs.
- Repair of damaged tissues.
- Normalization of immune responses.
- If sepsis is a potential problem, large quantities of HMGB1 inhibitors should be used.

Treatment of moderate to severe influenza is composed of three main formulations, to which others can be added if necessary. These are an antiviral tincture formulation, an antiviral ginger juice tea, and an immune complex tincture formulation.

ANTIVIRAL TINCTURE FORMULATION

Equal parts of Chinese skullcap, isatis, licorice, houttuynia, lomatium, red root, yerba santa (*Eriodictyon* spp.), elephant tree (*Bursera microphylla*), osha (*Ligusticum porteri*), and either inmortal (*Asclepias asperula*) or pleurisy root (*Asclepias tuberosa*).

This formulation contains potent antivirals, specifically Chinese skullcap, isatis, licorice, houttuynia, lomatium. These are designed to kill the virus and inhibit its entry into the body. And of course many of them have alternate actions as well. Licorice, for example, is mucoprotective, strongly anti-inflammatory, and expectorant. Chinese skullcap is potently anti-inflammatory for the cytokine cascades that influenza creates, provides splenic protection and activation, will help lower fevers, and is an expectorant. All of these antiviral herbs have multiple functions in respiratory diseases.

The four herbs added to this protocol that are not discussed in depth in this book (yerba santa, osha, elephant tree, and inmortal or pleurisy root) do not have to be included in this formulation, though they do help considerably, primarily through helping with the tastiness of the formulation, thinning the mucus, stimulating expectoration, and promoting lymph drainage from the lungs.

Both yerba santa and osha are added for taste as well as their medicinal actions (isatis really does taste foul to me). Osha is a relative of lomatium and has its own antiviral and expectorant actions.

Complex Formulations

For nearly 30 years I tended to use formulations that contained only three herbs, occasionally five. With the emergence of more intense forms of influenza, and my increasing age, I have found that a more complex formulation works better. I do think a major factor in that is aging. There are, in myself and in many of the people I help, considerable age-related alterations in our physiology. There are preexisting inflammations in many parts of our bodies, from age-related memory dysfunction to arthritis. Our bodies are wearing out, biodegrading, and that deterioration makes them more susceptible to infections such as influenza, and in more severe forms. Further, our immune systems are not as vital as they once were and have a great deal more trouble counteracting the infection.

It has strong impacts on inflammation in the lungs and increases the degree of oxygen intake during respiration. It also has the added benefit of anesthesizing the throat tissues, helping reduce throat soreness. Yerba santa is a very good expectorant, bronchial dilator, and decongestant. Elephant tree is anti-inflammatory, thins and softens bronchial mucus, and stimulates expectoration. It is a major source of copal and a close relative of myrrh. (Myrrh can be substituted for elephant tree in this formulation if the tincture is stabilized with 20 percent glycerin.) I consider all three of these herbs to be specific for maintaining the mucous membranes of the lungs, thinning the mucus, and increasing expectoration. Inmortal (or, as an alternative, pleurisy root) improves cilia function and is a bronchial dilator, an expectorant, a febrifuge (lowering fevers), and most especially a potent medicinal for stimulating lymph drainage from the lungs.

Dosage needs to be high for two reasons. The first is that there are so many herbs in the formulation that each herb has a reduced presence in the formulation. The second is the nature of moderate to severe influenza infections. As the disease progresses up the scale of severity, the cytokine cascade increases in intensity. The body needs to be *bathed* in the plant compounds in high enough quantities that the cytokine cascade is potently inhibited. In addition, the body needs to be suffused with enough of the antiviral compounds that the viral entry into host cells and its presence in the body are severely curtailed.

For moderate influenza: 60 drops or 3 ml (a little over 1/2 teaspoon) every hour.

For severe influenza: 1–2 teaspoons every hour.

Dividing the formulation: You can if you wish divide the formulation in two. The first would contain Chinese skullcap, isatis, licorice, houttuynia, and lomatium and would be primarily an antiviral formulation (and would taste from okay to bad). The second would contain red root, yerba santa (*Eriodictyon* spp.), elephant tree (*Bursera microphylla*), and either inmortal (*Asclepias asperula*) or pleurisy root (*Asclepias tuberosa*) and would taste very good. (I would skip the osha if the formulation is split in two.) This second formulation would primarily be for lymph and spleen optimization and protection, expectorant and decongestant actions, mucus thinning, cilia protection, and lymph drainage from the lungs. The dosage for each would be half the dosage as when combined.

GINGER JUICE TEA

This is the same as discussed earlier, in essence: ginger juice tea, hot. Again, ginger is useful for the flu *only* if the juice of the fresh root is used. Dried ginger is useless.

Juice one to two pounds of ginger. (Squeeze the pulp to get all the juice out of it.) Keep it refrigerated. Pour 3 to 4 ounces of the juice into a mug, and add one-quarter of a lime (squozen), a large tablespoon of honey, ⅛ teaspoon of cayenne, and 6 ounces of hot water. Stir well. Drink 4 to 6 cups daily.

Ginger in this form is potently antiviral for influenza. The fresh juice tea will also thin the mucus, help protect mucous membranes from damage, *and* act as a potent diaphoretic, lowering fever during the infection.

IMMUNE COMPLEX TINCTURE FORMULATION

Equal parts of the tinctures of astragalus, cordyceps, and rhodiola. All of these herbs are active against influenza viruses. They are also potently adaptogenic, that is, they increase the resistance of organisms to stressors, whether microbial or external. Additionally, astragalus and cordyceps are highly specific for the cytokine cascades that are initiated by influenza. These herbs will help through their antiviral actions, modulate the overactive immune response, lower cytokine levels, and enhance a healthy immune response to the infection.

Again, dosage levels should be highish, for the same reasons as outlined above.

For moderate influenza: ½ teaspoon of the tincture 3x daily.

For severe influenza: 1–2 teaspoons of the tincture 6x daily.

Supportive Additions

There are a few additional things that can be very helpful during acute influenza episodes. These are treatments for high fever, severe headache, cough, high HMGB1 levels during cytokine storms, and protecting cilial structures and mucous membranes in the lungs. Two supplements have also been found to be helpful (in a number of studies). And essential oil inhalants can help with the infection in the lungs, coughing, and mucous flow and secretion.

For Fever

There are a number of interventions that can help. The ginger juice tea previously described (page 49) can often lower the high fevers that occur during influenza, but if you want more:

- **Boneset tea:** Boneset is specific for influenza and a number of the cytokines it stimulates. It is also highly specific for diseases that alternate fevers and chill episodes. If I am going to use boneset, and I am already ill, it is easier to make up a lot at one time. Getting out of bed over and over again is too difficult. So . . . add 3 ounces of dried boneset herb to 1 gallon of hot water, let steep 30 minutes, then drink 8 ounces every few hours. *The tea must be consumed hot for it to be effective for fever.* The herb will stimulate sweating, thus lowering the fever. It will help interrupt the chill/fever, chill/fever cycles. It's bitter, so add honey.

- **Pasque flower (*Pulsatilla patens*) tincture:** 10 drops each hour as needed.

- **Any diaphoretic (causes sweating) tea:** Peppermint is a good choice, children like it, and it will also help calm the stomach. Yarrow is more bitter but is also good for this. Both of them do have some antiviral activity against influenza.

- **Wet cloth:** A wet washcloth, applied regularly over the entire body, will mimic the action of sweat in helping lower a fever. The higher the fever, the more often you have to do it.

For Headache

- **Indian pipe (*Monotropa uniflora*) tincture:** The best I have found for the kinds of recalcitrant headaches that can sometimes occur during the flu. Dosage is from 30 drops to 1 teaspoon every few hours.
- **Coral root (*Corallorhiza* spp.) tincture:** Up to 1 teaspoon every few hours. It does help and for some people it is specific.
- **Tinctures of motherwort (*Leonurus cardiaca*) and American wood betony (*Pedicularis* spp.):** Combined, equal parts. Dosage is up to 1 ounce (yes, that's right) of the combination at a time, in water. I usually use ¼ ounce but the high dosage can help occasionally when nothing else does. Go slow and work up, every 4 hours or so.

For Cough

I make a cough syrup every fall just before the flu season. It comes in handy. The recipe varies all the time, depending on what I have on hand and what I have wild-harvested in any particular year. But the recipe below gives you a good idea of what kinds of herbs are in it. I do keep it refrigerated though it will last awhile if it is not.

Cough Syrup Recipe

INGREDIENTS

3 ounces horehound	1 ounce vervain
2 ounces cherry bark	1 ounce lomatium (or osha)
2 ounces elderberries	7 pints water
2 ounces elecampane	3 ounces glycerin
2 ounces licorice	Wildflower honey
2 ounces mallow (or marshmallow)	2 ounces mullein tincture
1 ounce Russian or slippery elm bark	1 ounce yerba santa tincture

Combine the horehound, cherry bark, elderberries, elecampane, licorice, mallow, elm bark, vervain, and half of the lomatium in 7 pints of water in a large pot. Bring to a boil. Stir frequently as it heats to prevent sticking. Once it boils, reduce the heat and let simmer, stirring constantly. Cook until the liquid is reduced by half. Remove from the heat and let cool. (You can put the pot in a bath of cold water to cool it faster. Don't let it tip over.) Strain the liquid, pressing the marc (the spent plant matter) through a cloth to get as much liquid as you can.

(With mucilaginous herbs — the licorice, mallow, and elm bark — as part of the mix, it can be hard for the liquid to pass through the weave of the cloth you are using. So, alternatively, you can keep the mucilaginous herbs out of the mix and once the marc is pressed, heat all the liquid again, adding the licorice, mallow, and elm to the pot in a muslin bag to keep them out of the liquid. Bring to a boil and simmer, stirring constantly, for 30 minutes. Remove the bag, let it cool, then squeeze out the liquid as best you can.)

Warm the liquid again, just enough to dissolve the honey and glycerin. Add the glycerin, then the honey to taste. Grind the remaining lomatium (or osha) to a fine powder—a nut or coffee grinder or mortar and pestle is good for this—then add it to the liquid. Let the mix cool, then add the mullein and yerba santa tincture. (Keep in mind that you can substitute similar herbs for any used in this recipe.)

The honey, glycerin, and two tinctures help stabilize the syrup, keeping it from going bad. I do keep the whole thing in the refrigerator though. It will last a year very easily. Generally, it is best to make this kind of a syrup in the fall, after the berries are ripe and ready for harvest, and just before flu season. It is very effective.

To use:

I keep this by the bed and take as desired. Really, none of that 1-tablespoon-at-a-time stuff, that won't help at all. Just drink it as needed, right out of the bottle. It will help soothe the mucous membranes, reduce coughing, and ease the aches and pains that come with the flu.

To Reduce HMGB1 Levels during Cytokine Storms

The herbs that are already being used will help this considerably. However, if the condition significantly worsens then the following specific intervention is warranted. Take both formulations.

Formulation 1: Tincture combination of *Angelica sinensis* and *Salvia miltiorrhiza,* in equal parts. Dosage: 1 tablespoon every hour. Or . . .

Formulation 2: Strong infusion of the two herbs, 4 ounces of each in 1 gallon of just-boiled water. Remove from the heat, let sit 4 hours, and strain. Dosage: Drink 12 ounces every hour.

To Protect Cilial Structures and Lung Mucosa

There are a number of herbs that are specific for protecting the cilia: cordyceps, olive oil and leaf, the berberine plants, and, my favorite, *Bidens pilosa*. Bidens is a very strong systemic antibiotic that is used in Asia and Africa for systemic bacterial infections (including respiratory) *and* influenza (though it has not been tested against that virus). If the mucous membranes have been infected by a microbe and you start to get well, relapse, start to get well, relapse, this is the herb to use. The herb is specific for healing and protecting mucous membrane structures, including the cilia. Tincture of the fresh herb should be used. The dry herb is not as antimicrobial though it will still help the mucous membranes' tone. Dosage: 1/4–1/2 teaspoon up to 6x daily.

Supplements

Zinc and selenium are very helpful during influenza infections. Both have been found to protect mice from severe influenzal strains. Dosage: 200 mcg daily of selenium; 25–40 mg daily of zinc.

Some Comments on Treating Severe Influenza

When people become severely ill with influenza, they often present with high fever, extreme lethargy, and significantly reduced vital energy. They are usually bedridden and very, very afraid.

The interventions in such cases need to be highly focused and attentive. It takes a lot of work. They need to be nurtured continuously, fed if they will eat (chicken broth is very good), helped to the bathroom (if they can even get out of bed), and ministered to. The fever will often need to be brought down and you will have to monitor the plant medicine intake. It needs to be constant (every hour at minimum), and in fairly high dosages in order to lower the cytokine cascade, reduce the viral load, and get the immune system back online. It will often take a week to begin to turn the situation around, and several more weeks before the person really begins to get well. It can be done. Of all the herbs useful for this, lomatium, licorice, Chinese skullcap, and cordyceps are the most essential.

Essential Oil Inhalants

Essential oils of thyme, eucalyptus, rosemary, and sage can all help. They are all antiviral for influenza (to varying extents), will help reduce the coughing reflex, thin and help expectorate mucus, and improve airflow in the bronchial tract. To use: Bring a gallon of water to a boil in a pot on the stove. Turn off the heat, add 20 drops of each of the essential oils to the pot, and bring the pot to a comfortable location where you can sit with your head over it. Hold your head over the pot and breathe in the steam for as long as you can take it, every few hours.

SARS and Coronaviruses

SARS is, in its impacts in the body, very similar to acute influenza and at first was thought to be an emerging influenzal strain. However, SARS (sudden acute respiratory syndrome) is a new, emerging viral pathogen that appeared suddenly in 2002 in China. The disease is characterized by fever followed by respiratory symptoms and, ultimately for some of those infected, progressive respiratory failure. The nature of the virus, at the time, was unknown but eventually it was found to be a coronavirus that had jumped species. Into us.

Coronaviruses are enveloped, positive-stranded RNA viruses. They possess the largest genome of all the RNA viruses. The viruses in this group engage in a very high frequency of RNA combinations, continually producing new variants. Of the dozen or so coronaviruses only three infect people. Among them, SARS is the most serious.

The virus takes about 6 days to develop in the body and, like influenza, is primarily spread by respiratory droplets — though direct contact with body secretions can also transmit it. The virus sheds particles in feces and urine, often for several weeks, and cleaning up after the severely ill can spread the infection. Fever, cough, and difficulty breathing are the first symptoms of the disease. Headache, muscular stiffness, myalgia, loss of appetite, malaise, chills, confusion, dizziness, rash, night sweats, nausea, and diarrhea occur for many.

With increasing age comes increasing fatality. Those under the age of 24 are not very susceptible. For those aged 25 to 44 the fatality rate is 6 percent. It is 15 percent in those 45 to 64 and greater than 50 percent in those over 65.

SARS, unlike influenza, attaches not to sialic acid linkages but to angiotensin converting enzyme 2 (ACE-2). This is an integral membrane protein on many cells throughout the body, including the heart, vascular cells, and kidneys. It is intimately involved in regulating the renin-angiotensin system (RAS). The RAS is intimately involved in vascular constriction and renal electrolyte homeodynamis, which is where its primary impacts were thought to be. But the RAS is also crucial to the functioning of most organs, including the lungs, spleen, and lymph nodes. ACE-2 converts angiotensin II to less potent molecular forms. Among other things angiotensin II is a potent vasoconstrictor but it also is highly bioactive along a range of cellular actions.

SARS viruses attach to ACE-2 on the surface of lung, lymph, and spleen epithelial cells. (Licorice, Chinese skullcap, luteolin, horse chestnut, *Polygonum* spp., *Rheum officinale*, and plants high in procyanidins and lectins such as elder and cinnamon block attachment to varying degrees.) Once the receptors on these cells are compromised there is enhanced vascular permeability, increased lung edema, neutrophil accumulation, and worsened lung function. In essence, once the virus begins attaching to ACE-2, ACE-2 function begins to be destroyed. ACE-2 function also tends to be less dynamic as people grow older, hence the more negative the effects of SARS infection on the elderly. (Kudzu, *Salvia miltiorrhiza*, and ginkgo all upregulate and protect ACE-2 expression and activity and lower angiotensin II levels.) ACE (in contrast to ACE-2) inhibitors increase the presence of ACE-2 and help protect the lungs from injury. (Hawthorn and kudzu, for example.)

Upon infection by the SARS virus, similarly to influenza, inflammatory cytokines are strongly upregulated. IFN-γ, CXCL10, IL-1ß, TNF-α, and IL-6 are primary, IL-6 particularly so. RANTES, MCP-1, and IL-8 are elevated in about half of those who are infected. The p38

MAPK pathway is highly stimulated and as the infection progresses levels of PGE2 (prostaglandin E2) and TGF-ß both rise (with a later elevation of IL-2). Lowering TGF levels is very helpful (*Angelica sinensis, Astragalus mongholicus*). HMGB1 levels during SARS cytokine cascades are high, especially in those who die. During the infection, the cytokine cascade initiates a massive immune cell migration, infiltration, and accumulation into lung tissues. The older the infected animal (human or otherwise), the greater the cytokine upregulation and the worse the outcome. Sharply reducing IL-1ß has been found to significantly decrease the impact of the disease on the infected and to inhibit mortality (Japanese knotweed — i.e., *Polygonum cuspidatum* — Chinese senega root, Chinese skullcap, cordyceps, kudzu, and boneset). Severe hypoxia occurs in the cells that are affected (and in the person so afflicted). The RAS-stimulated cellular hypoxia generates high levels of free radicals through the rapid increase of angiotensin II, i.e., a hypoxia-reoxygenation injury cycle. In essence an abundance of hydrogen peroxide and superoxide radicals is generated. The high levels of angiotensin II stimulate free radical formation from endothelial cells, vascular smooth muscle cells, and mesangial cells as well. In short the excessive angiotensin II levels (due to the destruction of ACE-2 cells by the virus) cause massive damage to the lung, lymph, and spleen tissue. Protecting the cells from the induced hypoxia significantly reduces the damage in the lungs. (Rhodiola is specific for this. It prevents hypoxia-induced oxidative damage, increases intracellular oxygen diffusion, and increases the efficiency of oxygen utilization.)

The virus specifically targets (and replicates within) ciliated cells, destroying the cells and their capacity to move mucus up and out of the lungs. (Cilia-protective herbs are cordyceps, olive oil and leaf, the berberine plants, and *Bidens pilosa*.) Autoantibodies are produced that begin to attack host epithelial and endothelial cells, increasing the destruction. Reducing the autoimmune response (rhodiola, astragalus, cordyceps) and protecting endothelial cells (Japanese knotweed) is crucial.

Autopsies of those who died revealed that the alveolar damage in the lungs was severe. There was massive damage to the lymph nodes in the lungs, as well as severe necrosis in the white pulp and marginal sinus of the spleen, destruction of the germinal centers in the lymph, apoptosis of lymphocytes, and an infiltration of monocytic cells. Protection of the spleen and lymph is essential (red root, poke root, Chinese skullcap).

SARS replicates primarily in ciliated epithelial cells but also in infected dendritic cells, both mature and immature. Dendritic cells exist abundantly just under the epithelium layers in the lung tissue. The cytokine upregulation makes the endothelium much more porous, allowing the virus to penetrate and infect the dendritic cells. It does not kill the dendritic cells but merely stops them from stimulating an effective adaptive immune response. The virus very powerfully upregulates IL-6 and IL-8 in the epithelial cells. These particular cytokines concentrate around the immature dendritic cells and strongly inhibit their maturation.. This in turn inhibits mature dendritic cells' ability to prime the production of active T cells and allows the virus to enter and severely damage the lymph organs in the lungs. Stimulating dendritic cell maturation (cordyceps) and increasing T cell counts (licorice, red root, elder, and zinc) will reduce the symptom picture and disease severity.

Medical Treatment

Ribavirin is only marginally effective against SARS but is still used in spite of the side effects. Corticosteroids are used to try and reduce inflammation. The nonsteroidal anti-inflammatory drug indomethacin has shown potent antiviral activity against the virus and should be used. Rimantidine and lopinavir have both been found active in vitro.

The SARS Protocol

The plants found specific for the SARS virus are Chinese skullcap, houttuynia, isatis, licorice, *Forsythia suspensa*, and *Sophora flavescens*.

I would use the exact same protocol as for influenza, outlined earlier, with two exceptions:

- Because *Salvia miltiorrhiza* is so specific for the virus and due to the fact that HMGB1 is usually present, I would use one of the HMGB1 formulations (see page 52) from the day the infection begins.
- Because kudzu is so specific for this virus, I would add kudzu to the HMGB1 formulation. For the tincture formulation, add an equal part of kudzu tincture and increase the dosage by one-third; for the aqueous infusion, add an equal amount of the dried root to the formulation.

Other Anti-SARS Herbs

Other plants found active against SARS are:

Artemisia annua	*Lycoris radiata* (stem extracts are
Cassia tora	extremely potent)
Cibotium barometz	*Panax ginseng*
Dioscorea batatas	*Polygonum cuspidatum*
Eucalyptus spp.	*Polygonum multiflorum*
Gentiana scabra	*Pyrrosia lingua*
Lindera aggregata	*Rheum officinale*
Lonicera japonica	*Taxillus chinensis*

A Few Other Respiratory Viral Infections

The main ones that people encounter are the adenoviruses, parainfluenza viruses, respiratory syncytial virus, and rhinoviruses.

Adenoviruses

Adenovirus infections tend to be mild and are generally easy to treat. However, acute conditions such as pharyngoconjunctival fever, acute respiratory disease, pneumonia, and meningitis can also occur.

Adenovirus 14 is an emerging serotype that can cause serious infection, essentially acute respiratory disease, which can sometimes lead to death. Conjunctivitis, high fever, pneumonia, and gastrointestinal involvement can all occur. The virus sheds in both respiratory droplets and feces and can remain highly infective in feces for long periods.

The herbs specific for adenovirus infections are astragalus, Chinese skullcap, elder, isatis, and licorice. Other herbs that are active are *Ardisia squamulosa, Artemisia princeps, Boussingaultia gracilis, Caesalpinia pulcherrima, Ocimum basilicum,* and *Serissa japonica.*

Treatment: The same as for mild influenza. If it becomes serious, the same as for moderate to severe influenza.

Parainfluenza Viruses

Parainfluenza viruses generally cause what is called croup. It is an acute infection of the upper respiratory tract accompanied by barking cough (the croup part) and hoarseness. The throat is often swollen, which can interfere with breathing. The herbs specific for parainfluenza are Chinese skullcap, elder, and licorice. *Allium sativum* and *Cicer arietinum* have also been found active.

Treatment: Tincture combination of elderberry, Chinese skullcap, and licorice tinctures, in equal parts. Dosage: 30 drops every hour.

Respiratory Syncytial Virus

Respiratory syncytial virus is also a single-strand, enveloped RNA virus with high variation in its genome. It is a very common infection, especially in young children, throughout the world. It causes bronchiolitis and other types of respiratory infections, especially in the lower respiratory tract. It generally presents as a common cold but can sometimes become serious, turning into pneumonia if left untreated.

The herbs specific for respiratory syncytial virus infections are Chinese skullcap, *Eleutherococcus senticosus*, elder, isatis, licorice, and *Sophora flavescens*. Other herbs found active are *Barleria prionitis, Blumea laciniata, Elephantopus scaber, Laggera pterodonta, Markhamia lutea, Mussaenda pubescens, Narcissus tazetta, Selaginella sinensis, Scutellaria indica*, and *Schefflera octophylla* (in vitro).

Treatment: The same as for mild influenza. If it becomes serious, the same as for moderate to severe influenza.

Rhinoviruses

These viruses cause the common cold. The herbs/supplements specific for rhinovirus infections are ginger, *Echinacea angustifolia*, elder, *Eleutherococcus senticosus*, quercetin, *Papaver pseudocanescens*, and *Raoulia australis*. A Japanese traditional formulation, hochu-ekki-to, has been found highly effective, as has *Prunus mume*.

Treatment: I have found the use of an *E. angustifolia*, licorice, and red root tincture combination, as outlined earlier (see page 43), *and* the prolific use of the ginger juice tea, also discussed earlier (see page 44), to be very effective.

3

VIRAL ENCEPHALITIS INFECTIONS AND THEIR TREATMENT

Emerging RNA viral pathogens such as West Nile virus (WNV), Japanese encephalitis virus (JEV), Australian bat Lyssavirus, retroviruses, and Nipah virus have become increasingly important causes of encephalitis.... Worldwide, the flavivirus JEV is the most common cause of arthropod-borne encephalitis with over 50,000 cases reported per year in China, Southeast Asia, and India. Epidemics due to this arbovirus result in a mortality rate that ranges from 30 to 50% with death usually occurring within the first week, and the development of sustained neurological deficits in approximately half of the survivors. Another flavivirus, WNV, is also transmitted by Culex spp. mosquitoes and can cause fatal encephalitis or long-term neurological sequelae. Once inside the CNS, JEV and WNV infect neurons leading to neuronal apoptosis and causing severe immunopathology.

— **Samantha Furr and Ian Marriott, "Viral CNS Infections"**

West Nile virus (WNV) has expanded in the last 12 years worldwide, and particularly in the Americas, where it first occurred in 1999. It has extended throughout the Americas relentlessly since then, causing a severe epidemic of disastrous consequences for public health, wildlife, and livestock.

— **M. A. Jiminez-Clavero, "Animal Viral Diseases and Global Change"**

Encephalitis **sounds like a technical term** but it isn't really. It simply means inflammation (the "itis" part) of the brain ("encephal," meaning brain, from an ancient Greek root). As with hepatitis, whose name merely means inflammation of the liver, there are many things that can cause such inflammations; the term refers not to a disease per se but merely to a primary symptom that occurs during the disease process.

There are a range of viruses that can cause encephalitis; many of them are known by that particular symptom — West Nile encephalitis and Japanese viral encephalitis are some examples. The viruses that cause these conditions have an affinity for the brain; it's their preferred habitat. Many of them, such as the Japanese encephalitis virus (JEV), have a tropism for neurons in the brain; they reproduce most easily inside them. So once they infect a person, that is where they like to go. Once established in the brain or central nervous system (CNS), they begin to release (or stimulate the release of) unique compounds called cytokines. Cytokines cause particular cells in the brain to swell and burst apart (the inflammation aspect of things). This gives the viruses the nutrients they need and facilitates their spread. (If the meninges, the sheath covering the brain and spinal cord, also inflames, which it sometimes does, the infection is called meningitis.) Unfortunately, the damage to the brain neurons causes a number of problems, some serious, in whomever the virus has infected. One of the most difficult is the inflammation itself. The brain is encased in a solid shell that, itself, cannot expand. So, if the inflammation is such that the brain is forced to swell beyond the size of its container, well . . . things get dicey.

Technological medicine has a limited capacity to respond to this kind of infection. During a minor infection, the usual response is to tell the person to stay at home and rest in bed. If the condition is severe, as it becomes for many of the viral encephalitides, there is no accepted pharmaceutical treatment. In some cases, but not most, antivirals will help. In others, the treatments are new and rather experimental, and only offer limited help. If the swelling becomes threatening, intravenous steroids to reduce the inflammation may be used, though there are a number of very serious side effects to their use if they are needed long term.

Plant medicines, on the other hand, offer a much more elegant intervention, especially for this kind of condition. With plant medicines, each aspect of the disease can be addressed. Antivirals can be used to kill the organism (or limit its ability to infect the body's cells). Anti-inflammatories, specific for the brain, can be used to reduce inflammation. Neural protectors can be used to safeguard brain structures from damage (or to restore damaged structures). Immune facilitators (adaptogens) can be used to enhance immune function so the body is more able to fight the infection on its own. And the unique symptom picture that emerges for the infected person can be addressed through the use of plant symptomatics. Too, most of these plant medicines tend to be synergistic with one another (as many of the individual plant compounds are with one another) and, together, produce outcomes that can be very potent. With time, the ability to respond to viral infections can become tremendously sophisticated.

This is an initial exploration of how such an approach can be applied to viral encephalitis.

The Encephalitis Viruses

There are some viruses that specifically infect the brain and cause encephalitis (West Nile) and there are others that sometimes get into the brain and cause encephalitis (herpes simplex). Many of them are spread by insect vectors (mosquitoes and ticks). For some of them, there are vaccines (tick-borne encephalitis — TBE). Others will sometimes respond fairly well to pharmaceuticals (acyclovir for instance for nonresistant herpes encephalitis). Most of the viruses that cause encephalitis show similar initial symptoms; all of them can be treated with plant medicines. (And yes, pharmaceuticals can be used along with plant-based protocols. The plant protocol tends to *increase* the effectiveness of the pharmaceutical protocol while at the same time significantly relieving the symptom picture.)

Here is a look at the most common encephalitis viruses and their geographical distribution:

- **Togaviruses, the alphavirus complex:** eastern equine encephalitis (eastern and Gulf coasts of the United States, Caribbean, South America), western equine encephalitis (western United States and Canada), Venezuelan equine encephalitis (South and Central America, Florida, southwest United States). All are spread by mosquitoes.

- **Flaviviruses, the West Nile complex:** St. Louis encephalitis (United States), Japanese encephalitis (Japan, China, southeast Asia, India, southeast Russia, northern Australia, New Guinea), Murray Valley encephalitis (Australia and New Guinea), West Nile (United States, Africa, Europe, Middle East, Asia), Ilhéus (South and Central America), Rocio (Brazil). All are spread by mosquitoes.

- **Flaviviruses, the tick-borne complex:** Far Eastern tick-borne encephalitis (eastern Russia), central European encephalitis (central Europe), Kyasanur forest disease (India), louping ill (England, Scotland, northern Ireland), Powassan (Canada and northern United States), Negishi (Japan). All spread by ticks. In general, this group is usually just referred to as TBE or tick-borne encephalitis virus and treated accordingly.

- **Bunyaviruses, the bunyavirus complex:** California encephalitis (western United States), La Crosse encephalitis (mid- and eastern United States), Jamestown Canyon (United States, including Alaska), snowshoe hare (Canada, Alaska, northern United States), Tahyna (Czech Republic, Slovakia, former Yugoslavian states, Italy, southern France), Inkoo (Finland). All spread by mosquitoes.

- **Phlebovirus:** Rift Valley fever (eastern Africa). Spread by mosquitoes.

- **Reovirus, orbivirus:** Colorado tick fever (Rocky Mountains, western United States and Canada). Spread by ticks.

The most common, in the United States, are West Nile, St. Louis encephalitis, La Crosse encephalitis, and California encephalitis. Japanese encephalitis virus (JEV) is the most common in Asia (estimates are that in some areas the infection rate is 100 percent). From all reports, it is the main member of the common viral encephalitides that causes the most damage. The most common viral encephalitis in Europe and Russia is West Nile and TBE; West Nile is, in fact, becoming a worldwide phenomenon and is present in most of the world. Most of the other encephalitis viruses are somewhat uncommon in people. Vaccines have been created for both Japanese viral encephalitis and TBE but they can't be used on those younger than 15 to 17 years of age.

In spite of the existence of vaccines, there are large outbreaks of both Japanese viral encephalitis and TBE every year, especially in the young. The vaccine needs to be repeated every year (Japanese) or every 3 years (TBE). For many cultures, the cost is often prohibitive and many people simply never get the vaccines. There are also certain groups of people for whom it is considered risky to give the vaccine, primarily the old and the young. Specifically: 1) those over 60 years of age; 2) those allergic to formaldehyde, neomycin, gentamycin, protamine sulfate, latex, eggs, or chickens; 3) those with a brain or central nervous system problem; 4) those with high temperatures; 5) those with weakened immune systems; 6) those with autoimmune conditions; 7) women who are pregnant; 8) those under 15 years of age (17 for the Japanese viral encephalitis vaccine). There remain a large number of people who can't be vaccinated, many of whom succumb to the infections each year.

Symptoms

Nearly all, 90 percent, of people infected by an encephalitis virus have flu-like symptoms: fever, sore throat, cough, general ill feeling, aches and pains, weakness, and malaise. About 10 percent have no symptoms at all. And for most people the infection passes, just like the flu; they really have no idea that they were infected with viral encephalitis.

If the infection is severe, the symptom picture alters accordingly: Headache, confusion, disorientation, photophobia, agitation, optic neuritis, myelitis, personality alterations, seizures, coma, and death can all occur, depending on the severity of the infection. Depending on which part of the brain is affected, language skills may be impaired and voluntary movement affected, and severe muscle weakness, uncontrollable tremors, partial paralysis, involuntary movements, and loss of ability to regulate body temperature may occur.

Medical Treatment

Most neural encephalitis infections such as Japanese viral encephalitis and West Nile encephalitis have no established pharmaceutical treatment approaches — though there are a few treatments that are showing promise. Minocycline does work to some extent in Japanese viral encephalitis. It modulates the degree of infection and the persistence of the virus, reduces the inflammatory cytokines in the brain, and is neuroprotective. It also reduces viral replication. Although not yet in common use, it is probably the best treatment approach for severe JEV infections.

Immunoglobulin therapy has helped with a number of different viral encephalitides including West Nile. Interferon-alpha and ribavirin have also been used, though with mixed to moderate success for West Nile. Minocycline has been found effective in West Nile encephalitis and I think it a good treatment approach if the disease becomes serious. Erythromycin can significantly reduce the endothelial hyperplasia that sometimes occurs during West Nile encephalitis.

Anticonvulsant medications are sometimes used to treat seizures. Steroid medications, IV, are used for inflammation in severe cases.

Some of the nonspecific viruses that can sometimes infect the brain, such as herpes, do respond to pharmaceuticals. The usual treatment for them is antivirals: acyclovir (for herpes simplex, Epstein-Barr, and varicella zoster encephalitis) and ganciclovir (for cytomegalovirus and herpes simplex 1 encephalitis).

Mechanisms of Viral Infection

Japanese encephalitis virus (JEV), West Nile virus (WNV), tick-borne encephalitis virus (TBE), St. Louis encephalitis virus, and dengue virus are all flaviviruses, they are closely related, and they have very similar impacts in the body. In other words, with slight differences, what they do once they are in the body, how they affect brain structures, and the kinds of cytokines they stimulate are all very similar. (The treatment protocol for each, in consequence, is also very similar.) I will look in the most depth at JEV and WNV, then just a bit at TBE (which, being tick spread, has some unique features) and a bit at La Crosse, the most common nonflavivirus encephalitis virus. I take a brief look at dengue in general in the next chapter with just a touch on its encephalitis aspects in this one.

Japanese Encephalitis Virus: Initial Infection

Japanese encephalitis virus (JEV), sometimes called encephalitis B, is the best studied of these viruses. At the time of this writing there are over 4,300 journal articles about it in the online medical database PubMed and another 1,600 at the fledgling Chinese database CNKI. It has been rather intensively studied since the 1930s. It's spread, as most viral encephalitides are, by mosquitoes.

Once the mosquito bites a person, the virus enters the body while the mosquito feeds, then travels to the liver, spleen, and lymph system over the next 5 to 15 days (the incubation period). As with tick-borne infections, the virus uses the saliva of the arthropod vector to facilitate its entry into the body. The chemicals in mosquito saliva interfere with host immune responses, downregulating interferon responses and T cell activation and immune cell numbers. This allows the virus to bypass the immune system, get into the lymph system, and spread throughout the body.

Once inside the spleen it begins infecting dendritic cells and monocytes/macrophages. It is able to replicate, slowly, inside these cells even though they are not its preferred habitat. It uses the cells primarily to foster its invasion of the body.

JEV uses the dendritic cells to begin its subversion of the host immune system, essentially by inhibiting the ability of the dendritic cells to mature. Dendritic cells mature or develop in specific ways when they detect infections in the body. In this particular instance the lack of maturity stops dendritic cell activation of T cells; activated T cells and immunoglobulin M (IgM) play a major role in relieving the body of viral infection and reducing neuronal damage. The most active T cells for this kind of viral infection are those that express CD8+ proteins on their surface. These cytotoxic T cells, or killer lymphocytes, are a type of white blood cell that is very good at killing cells infected with viruses.

While inhibiting the activation of these T cells, the virus begins to infect monocytes/macrophages. These essentially act as transport mechanisms for the virus, taking it into the brain, where it can more easily spread. JEV releases a number of specific compounds to increase the permeability of the blood-brain barrier, thus easing its passage into the brain. Once inside the brain it moves outside the macrophage/monocyte cells and begins to attach itself to brain neurons. JEV has the strongest tropism for neurons in the thalamus, cortex, striatum, hippocampus, and midbrain, which are the parts of the brain impacted most severely by the infection. The virus reaches peak levels in the brain on the sixth day (11 to 20 days postinfection).

Once attached to the surface of a neuronal cell, the viruses stimulate endocytosis — the process by which cells take molecules into themselves (engulfment). Once inside the neurons, the viruses begin to replicate. The viral particles also begin attaching themselves to microglia, the resident macrophages of the brain and spinal cord. These are the primary immune defensive forces of the CNS. Microglia, like most macrophages, release a number of chemicals during infection that are designed to kill invading organisms. But many microbes have learned to use the host defense system for their own purposes. These kinds of encephalitis viruses are no exception. JEV attaches to the surface of the microglia, stimulating them to release cytokines and chemokines. The virus uses the microglia primarily as a source of inflammation *and* as a reservoir site in the brain.

The astroglia (astrocytes) are often infected as well. These cells are tremendously abundant in the brain and do a number of things, among them keeping the blood-brain barrier intact, providing nutrients to neurons, maintaining ion balance, and, most importantly, repairing damaged neurons. JEV infection of the astroglia inhibits their repair functions and stimulates them, as well, to release a number of cytokines: IL-6, RANTES, and MCP-1. The primary purpose of their infection appears to be inhibition of their maintenance and repair functions. However, more sophisticated research has found that there is considerable virus-stimulated synergy between the cytokine cascades from the astrocytes and microglia. A sort of cross-talk occurs that promotes what researchers call a "fulminate inflammation," which the virus uses to its advantage.

> A defining feature of viral CNS infection is the rapid onset of severe neuroinflammation and overzealous glial responses. [These] are associated with significant neurological damage or even death. . . . [There is] the possibility that cross-talk exists between these disparate viral sensors and their signaling pathways [and that they can] act in a cooperative manner to promote the fulminate inflammation associated with acute neurotropic viral infection.
>
> — *Samantha Furr and Ian Marriott,*
> "Viral CNS Infections"

NEURONAL DAMAGE

After JEV is established in the brain, it begins to cause the death of neurons. This is the main source of the symptoms that occur from infection and it results from two factors: 1) direct infection of neurons by the virus, and 2) the overactive immune responses initiated by the virus after it attaches to the microglia.

Once attached to a neural cell, the virus stimulates the production of sphingomyelinase. This is an enzyme that breaks down sphingomyelin, a kind of lipid that makes up some of the structural elements of cells, especially the myelin sheath that surrounds nerve cells. This causes a variety of neurological problems; for example myelin sheath degradation is common in diseases such as Parkinson's disease. Sphingomyelinase inhibitors (such as cordyceps, which is a very potent sphingomyelinase inhibitor) can reduce or eliminate the damage. As the sphingomyelin is broken apart the cellular membrane becomes more porous but, as well, one of sphingomyelin's major consituents, ceramide, is released.

Ceramide has a number of functions in the cell and body. Its release is intimately involved in apoptosis, or cellular death. It also is deeply involved in the creation of lipid rafts. These rafts can cross the entire lipid bilayer of cells, allowing things from outside the cell (usually molecules) to enter into the cell. The virus attaches itself to the lipid rafts and rides them into the cell.

Once inside the cell, the virus begins reproducing in the cytoplasm, the space inside the cell. The rough endoplasmic reticulum (RER), which covers the outer surface of the nucleus, is used as a sort of uterus for the newly developing viruses; they bud from its membranes as they develop. The RER is also stimulated to proliferate and the resulting hypertrophy makes more space for the viruses to create offspring. Most of the viruses (about 60 percent) remain in this location, while another 20 percent invade the Golgi apparatus that lies between the inner side of the cell and the nucleus. The Golgi apparatus's primary function is to modify proteins delivered from the RER. It generates glycosaminoglycans and proteoglycans. These are forms of sugar molecules that are used structurally in the body. The Golgi apparatus also generates and stores Bcl-2.

The remaining 20 percent of the viruses invade the nucleus of the cell, specifically the nucleolus. In this location, they scavenge RNA particles from the nucleus to facilitate their reproduction. There is a constant movement between the viral particles in the nucleus and those in the cytoplasm where the scavenged RNA is exchanged and used to form new viral particles.

All the infected cell's functions are tightly controlled by the virus. It controls cell life and cell death. Initially it slows the ability of the infected cell to die but once enough virus particles have been reproduced, it stimulates cellular death. The cell bursts apart and a swarm of viral particles is released and the process begins again. The virus uses a highly elegant control of cellular signaling molecules to accomplish this.

The infected cell is stimulated to begin a signaling cascade of highly bioactive molecules: p38 MAPK and a number of caspases are activated. These stimulate the production of CHOP (C/EBP homologous protein), which ultimately is used by the virus to cause cell death. The death of these neuronal cells is the main cause of the damage the disease does and the source of many of the symptoms. (The use of p38 MAPK inhibitors — Chinese skullcap, houttuynia, cordyceps — significantly reduces neuronal cell death, slows the proliferation of new viral particles in the brain, and reduces the damage the disease does.)

The virus specifically downregulates Bcl-2, inhibiting its release by the Golgi apparatus. This stimulates the release of cytochrome c from the mitochondria, initiating a mitochondrial-controlled cellular death process that is tightly controlled by the virus. Bcl-2 downregulation causes the subsequent activation of caspase-8 and caspase-9 (caspases are sometimes referred to as the "central executioners" of cell death), a burst of free radicals, and significant depletion of intracellular glutathione in the cell. (Upregulation of Bcl-2, by such plants as Chinese skullcap, licorice, and rhodiola, can inhibit the process.) All this is part of the sudden cell death the virus causes once its numbers have reproduced sufficiently. (The use of mitochondrial protectors, such as kudzu root, can also interfere with Bcl-2 downregulation, subsequent cytochrome c release, activation of caspase-8 and caspase-9, the intracellular depletion of glutathione, and free radical production.)

MICROGLIAL CYTOKINE CASCADES

Once the virus reaches the brain, microglia are strongly stimulated by virus attachment and tremendously overactivated. The microglia begin producing an overabundance of IL-6, TNF-α, monocyte chemoattractant protein-1 (MCP-1), and RANTES (CCL5). This causes a massive leukocyte migration and infiltration into the brain. (The activated astrocytes produce upregulated levels of IFN-γ and RANTES, also contributing to the problem.) Manganese superoxide dismutase (SOD), IL-8, IL-12, IL-1ß, p38 MAPK, iNOS (inducible nitric oxide synthase), COX-2 (cyclooxygenase-2), IFN-γ, and NF-κB are also upregulated, making the problem worse. Levels of IL-10 and IL-4 (cytokine regulators) are initially high (which reduces the normal, initial antiviral response) and then are inhibited (to keep their balancing effect on inflammatory cytokine upregulation in check) and decline over the course of the illness.

The virus interferes with interferon signaling during infection, reducing the impacts of immune interferons alpha and beta on the infection. The virus also stimulates the production and activity of tyrosine kinase, which is one of the factors behind the production of TNF-α and IL-1ß cytokines.

The greater the levels of induced cytokines in the brain, the worse the outcome. The degree of long-term damage and incidence of mortality are directly proportional to the cytokine levels induced by the virus. Additionally, the cytokine cascade, especially NF-κB, TNF-α, IL-1ß, and IL-6, can stimulate the release of HMGB1 protein (see page 37). The damage to neuronal cells by the virus also causes HMGB1 release into the brain. This induces the release of inflammatory cytokines and excitatory amino acids such as glutamate, stimulates fever, and exacerbates ischemic injury. (The use of HMGB1 inhibitors such as licorice, *Angelica sinensis*, and *Salvia miltiorrhiza* is essential to stop the disease's progression to a generalized sepsis.)

Reducing the cytokine and chemokine cascades has been found to inhibit the course of the disease and reduce neural damage. Studies have shown that ERK and glutaminase inhibition helps prevent cytokine damage in the brain. And rosmarinic acid from *Rosmarinus officinalis*, which has been studied in some depth, has been found to be highly effective in reducing major elements of the cytokine cascade (IL-12, IL-6, MCP-1, IFN-γ, and IFN-α), thus protecting the brain and reducing the mortality levels in mice.

Comment: Rosmarinic acid is not very systemic; it is usually injected to get this impact in the CNS. As such systemic inhibitors of the cytokines are much preferred since they don't need to be injected. These include inhibitors of ERK (kudzu, Chinese skullcap, cordyceps); MCP-1 (houttuynia); RANTES (licorice, isatis); IL-6 (Chinese skullcap, astragalus, cordyceps); TNF-α (kudzu, Chinese senega root, Chinese skullcap, elder, ginger, houttuynia, licorice, boneset, cordyceps); NF-κB (Chinese senega root, Chinese skullcap, ginger, houttuynia, kudzu, licorice, boneset, astragalus); IL-1ß (Japanese knotweed, Chinese senega root, Chinese skullcap, cordyceps, kudzu, boneset); and IL-8 (cordyceps, isatis, Japanese knotweed).

In essence, flooding the CNS with inhibitors of the stimulated cytokines stops the progression of the disease and significantly reduces long-term impacts on the brain. Many of these herbs are known for their brain protective effects; they are systemically disseminated, cross the blood-brain barrier, and are specifically protective, in many instances, for brain neurons. Many of them also possess antiviral actions. Because they hit in so many areas of activity, they are the specifics to use for these kinds of viral diseases.

Of additional use are tyrosine kinase inhibitors (such as cordyceps and Japanese knotweed), which have been found to attenuate JEV-induced neurotoxicity. This does not stop JEV replication in neuronal cells but does stop the neuronal damage caused by cytokines. Sphingomyelinase inhibitors (such as cordyceps) slow the movement of viral particles into cells. Alpha-glucosidase inhibitors of the endoplasmic reticulum (strongly present in such plants as Chinese skullcap and rhodiola) have been found to stop the replication of the virus. And this is, in fact, one of the approaches the body itself uses eventually.

The body, in challenging the virus, ultimately does activate T cells in the spleen. Once activated, the T cells begin production of a T-cell-specific alpha-glucosidase inhibitor. This actively suppresses the replication of the virus but also tends to produce a lingering hypoglycemia during the postinfection stage of Japanese viral encephalitis.

Higher IL-4 and IL-10 levels (Chinese skullcap, elder, houttuynia, licorice, cordyceps) and splenic activation of T cells (red root, poke root, Chinese skullcap, houttuynia, astragalus, cordyceps) have both been found to produce milder infections. IL-10 has neuroprotective effects and helps reduce inflammatory damage.

POSTINFECTION DAMAGE

Survivors of severe Japanese viral encephalitis often have long-term neurological damage. This can include major cognitive impairment and motor and behavioral problems. Part of this comes from the damage to neural structures in the brain, but the virus also significantly reduces the levels of neural progenitor cells in the body. This significantly impairs recovery after the disease since the brain cannot use the progenitor cells to repair the viral damage. The virus initiates the activation of phosphoinositide 3-kinase/Akt signaling during the early stages of infection, which leads, in part, to this effect on progenitor cells. Inhibitors of this (cordyceps) can help alleviate the emergence of this long-term problem. The use of herbs that stimulate neural growth and contain nerve growth factor (Chinese senega root, lion's mane, *Knema laurina*) will help stimulate the production of new neural structures in the brain and significantly reduce postinfection damage.

West Nile Encephalitis

West Nile, in contrast to Japanese encephalitis, and in spite of the concern about it, has been much less explored by researchers. Although discovered in 1937 the first large outbreak did not occur until the 1990s; research did not begin in earnest until the latter part of that decade — after outbreaks occurred in the United States. Thirty-two hundred of the 3,600 studies on the virus have occurred since then; the Chinese database CNKI has a mere 74 journal articles on the virus. Oddly enough, in contrast to the Japanese encephalitis virus, there has been much less work on the cytokine cascade caused by West Nile virus (WNV). The virus is much more poorly understood and its exact dynamics inside the body and brain are less clear.

Nevertheless, WNV follows almost the same process during infection as JEV though it is not nearly so dangerous. Four in five of those infected have few or no symptoms at all. One in five experience a flu-like febrile illness of limited duration. One in 150 develops encephalitis or meningitis or both. In contrast to JEV, which is most active in the young, WNV has the most damaging effects in the aged. The older a person is, the worse the outcome and the greater likelihood they will be seriously ill. The virus seems to specialize in attacking the aging brain (JEV, in contrast, has a preference for immature and developing neural structures). The younger the person, the younger the neural structures, the less likely the disease is to be severe, or even to be symptomatic. Children and young adults tend to be asymptomatic. The median age of those who present with just fever and flu-like symptoms is 43; the median age of those who develop severe symptoms is 59. The old are also especially at risk because the aging immune system is less strong (immune senescence) and, at the same time, they tend to have preexisting conditions that affect brain function (such as higher reactive oxygen species and other cytokines already active in the brain from Alzheimer's and similar conditions). The incubation period is about the same as for JEV, 3 to 11 days, with the average at 5 days.

Most of the people who experience severe infection have similar symptoms: muscle weakness, gastrointestinal symptoms, fever, headache, alterations in mental status, and movement disorders such as tremors, myoclonus, Parkinsonism. A smaller proportion have an erythematous macular rash of one sort or another that can appear in various places on the body. Meningoencephalitis is common. A polio-like paralysis appears in a small subset of those infected. If meningitis occurs, neck stiffness, headache, hypothermia, photophobia, and/or phonophobia are common. With encephalitis, especially severe, depressed or altered consciousness, lethargy, personality alterations, fever, and hypothermia are common.

Ribavirin and interferon-a2b are the most common pharmaceuticals used, but they show a very mixed success rate. The main intervention is hospitalization ("supportive" treatment, as most journal articles refer to it) and observation; there is little medical intervention. Mostly the people just get well on their own . . . or don't.

INFECTION PROGRESSION

After infection (by mosquito bite) nothing appears amiss for about 5 days or so but on day 6 or 7 lethargy sets in, food intake slows, weakness begins to develop. By days 7 to 10 (in severe cases) tremors and difficulty walking, thinking, and communicating start to occur.

As with Japanese encephalitis, the virus travels first to the spleen and thence to the CNS. The blood-brain barrier is made more permeable (as with JEV) and once into the brain the virus begins to seek out its preferred areas. Those are the cerebral cortex, cerebellar cortex, subcortical gray matter, hippocampus, and basal ganglia. As the infection progresses the cerebral cortex and the hippocampus are more heavily affected; severe degeneration begins in the neurons in those areas, then escalates as the virus reproduces. The virus then spreads to the brain stem and spinal cord (which is when a general paralysis can occur).

There is direct infection of neurons and an inflammatory stimulation of the host immune system, which the virus uses during the disease process. In essence, it stimulates an autoimmune response to break down cellular structures in the CNS. The microglia are infected, and microglial nodules form, filled with lymphocytic infiltrate, the nodules surrounded by degenerated (exploded) neurons. As the disease progresses, the brain stem is more deeply affected and begins showing tremendous neuronal degeneration and the inflammation in the spinal cord is much more developed. The lumbar region of the spinal cord can become severely affected, with inflammatory infiltrates along the entire length of the cord. The brain stem, temporal lobes, and basal ganglia are, generally, the most severely affected regions of the brain.

In those who survive the illness, persistent neurological problems can remain. The virus can, in some, develop into a long-term, chronic infection that does not heal. Long-term chronic infection with West Nile is almost totally dependent on the failure of CD8+ T cells to become active or highly present in the body. As with Japanese viral encephalitis, the higher the CD8+ T cell activity prior to infection, the less chance there is for infection, especially serious infection, to occur.

THE CYTOKINE/CHEMOKINE CASCADE

The cytokine and chemokine profiles in the CNS are similar to those of Japanese viral encephalitis but there are differences. The cytokines TNF-α, IL-1ß, IL-5, IL-6, IL-8, IL-13, interferon-inducible protein-10 (IP-10), matrix metalloproteinase-1 (MMP-1), MMP-3, MMP-9, NF-κB, COX-2, and the chemokine MCP-1 are all increased. Interferon-gamma levels are strongly increased, as are the levels of IDO (indoleamine 2,3-dioxygenase), ICAM-1 (intercellular adhesion molecule-1), VCAM-1 (vascular cell adhesion molecule-1), E-selectin, p38 MAPK, RANTES, and PGE2 (prostaglandin E2).

Researchers have looked intensively at the presence of a number of chemokines in West Nile encephalitis (not explored in the development of Japanese viral encephalitis); CCR1, CCR2, CCR5, CCL2, CCL3, and CCL4 all showed increases. IL-10 levels are initially upregulated by the virus upon infection in order to keep the innate immune response as low as possible. Once the virus is established in the body and cytokine levels begin to rise, the levels of IL-4 and IL-10 are inhibited in order to stop their cytokine regulatory actions. The longer the infection, the lower the levels become. Perforin levels are reduced as well. Perforin is a protein in cytotoxic T cells that creates pores in target cells that allows the T cells to enter the infected cells and kill them.

All in all, the infection cytokine dynamic is very similar to that of Japanese viral encephalitis. Three of the main differences, however, are the generation of matrix metalloproteinases (MMPs), cellular adhesion molecules, and IDO.

The virus stimulates the production of MMPs (MMP-1, MMP-3, and MMP-9) once it enters the spleen. The MMPs are a kind of enzyme that especially degrade extracellular matrix proteins. These proteins make up much of the connective tissue in animals, including crucial elements of the blood-brain barrier. In essence, once MMPs are activated in a location, the connective tissue in that location begins to degrade. West Nile uses these to degrade the blood-brain barrier enough that it can gain entry to the brain and spinal cord. The tight junction protein bonds are weakened, making the barrier more permeable. Once inside the brain the virus attaches much more strongly to astrocytes than JEV does and stimulates them to continue releasing MMPs. Astrocytes are, in fact, the main source of these compounds in the brain. (The endothelial cells of the brain's microvascular are also activated to produce MMPs.) This makes the blood-brain barrier significantly more porous, and keeps it that way. This creates an enhanced infiltration of immune cells into the brain, and they cluster around the sites of viral infection and contribute to the inflammation in those locations. The cellular structures are weakened, helping the virus gain entry to their host's cells. In other words, the virus makes the blood-brain barrier porous and actively damages neural structures, which stimulates the production of cytokines and chemokines, which then call to themselves a variety of immune cells at the specific neural locations the virus wants them. The use of MMP inhibitors (such as Japanese knotweed root, Chinese skullcap, cordyceps) has been found to stop the process by inhibiting astrocyte production of MMPs and restoring blood-brain barrier integrity.

WNV also manipulates cholesterol content in cellular membranes. It upregulates host cell cholesterol biosynthesis and redistributes the produced cholesterol into viral replication membranes.

The cytokines stimulated by the virus (specifically TNF-α and IL-1ß) in turn stimulate the production of ICAM-1, VCAM-1, and E-selectin by both astrocytes and endothelial cells in the brain. These are chemotactic for immune infiltrates that form the microglial nodules. Basically, they act like magnets, calling the immune cells to them. The leukocytes that are called to those locations bind to cells and then transmigrate into tissues, in this instance making the cells more accessible to the viral particles. PGE2, which is stimulated by COX-2, is strongly involved in the inflammation process and the aggregation of platelets; it has a number of potent impacts on spinal neurons and is a stimulant of IDO in the body. TNF-α inhibitors (kudzu, Chinese senega root, Chinese skullcap, elder, ginger, houttuynia, licorice, boneset, cordyceps) and IL-1ß inhibitors (Japanese knotweed, Chinese senega root, Chinese skullcap, cordyceps, kudzu, boneset) have all been found to stop this process. Inhibitors of ICAM-1 (Japanese knotweed, elder, cordyceps), VCAM-1 (Japanese knotweed, kudzu, elder, licorice), and E-selectin (Japanese knotweed, kudzu, licorice) can significantly reduce leukocyte infiltration and congregation.

The stimulation of the endothelial cells in the brain's microvascular network also causes a hypertrophy of those cells, interfering with blood flow to the brain. A central nervous system vasculitis can occur that can, sometimes, lead to stroke or other complications. Plants such as Japanese knotweed (or compounds such as EGCG and resveratrol), which are specific inhibitors of endothelial hypertrophy, can not only reduce MMP production but also inhibit this process. (Erythromycin is also specifically indicated for this.) Cerebral vasculitis from West Nile infection is somewhat more common than understood. In severe cases endothelial cell normalizers (Japanese knotweed root, EGCG, hawthorn berry, *Salvia miltiorrhiza*, licorice) really should be used. COX-2 (and PGE2) inhibitors are also helpful, especially because they help reduce IDO levels (Japanese knotweed, kudzu, Chinese skullcap, Chinese senega root, elder, ginger, houttuynia, isatis, cordyceps). COX-2 inhibitors also specifically block the production of WNV-induced cytokines in astrocytes (essentially the same herbs).

One of the first things that the virus does is to, in a specific process, increase levels of interferon-gamma (and TNF-α) in order to stimulate the production of indoleamine 2,3-dioxygenase (IDO). During WNV infection, high levels of IFN-γ, TNF-α, IL-1ß, and IL-2 are present in the brain. (TNF-α is synergistic with IFN-γ in stimulating IDO production.) Additionally, once the virus enters the spleen and infects dendritic cells it begins stimulating them to produce IDO (which reduces T cell proliferation, thus protecting the virus from the most effective immune response). This is one of the main differences between this virus and JEV. IDO is an enzyme that breaks apart (catalyzes) the amino acid L-tryptophan. There are a number of wide-ranging effects from this, all of which have deleterious effects in the body.

Normally, when infection occurs, the body creates IFN-γ to catalyze tryptophan because tryptophan degradation limits protein biosynthesis by depriving cells of an essential amino acid. But West Nile doesn't need tryptophan. It, instead, uses this natural immune response to limit T cell proliferation and to create specific, and very potent, inflammations in the brain. IDO is a potent inhibitor of T cells (it also induces apoptosis of competent T cells) and through its degradation of tryptophan creates powerful inflammatory molecules in the brain. The degree of tryptophan degradation is a specific indicator of the progression, and seriousness, of the infection.

L-tryptophan is normally degraded into L-kynurenine and then into three intermediary compounds that are highly neuroactive in the brain: 3-hydroxykynurenine (3-HK), quinolinic acid (QUIN), and kynurenic acid (KYNA).

High QUIN levels in the brain will cause an overstimulation of neurons, excitotoxic lesions, degradation of brain tissue, high levels of reactive oxygen species in the brain, and convulsions. The precursor to QUIN, 3-HK, is highly neurodestructive, causing cellular disintegration, primarily through the generation of free radicals. Neurons are particularly vulnerable to its actions. KYNA, on the other hand, is neuroprotective, and ameliorates the impacts of QUIN and 3-HK. Unfortunately, the amount of KYNA depends on healthy neuron function, which in WNV infection is inhibited severely. Compromised cellular energy metabolism (i.e., mitochondrial function) will also significantly reduce KYNA levels. In WNV infection 3-HK and QUIN levels are very high, and KYNA levels are very low. Upon microglial and astro-cyte activation 3-HK and QUIN levels can increase 100 to 1,000 times; this is especially true if there is the kind of macrophage infiltration that occurs during West Nile encephalitis. The number and serious-ness of seizures, convulsions, and paralysis that people with West Nile experience are directly proportional to the level of IDO generated in the brain (and its subsequent generation of QUIN and 3-HK).

IDO stimulation also has the regrettable ability to significantly inhibit serotonin and melatonin production in the brain. Melatonin, besides its potent sleep regulatory actions, is also an incredibly strong antioxidant, more powerful than most. It very specifically deactivates the oxidants that 3-HK and QUIN create. During WNV infection, how-ever, melatonin levels fall very low in the brain. (Keeping melatonin levels high will reduce, or eliminate, the ability of West Nile — and other encephalitis viruses — to cause infections. Increasing melatonin levels, by using plants such as Chinese skullcap that are very high in melatonin, will reduce vulnerability to infection, symptom picture, and mortality. It specifically reduces paralysis and convulsions and is highly protective of the brain's neural structures.)

IDO inhibitors (and exogenous melatonin) can stop this process (*and* reduce IFN-γ and TNF-α levels), thus protecting brain tissues and reducing symptom severity, postinfection complications, and mortality. The most potent inhibitors of IDO are Chinese skullcap, Japanese knotweed, isatis, and, most especially, *Crinum latifolium*.

The high levels of IDO also create tryptophan depletion in the body. Tryptophan is an essential amino acid that cannot be synthesized by the body; it has to come from outside sources. During severe West Nile encephalitis, tryptophan supplementation should occur. (This will *not* feed the viruses, making the disease worse, but will, in fact, help repair CNS damage.) Studies have found that exogenous tryptophan can help restore healthy T cell function and responses.

There are several other interventions that have been found to reduce WNV impacts in the body. The inhibition of p38 MAPK (Chinese skullcap, houttuynia, cordyceps) significantly decreases chemokine production in response to WNV. CD8+ T cells require perforin to clear West Nile virus from infected neurons. Low perforin levels correlate to a much higher viral load, worse symptom picture, and increased mortality. Increasing perforin levels (by using plants such as astragalus) stimulates clearance of the virus and reduces symptoms.

Tick-Borne Encephalitis

TBE is very similar to the other members of this group. It has a higher affinity for the lymph system, with subsequent involvement of the nodes. And this is where it first replicates before traveling to the brain (via the spleen and lymph system). The spleen is particularly infected (making the use of spleen herbs essential) and the virus can remain in the body, including the spleen, for months, perhaps years. Acute symptoms (beyond the initial flu symptoms) are hyperemia, petechial hemorrhages, inflammatory infiltration, necrosis of microglial cells, hyperplastic and hypertrophic glial nodules. Lesions are most common in the periventricular regions of the brain stem, including the cerebellum and reticular formation. The cerebellar cortex and basilar portions of the pons, thalamus, and olivary nuclei can also be affected. Perivascular inflammation around the blood vessels and cerebral interstitial edema are common. Laminar necrosis can occur. The cranial nerve and cervical anterior horn motor neuron cells are commonly affected during deeper progressions of the disease. Meningitis is common.

The cytokine/chemokine profiles are similar to those of other encephalitides: IL-6, TNF-α, IL-1ß, IL-1α are all high; IL-10 is initially high, then decreases substantially — as usual with these kinds of viruses. One difference is that if the pH of the blood moves from its normal alkaline state (around 7.3) to an acidic state, it strongly facilitates the ability of TBE virus to infect the body. Sodium bicarbonate, calcium citrate, magnesium citrate (and isatis) supplementation will reliably increase pH and reduce the ability of the virus to fuse with host cells.

Presenting symptoms in serious cases are high fever, headache, vomiting, and vertigo. Then tremors, profuse sweating, paresis, delirium, psychosis, coma, and death. There is no pharmaceutical treatment for TBE though tetracycline hydrochloride has been found to significantly reduce the inflammatory cytokines during infection. Corticosteroids have as well been found to inhibit inflammation, decreasing the severity of symptoms.

There are two specific physiological differences during TBE (when compared to West Nile and Japanese viral encephalitis): edema is often pronounced in TBE and the microglia are often necrotic.

La Crosse Encephalitis

La Crosse encephalitis virus (LCEV) infections decrease with the age of the host; the younger the person, the more susceptible they are to infection, and the more likely the disease is to be severe. Those under age eight are the most affected.

There are about 300,000 new LCEV infections each year in the United States. As with most encephalitis infections, many cases are asymptomatic or present as a mild to moderate flu that passes without serious effects. In severe cases, the same kinds of inflammatory lesions that are seen in TBE are found, either diffuse or as microglial nodules. The cerebral cortex is most adversely affected, including the frontal, parietal, and temporal lobes. Inflammatory foci are also present in the pons and basal ganglia. Unlike in TBE the spinal cord is rarely affected, but if the infection travels down the spinal cord from the brain it will cause perivascular cuffs of lymphocytes and nerve degeneration.

There has been, oddly, little study of the cytokine profile of the disease. Though what has been done shows that it is similar to most viral encephalitis infections. LCEV stimulates the production of IL-1ß, TNF-α, and IL-6. Bcl-2 is downregulated as well.

Symptoms during severe infection are meningoencephalitis, high fever, seizures, vomiting, photophobia, stiff neck, confusion, paresis, aphasia, chorea, dysarthria, ataxia, and coma. Fever, headache, behavioral changes, and vomiting are the most common symptoms. Those who recover often show lower IQ scores and a high proportion show ADHD behaviors. Some continue to experience seizures.

The virus is spread by mosquitoes. Once in the body the virus begins replicating in the muscle tissue and spreads to the blood, lymph, and spleen and thence to the brain, where it begins to infect neurons, its preferred replication site. It, like the other encephalitides, is present in high quantities in both the spleen and lymph. There are sometimes areas of necrosis in the spleen. Unlike other such viruses, it also infects the respiratory passages.

Although there is no accepted pharmaceutical treatment, ribavirin and recombinant glycoproteins have been found to help. Corticosteroids are sometimes used to reduce the inflammation.

The infection is considered to most closely resemble herpes simplex encephalitis, with which it is often confused. However, I think the infection dynamics are very similar to those of Japanese encephalitis and natural treatment should follow that protocol with one addition: Endothelial swelling can commonly occur with La Crosse viral encephalitis; Japanese knotweed (or an equivalent) should be added to the protocol to help alleviate it.

Natural Treatment for Encephalitis

This treatment protocol is specific for all viral encephalitis infections. Some adjustment is needed for West Nile, TBE, and dengue, and those adjustments are detailed at the end of the protocol.

If seizures occur, Chinese skullcap and lion's mane should be used, in large doses. If cerebral edema, ischemia, or hypoxia are present, *Ligusticum wallichii* (or the extract ligustrazine) is specific. Rhodiola is also specific for hypoxia.

Note: Chondroitin sulfate has been found to enhance the infection of brain cells by JEV and the damage it causes in the brain. This supplement should be avoided during active infection.

The treatment protocol is followed by a brief look at some of the more important herbs that are neuroprotective and neuroregenerative: Chinese senega root, Japanese knotweed root, kudzu root, lion's mane, and *Crinum latifolium*.

The Protocol Overview

Treatment approaches that can reduce the impacts of the encephalitis infections consist of the following steps:

1. Antiviral systemics
2. Stimulation of the spleen and lymph system to actively attack the infection, thus reducing movement into the brain by the virus and promoting the induction of splenic T cell activation
3. Reduction of cytokine/chemokine cascades through the use of specific inhibitors
4. Protection of neural cells and neural mitochondria
5. Inhibition of viral infection of neural cells
6. Regeneration of damaged neural structures
7. Enhancement of healthy immune system responses through the use of adaptogenic agents
8. Inhibition of HMGB1 if sepsis appears likely

Protocol Specifics

The protocol contains elements to address all these aspects of the infection.

1. ANTIVIRAL SYSTEMICS

Specific antivirals for encephalitis viruses are licorice, Chinese skullcap, isatis, houttuynia. I personally also use lomatium for West Nile and consider it specific.

Formulation: Equal parts of the tinctures of each herb, combined.

Dosage: Depending on the severity of condition, from 1/4 teaspoon to 1 tablespoon of the combination tincture up to 6x daily. My normal use for mild to moderate West Nile, for example, is 1 teaspoon 4–6x daily for 2–4 weeks. Note: The dosage needs to be moderated for children, depending on their weight.

2. STIMULATION OF THE SPLEEN AND LYMPH SYSTEM

Red root (or poke if you can't find red root) will stimulate spleen function, reduce inflammation in the spleen, and enhance T cell counts.

Formulation: Red root tincture. Dosage: $1/4$–1 teaspoon up to 6x daily depending on the severity of the condition.

3. REDUCTION OF CYTOKINE CASCADES

The herbs specific for this are Chinese skullcap, licorice, isatis, houttuynia, cordyceps, rhodiola, astragalus. They're all included in antiviral and immune formulations (steps 1 and 7, respectively).

4. PROTECTION OF NEURAL CELLS AND NEURAL MITOCHONDRIA

The main herbs for this are Chinese skullcap, cordyceps, Japanese knotweed, rhodiola, kudzu, olive oil (oleorupin). They're all included in the antiviral and immune formulations (steps 1 and 7, respectively).

5. INHIBITION OF VIRAL INFECTION OF NEURAL CELLS

The main herbs for this are cordyceps, licorice, Chinese skullcap. They're included in the antiviral and immune formulations (steps 1 and 7, respectively).

6. REGENERATION OF DAMAGED NEURAL STRUCTURES

The best herbs are Chinese senega root (*Polygala tenuifolia*) and lion's mane (*Hericium erinaceus*). Both contain substantial amounts of nerve growth factor.

Formulation and dosage:
- **Chinese senega root:** 30 drops of the tincture 3x daily for 30 days, and . . .
- **Lion's mane:** 3–8 grams per day or 1 teaspoon of the tincture 2x daily.

7. IMMUNE HERBS/ADAPTOGENS

The best for this are astragalus, cordyceps, rhodiola.

Formulation: Tincture combination of all three herbs, with 1 part astragalus, 1 part rhodiola, and 2 parts cordyceps. Dosage: 1 teaspoon of the combination tincture 6x daily during active infections.

Note: Cordyceps is very specific for the kinds of neuroinflammation that occur in the brain during encephalitis infections. In severe cases the dosage of cordyceps can be substantially increased. There is no toxic upper range to the herb.

8. INHIBITION OF HMGB1

The best herbs for this are licorice, *Angelica sinensis*, *Salvia miltiorrhiza*.

Formulation: Equal parts of the tinctures of *Angelica sinensis* and *Salvia miltiorrhiza*, combined. Dosage: 1 teaspoon to 1 tablespoon of the combination tincture up to 10x daily (or more) depending on the degree of inflammation occurring.

Strong infusions of these herbs will also work just fine. Formulation: 8 ounces of herb per gallon of water; pour boiling water over the herb, cover, and let stand for 4 hours. Strain and use. Dosage: An entire gallon should be consumed daily as the primary liquid source.

Note: There is no upper dosage range for these herbs. The inhibition is dose dependent.

For West Nile Encephalitis

Add the following to the basic protocol described above:

- **Astragalus:** Increase the dosage of astragalus by taking 3,000 mg daily or ¹/₂ teaspoon of the tincture 3–6x daily.
- **Japanese knotweed (*Polygonum cuspidatum*):** Tincture, ¹/₂ teaspoon 3–6x daily (or resveratrol, from knotweed root, 4,000 mg daily).
- ***Crinum latifolium* leaf:** Tea, 4–6 cups daily, or, if you wish, capsules, 8,000 mg daily. (Aqueous extracts are best.)

For Tick-Borne Encephalitis

Add the following to the basic protocol described above:

- **Greater celandine (*Chelidonium majus*) tincture:** $1/4$ teaspoon 3x daily (not to exceed 30 days).
- **Motherwort (*Leonurus cardiaca*) tincture:** $1/4$–$1/2$ teaspoon up to 6x daily.
- *Ligusticum wallichii* **tincture (for edema):** $1/4$–$1/2$ teaspoon up to 6x daily, or a strong infusion 6x daily. (This herb will also reduce many of the cytokines TBE induces; the related herbs *Ligusticum porteri* and *Lomatium dissectum* may possibly be legitimate substitutes.)
- **Reduce blood acidity:** Reduce purine intake in the diet, explore acid/alkaline diet modification, supplement with beta-alanine (750–2,250 mg daily).

For Dengue Encephalitis

To the basic protocol described above, add velvet leaf (*Cissampelos pareira*), which is active against all four serotypes of the virus (see the discussion of dengue on page 98 for more). Sea buckthorn leaf (*Hippophae rhamnoides*), boneset, and cat's claw (*Uncaria tomentosa*) are all antivirals specific for dengue as well. Cat's claw is also a decent immune-enhancing herb. The specifics:

- **Velvet leaf tea:** A strong decoction of velvet leaf. Take 2 ounces 4x daily.
- **Tea from sea buckthorn and boneset leaves:** Add 1 ounce each of sea buckthorn leaf and boneset leaf to a quart jar (that can take heat), add boiling water, cover, and let steep 1 hour. Drink throughout the day, every day, for 2 weeks.
- **Sea buckthorn oil:** $1/2$–1 teaspoon 3x daily.
- **Cat's claw:** Tincture, 1 teaspoon 3–6x daily, or capsules, 1,200 mg 3–6x daily, for 2 weeks.

For Some Other, Rarer Encephalitis Infections

Aqueous extracts of *Achyrocline satureioides* are specific for western equine encephalitis virus. *Nyctanthese arbor-tristis* is specific for Semliki Forest virus and encephalomyocarditis virus.

A Brief Look at Some Neural Herbs for Encephalitis Treatment

There are a few herbs that are very specific for protecting or stimulating the regrowth of the neural structures of the brain. They are Chinese senega root, Japanese knotweed, kudzu root, lion's mane, and pink-striped trumpet lily.

Chinese Senega Root (*Polygala tenuifolia*)

This is one of the 50 fundamental herbs of Chinese medicine and is known there as *yuan zhi*. It is used in China primarily as an expectorant and to help lung inflammations. But it also has strong impacts on cognitive function, enhancing memory, alleviating neurotoxicity, and producing positive impacts in the treatment of Alzheimer's, dementia, depression, and degenerative diseases. It is a very good anti-inflammatory and inhibits NF-κB, nitric oxide, iNOS, COX-2, PGE2, TNF-α, and IL-1ß in microglial cells. One of the more important activities of the herb is that it enhances the secretion of nerve growth factor (NGF) in the brain, spinal cord, and peripheral nervous systems. NGF is a small protein that is crucial for the growth, maintenance, and survival of neurons. When neuronal damage occurs, higher levels of NGF are essential in stimulating axonal regeneration. This is perhaps the best plant for stimulation of NGF.

PREPARATION AND USE

Take 30 drops of the tincture 3x daily for 30 days. It is contraindicated in those with ulcers or gastritis.

Japanese Knotweed (*Polygonum cuspidatum*)

Japanese knotweed is a world-class invasive originally native to Japan, north China, Taiwan, and Korea. It is another significant invasive that is specific for emerging infections. The root is the part of the plant used for medicine.

The herb has a wide range of actions; among other things, it is an antiviral, antimicrobial (widely), antifungal, immunomodulant, anti-inflammatory, angiogenesis modulator, central nervous system relaxant, central nervous system (brain and spinal cord) protectant and anti-inflammatory, antioxidant, inhibitor of platelet aggregation, inhibitor of eicosanoid synthesis, antithrombotic, tyrosine kinase inhibitor, antipyretic, cardioprotective, analgesic, hemostatic, and astringent.

A broadly systemic plant, Japanese knotweed modulates immune function, reducing and balancing cytokine cascades; is anti-inflammatory for arthritic, viral, and bacterial inflammations; protects the body against endotoxin damage; and is a potently strong angiogenesis modulator, highly protective of the endothelia of the body. It is specifically inhibitive of endothelial hyperplasia. It crosses the blood-brain barrier and is potently anti-inflammatory in the brain and CNS. It is highly specific for all CNS infections.

Knotweed is a very strong inhibitor of cytokine cascades initiated by pathogens, especially MMP-1, MMP-3, and MMP-9. These can be stimulated through various pathways but knotweed is highly specific for reducing MMPs *and* mitogen-activated protein kinases (MAPKs), specifically c-Jun N-terminal kinase (JNK), p38 mitogen-activated protein kinase (p38 MAPK), and extracellular-signal-regulated kinase 1 and 2 (ERK-1 and ERK-2). Resveratrol (one of the plant's constituents) is also directly active in reducing MMP-9 levels through both the JNK and protein kinase C-delta pathways; it has been found to specifically inhibit MMP-9 gene transcription. The plant root is so high in resveratrols that it is the main source of the supplement throughout the world. Another component of the plant, rhein, inhibits the JNK pathway for MMP-1, MMP-3, and MMP-9 expression. The plant is also high in emodin, a constituent that has been found specifically active against a range of encephalitis viruses. Knotweed is also a formidable inhibitor of NF-κB, TNF-α, ICAM-1, VCAM-1, IL-1ß, IL-6, COX-2, IL-8, PI3K (phosphoinositide 3-kinase), E-selectin, IDO, and VEGF (vascular endothelial growth factor).

Polygonum cuspidatum's constituents cross the blood-brain barrier, where they act on the central nervous system as antimicrobials, anti-inflammatories, protectants against oxidative and microbial damage, and calming agents. The herb specifically protects the brain from inflammatory damage, microbial endotoxins, and bacterial infections. The compounds easily move across the gastrointestinal mucosa and circulate in the bloodstream.

The whole herb and its constituent, resveratrol, are both strong antioxidants. People who consume the herb (or constituent) have been found to have significantly increased antioxidant activity in their blood. This potent antioxidant action has been detected throughout the body. Interestingly, resveratrol seems to be an antioxidant modulator in that it will increase antioxidant action when needed (most of the time) but will lower it in instances where necessary, e.g., in leukemia cells.

Another component of knotweed, emodin, is highly protective of brain neurons and reduces pain by inhibiting the activation of the P2X7 receptors in the brain. It reduces impacts on the P2X2/3 receptors as well.

The herb, in fact, is a potent immunomodulator. It normalizes immune response, especially in diseases where autoimmune reactions are stimulated (such as Lyme disease and lupus). It seems able to bring up immune function when necessary and reduce its local manifestations when overstimulated, e.g., in rheumatoid arthritis. This is a very strong aspect of the plant's actions.

The herb and its constituent have also been found to enhance and potentiate the action of other drugs and herbs when taken with them.

Japanese knotweed and its constituents also possess strong actions in the central nervous system and brain, and this range of activity is where a great deal of interest in the plant is being generated.

Knotweed and the constituents trans-resveratrol and resveratrol have been found to be strongly neuroprotective through a variety of actions in numerous studies. One of the herb's mechanisms of action in this regard is as an antioxidant. Resveratrol and trans-resveratrol have been found to protect rat embryonic mesencephalic cells from a powerful pro-oxidant, tert-butyl hydroperoxide. Another study found that regular use of trans-resveratrol prevented streptozotocin-induced cognitive impairment and oxidative stress in rats (an Alzheimer's-like condition). And yet another found that trans-resveratrol protected and reversed many of the impacts of induced stroke in rats.

While the herb's antioxidant actions are important, trans-resveratrol, for example, has been found in a number of studies to strongly protect neuronal structures from damage through mechanisms other than antioxidant activity alone. Resveratrol has been found specific for protecting the brain from neurotoxic substances such as the beta-amyloid peptides, which are associated with Alzheimer's disease.

Resveratrol and trans-resveratrol are specific for reducing inflammation in the brain and central nervous system. In spinal cord injuries resveratrol "remarkably" reduced secondary spinal cord edema, significantly suppressed the activity of lactate dehydrogenase, reduced malondialdehyde content in the injured spinal cord tissue, and markedly improved NA+/K+-ATPase activities. It immediately stimulated microcirculation to the injured tissues.

Low-level, chronic inflammation in the brain and central nervous system plays a major role in many neurodegenerative conditions. Both the herb and its constituents are specific for such inflammations. They have been found active for such things as amyotrophic lateral sclerosis and other motor neuron diseases, Parkinson's disease, Alzheimer's disease, bulbar atrophy, dementia, Huntington's disease, myasthenia gravis, stroke, multiple sclerosis, frontotemporal dementia, encephalomyelitis, traumatic brain injury, cerebral ischemia, and so on. The resveratrols specifically protect brain cells from assault, whether chemical or microbial in origin. The herb and its constituents, as well, stimulate microcirculation in the brain.

PREPARATION AND USE

Capsules or tincture can be used. Capsules of pure knotweed root can be had from Green Dragon Botanicals (see the resources) or you can buy "resveratrol," which is in fact only a standardized knotweed root formulation. That is, it is knotweed root standardized for the presence of a certain percentage of resveratrols. Most of the brands on the market are usable. Just make sure they are made from knotweed root (it will say on the package someplace in tiny print) and not grapes. As for dosage:

- **Capsules:** 3 or 4 capsules 3 or 4x daily (or 1 tablespoon of the powdered root in juice 3 or 4x daily).
- **Tincture:** $1/4$–$1/2$ teaspoon 3–6x daily.

The major side effect, in about 0.5 percent of those who use it, is loss of taste. This corrects upon discontinuance of the herb (in a week or so). Metallic or odd taste is moderately common. GI tract disturbances are rare but do occur. Note: Some people have reported rather strong negative physical responses to the Source Naturals resveratrol. I am not sure why this is; however, those who do, having switched to another product by Paradise Herbs, report a better outcome. Just an FYI on that one.

Japanese knotweed should not be used with blood-thinning agents. Discontinue use of the herb 10 days prior to any surgery. The plant is a synergist and may potentiate the effects of pharmaceuticals and other herbs.

Kudzu Root (*Pueraria lobata*)

Kudzu root and its major constituents (puerarin and kakkalide and irisolidone — a metabolite of kakkalide produced by intestinal microflora that is more potent than kakkalide) inhibit TNF-α, IL-1ß, NF-κB, ERK, iNOS, PGE2, COX-2, AP-1 (activator protein-1), ICAM-1, VCAM-1, E-selectin, C-reactive protein (CRP), and the phosphorylation of the 1κB-α protein. It has targeted and potent effects on cytokine-activated microglial cells and will reduce damage by cytokines in the CNS.

Kudzu (and puerarin) are strongly protective of the brain and CNS, especially in ischemia/reperfusion injury. They have a strong protective effect against beta-amyloid-induced neurotoxicity in hippocampal neurons, protect mitochondria from reactive oxygen species (ROS), and stimulate peripheral nerve regeneration. Neuron pain receptors P2X3 and P2X2/3, similar to P2X7, in the brain are inhibited by puerarin, making this a very good companion herb to use with greater celandine. The root is, in fact, strongly anti-inflammatory in the brain and CNS. It significantly inhibits neutrophil respiratory bursts, reducing autoimmune dynamics in the brain. It modulates Bax/Bcl-2 actions in the mitochondria in the brain and inhibits caspase-3 and iNOS expressions. It is strongly neuroprotective during inflammation disturbances in the brain and CNS.

It is a good herb for viral encephalitis types of cytokine cascades, especially so since it is invasive and there is no dearth of supply. *Anywhere* encephalitis occurs and kudzu grows, use kudzu.

PREPARATION AND USE

In traditional Chinese medicine the usual dose is 6–12 grams per day of the powdered root. Normally dosing in the West is 1 gram per day. The tincture dosage in encephalitis infection is $1/2$ teaspoon 3 or 4x daily.

Lion's Mane (*Hericium erinaceus*)

Lion's mane is a highly edible mushroom, a member of the tooth fungus group of mushrooms. (It should look sort of like a waterfall of beautiful white threads. If it does not, be suspicious.) The mushroom has a long history of use in Asia. Like most mushrooms, it is high in polysaccharides and possesses strong immunomodulating and immune-activating properties. It strongly activates T cells and strongly downregulates iNOS, nitric oxide, ROS, PGE2, COX-2, NF-κB, and JNK during inflammatory overreactions.

However, its strongest actions are in its effects on nerve cells and brain function. The herb stimulates peripheral and CNS nerve regeneration after damage (specifically by inducing nerve growth factor in the body), increases remyelination of nerve sheaths, improves cognitive impairment after neural damage (including amyloid peptide-induced), and significantly alleviates depression and anxiety.

PREPARATION AND USE

The herb can be used as either an aqueous or alcohol preparation; I tend to prefer the alcohol tincture made from the fresh mushroom. Dosage for encephalitis is $1/4$–$1/2$ teaspoon 3–6x daily, depending on the severity of the condition. I think the herb highly indicated to alleviate or in the treatment of postencephalitis conditions.

Pink-Striped Trumpet Lily (*Crinum latifolium*)

Pink-striped trumpet lily is a typical-looking lily, a perennial that grows from a bulb. The herb is commonly used in Asia as a medicinal for inflammatory problems of various sorts, especially rheumatoid complaints. It is most commonly used in the West now to reduce prostate enlargement, either benign prostatic hyperplasia or prostatitis.

The herb is a potent inhibitor, perhaps the best currently known, of indoleamine 2,3-dioxygenase (IDO). In consequence it is a potent stimulant of T cell activation in cases where IDO has been overexpressed by pathogens. It is strongly inhibitive of IFN-γ, stopping the particular cytokine cascade that it starts during infections. It also inhibits NF-κB. The plant is a pretty good free radical scavenger, reducing ROS in the body and CNS. The herb is anti-angiogenic, protecting the endothelial cells from inflammation, hyperplasia, and overstimulation by cytokines. It has been found to possess antiviral activity against some vaccinia viruses. And it is active, in vitro and in vivo, against a variety of cancers, including prostate.

PREPARATION AND USE

The leaf, prepared as a tea (aqueous extracts are best), 4–6 cups daily, or, if you wish, in capsules, 8,000 mg daily. The bulbs are easy to find and the herb grows easily. You can find the tea most easily on the online site eBay.

4

A BRIEF LOOK AT SOME OTHER VIRUSES

From Cytomegalovirus and Dengue to Shingles and Their Treatment Protocols

The underlying causes for the emergence of infectious diseases are anthropogenic social and environmental changes. These result from the combined weight of human numbers and their consumption patterns that are overloading the planet's biophysical and ecological capacity.... If the human impact on the ecosphere continues to escalate, the rate of emergence of infectious diseases will only increase in the future.
— Thijs Kuiken et al., "Emerging Viral Infections in a Rapidly Changing World"

There is currently a large and ever-expanding global population base that prefers the use of natural products in treating and preventing medical problems.
— R. Hafidh et al., "Asia Is the Mine of Natural Antiviral Products for Public Health"

There are many other viruses that cause human illness that either are becoming resistant or are emerging more strongly into the world's population of people. In this section I will look at cytomegalovirus, dengue virus, enterovirus 71, Epstein-Barr virus, herpes simplex viruses, varicella zoster (shingles), and a few gastrointestinal viruses such as rotavirus and norovirus. I am not going to explore the Coxsackie or ECHO viruses in this book at this time, nor am I going to look at the five hepatitis viruses or HIV. Viral hepatitis and HIV need, for the most part, highly involved treatment protocols that are beyond the scope of this book; they each need in-depth books of their own.

Cytomegalovirus

Cytomegalovirus (CMV) is a member of the Herpesviridae family of viruses, a very large group of DNA viruses that also includes the herpes simplex viruses, Epstein-Barr virus, and varicella zoster virus (chicken pox/shingles). It is sometimes referred to as human herpesvirus 5 (HHV-5). It usually causes minor problems in people with healthy immune systems but if immune function drops (especially in those with AIDS, those taking immunosuppressive drugs, or those whose immune function is simply becoming weak from either age or illness) or if the immune system has not yet developed fully (babies, in and out of utero) it can cause severe problems up to and including death.

Infection rates are high. In the United States somewhere between 50 and 80 percent of the adult population are asymptomatically infected. When people first become infected the usual signs are fever, fatigue, muscle tenderness, and tender and enlarged lymph nodes. Just like the flu. Then it passes, you feel fine, and you are an asymptomatic carrier.

As the years go by the virus periodically blooms, sending viruses to body fluids: saliva, tears, urine, blood, semen, vaginal secretions, and breast milk. From there it spreads to new hosts. It is a pretty good parasitic virus, and it usually doesn't cause much trouble. However, in people whose immune function is impaired, the virus can cause a wide range of symptoms: encephalitis, myelitis, seizures, coma, psychosis, dysphagia, weakness, numbness in the legs, retinitis, visual impairments including blurred vision or blindness, pneumonia, gastritis, enteritis, colitis, diarrhea, ulcers in the GI tract, and hepatitis.

In babies, CMV is the most common congenital infection in the United States. For most it will not be a problem but for some it can cause severe and long-term difficulties: neurological problems, hearing impairment or loss, visual problems, seizures, or mental and physical disabilities. The worst problems occur in infants whose mothers become infected while the infants are in utero.

CMV is normally treated with the intravenous antibiotic ganciclovir (or valganciclovir), usually along with CMV-specific immune globulin. Treatment usually lasts 2 to 4 weeks, followed by a transition to oral valganciclovir. Unfortunately the virus is becoming fairly resistant to ganciclovir. Generally, this drug will not cure the infection but only lessen its effects. Again, the search is for a vaccine; however, early trials show that the vaccines in development only tend to lessen the effects of the disease, not eliminate it, for the majority of people using them.

Dengue Fever

Dengue viruses (DENVs) are single-stranded RNA viruses in the Flaviviridae family, specifically in the *Flavivirus* genus. This genus includes many of the encephalitis viruses such as West Nile, tick-borne encephalitis, Japanese encephalitis, Murray Valley encephalitis, St. Louis encephalitis, and so on. Yellow fever virus is also in this group. There are various serotypes of dengue (1, 2, 3, and 4). Each one produces a slightly different spectrum of symptoms. DENV-3 produces more musculoskeletal and gastrointestinal symptoms, DENV-4 has more respiratory and cutaneous symptoms.

Dengue fever, a.k.a. breakbone fever, is a mosquito-transmitted disease and is not infectious except through that route. There are about 100 million people infected with dengue each year; several hundred thousand develop dengue hemorrhagic fever, which is very serious, and about 22,000 die.

The disease is endemic pretty much everywhere, including the southern United States. Outbreaks have occurred in recent years throughout the Caribbean including Puerto Rico, the U.S. Virgin Islands, and Cuba. The disease is common in Tahiti, Singapore, the South Pacific, Southeast Asia, the West Indies, India, and the Middle East as well as throughout South America. The incidence of the disease is growing each year.

Once a mosquito bites a person, the virus enters the body and begins seeking out monocytes and macrophages, the primary parts of the body it infects. The symptoms develop in 3 to 15 days (normally 5 to 8). The symptoms are sudden-onset fever, headache, pain on eye movement, and low backache. Muscle and joint pain (which is often very severe — it's called "breakbone" fever for a reason) occurs soon after, a fever, often as high as 104 degrees Fahrenheit, develops, heart rate and blood pressure drop. The eyes redden, a rash may occur on the face, lymph nodes often swell.

The fever tends to last several days, then a sudden drop in body temperature occurs accompanied by extreme sweating. This passes, you feel fine, then it starts all over again. This time the rash covers the whole body except for the face.

Dengue hemorrhagic fever (DHF) usually affects children under 10 years of age. It causes severe abdominal pain, hemorrhage, and shock. Sore throat, cough, nausea, vomiting all occur. Somewhere from 2 to 6 days after symptoms begin there is sudden collapse, with cool, clammy extremities, weak pulse, and cyanosis around the mouth. The skin bruises easily; there is bleeding, spitting up of blood, blood in the stool, bleeding gums, nosebleeds. Pneumonia is common; inflammation of the heart may occur. The disease is associated with high levels of circulating von Willebrand factor. Normal treatment for DHF is transfusions, oxygen, and fluid replacement.

There are no pharmaceutical treatments for either form of dengue fever. There is no vaccine. However, recent research has shown that the antibiotic Geneticin is active against the virus. Its effectiveness in practice is unknown.

Enterovirus 71

Enterovirus 71 (sometimes called hand, foot, and mouth disease) is a single-stranded, nonenveloped RNA virus in the Picornaviridae family. Rhinoviruses (common cold), hepatitis A, and the polio virus are some of the better-known members of the family.

Enterovirus 71 was first identified in 1965; the first known outbreak was in 1969 in the United States. There are severe outbreaks every 3 to 4 years throughout the world with smaller annual episodes here and there. A huge outbreak in Taiwan in 1998 infected over 130,000 people, mostly children. The virus is usually spread by respiratory droplets or contact with an infected person's body fluids. It is excreted in feces for weeks or months after infection.

The virus initially colonizes the GI tract and from there, if the disease does increase in severity, it invades the spinal cord and ascends to the brain. In the CNS and brain it produces high levels of cytokines: IL-1ß, IL-6, IL-8, and TNF-α. Enterovirus 71 is considered to be an emerging pathogen, with the number of cases increasing each year.

The most common symptoms of infection are fever, headache, fatigue, malaise, ear pain, sore throat, body rash, blisters on the palms of the hands or soles of the feet (they may also occur in the nostrils and buttocks), oral ulcers, loss of appetite, diarrhea, vomiting. Fever and sore throat are usually the first signs.

Unfortunately, there are some more serious complications that can occur during infection: high fever, meningitis, encephalitis, paralysis, cardiopulmonary edema, and sometimes coma and death.

There is no pharmaceutical treatment or vaccine.

Epstein-Barr

Epstein-Barr is a member of the Herpesviridae or herpesvirus family; it's sometimes referred to as human herpesvirus 4 (HHV-4). It is the cause of mononucleosis and a very common cause of chronic fatigue syndrome. It is considered an oncovirus, meaning it can, under some circumstances, over long periods of time, cause certain forms of cancer. Most children become infected with it at a young age, in which case the symptoms are usually mild — it looks like a mild case of the flu. The older the person at infection, the more severe the symptoms. In teenagers it causes infectious mononucleosis. This is usually accompanied by a severe sore throat, fever, and extreme fatigue and malaise. The infected may also experience swollen throat, loss of appetite, enlarged lymph nodes, swollen spleen and liver, jaundice, petechiae. Some of the very serious complications are splenic rupture or hemorrhage, meningitis, peripheral neuritis, and pneumonitis. An autoimmune hemolytic anemia can occur as well, though it is much rarer.

There are no reliable pharmaceutical treatments for the disease. Acyclovir can help reduce viral shedding. Valacyclovir has been found to, sometimes, significantly reduce the viral load and thus the symptoms of the disease.

Herpes Simplex 1 and 2

Herpes is probably the most famous (or infamous) member of the Herpesviridae family of viruses. There are two types, herpes simplex virus 1 (HSV-1) and herpes simplex virus 2 (HSV-2). The most common sites of infection are around the lips (cold sores, fever blisters) and on the genitals (herpes). Cold sores are usually caused by herpes simplex 1, genital herpes by herpes simplex 2. A less common form is infection of the fingers, called herpetic whitlow. It is caused by either type. There are some more serious forms of infection: ocular herpes (which infects the eyes, causing a form of keratitis), herpes gladiatorum (which broadly infects the skin), herpes encephalitis (which infects the brain), Mollaret's meningitis (which infects the protective membranes covering the brain and spinal cord), and neonatal herpes (where the baby is infected as it is born or in utero).

Herpes, either oral or genital, is usually cyclic with long (or short) periods of remission between episodes. With genital herpes, once the virus enters a new host it travels along the nerve paths, where it takes up residence. For many people, after an initial outbreak, the virus may become dormant indefinitely. For others, every so often, the virus becomes active. It then travels back along the nerve paths to the surface of the skin, where it creates blisters that shed viruses, spreading the disease.

Just prior to a new episode, there may be a feeling of pain in the nerves in the genitals. Soon small blisters may appear; they eventually break open and produce very painful sores that scab over and heal after several weeks. Sometimes people with an active infection feel as if they have the flu, and the lymph nodes may be swollen.

Oral herpes and herpetic whitlow symptoms are similar but occur around the lips and fingers respectively.

There are generally three types of ocular, or eye, herpes. Herpes keratitis is the most common form; it's a viral infection of the cornea or surface of the eye. This usually heals without damage to the eye. Stromal keratitis is a deeper form, where the virus penetrates deeper into the layers of the cornea. It can cause scarring of the cornea and, sometimes, blindness. The final type is iridocyclitis. Here the iris and surrounding tissues of the eye are infected and become inflamed. There is often severe light sensitivity and blurred vision, and the infected eye is red. Sometimes this kind of infection can occur in the retina or inside lining of the back of the eye; it's then called herpes retinitis.

Signs and symptoms of herpetic eye infections are swelling, tearing, irritation, foreign body sensation, redness, eye sores, discharge, light sensitivity.

The normal treatment for eye herpes is ganciclovir as an ophthalmic gel, five drops daily. Sometimes steroid eyedrops are used to decrease the inflammation. The infected cornea is sometimes scraped away. There is no effective cure; these interventions reduce the impact of the episode and, hopefully, prevent permanent damage.

Herpes gladiatorum is tremendously infective and is transmitted by skin-to-skin contact. It is essentially a cutaneous form of herpes, usually herpes simplex 1 (the same form of the virus that causes cold sores). It is somewhat common in sports clubs (which is where it got its name). In this condition, the sores, instead of being confined to the genitals or lips, are found in clusters over the body: neck, chest, face, stomach, legs. The lymph nodes are often enlarged, with fever, sore throat, headache. The blisters are very painful and take weeks to heal.

Herpes encephalitis and meningitis are uncommon but severe complications of herpes infection. Herpes meningitis is usually caused by the HSV-2 serotype and is an inflammation of the meninges, the tissue surrounding the brain and spinal cord. The normal symptoms are stiff neck, headache, fever, light sensitivity, fatigue, nausea, appetite loss, vomiting (sometimes). It is usually a self-limiting disease and clears on its own. For some people it recurs at periodic intervals just as genital and oral herpes do. In rare instances it may cause minor mental dysfunctions, slight confusion, and difficulty in problem solving that fail to resolve.

Herpes simplex encephalitis is usually caused by HSV-1. During herpes simplex encephalitis the temporal and frontal lobes are usually infected when the virus travels along the nerve lines into the brain. The usual encephalitic processes occur: inflammation of the brain, confusion, psychological alterations, fever, and in anywhere from 30 to 70 percent of those infected seizures, coma, and death. The infection is usually treated with IV acyclovir but there is still a 30 percent mortality rate. There is often long-lasting brain damage.

The usual treatment for herpes infections is valacyclovir, acyclovir (a.k.a. aciclovir), or famciclovir. All are forms of guanosine analogue antiviral drugs that, when taken, are metabolized by the body into an active form. These drugs are widely used to help control outbreaks of herpes simplex viruses, chicken pox, shingles, Epstein-Barr, and cytomegalovirus, all of which are closely related herpesviruses. They are strongest against the simplex types and have no effect on the viruses in their latent form in the nerve sheaths; they are effective only when the viruses become active. The drugs can shorten the course of the disease to some extent and help prevent spread. They do not cure it.

Herpesviruses are becoming resistant fairly rapidly to acyclovir, especially in those with compromised immune systems.

Varicella Zoster Virus (Chicken Pox/Shingles)

Varicella zoster virus is also a member of the Herpesviridae family; it's sometimes referred to as human herpesvirus 3 (HHV-3). HHV-3 usually occurs first as chicken pox (i.e., varicella), later as shingles (herpes zoster).

During the initial infection, normally during childhood, spread via respiratory droplets in the air, the virus enters the bloodstream and travels everywhere, making spots all over the surface of the body. It takes about 2 weeks for the spots to appear and the infection period lasts for up to 3 weeks after that, until the spots crust over. At that point, still spotted, the child is no longer infected. ("Yes, you still have to go to school.")

Though the disease was usually self-limiting and fairly benign vaccines are now commonly used in the West for chicken pox. However . . .

Regrettably, the virus, once the initial infection has passed, settles in the dorsal ganglion, part of the nerve structure of the central nervous system. There it lives quite happily for decades, until in later age, usually as a result of lowering immune function, it sometimes reappears as shingles.

The virus leaves its happy home, travels along the nerves, and emerges at the surface of the skin, often on the face, and makes life intolerable. There is often hemorrhage, edema, and lymphocytic infiltration of the affected nerves. Usually, the person can feel the event beginning — as the virus travels along the nerves it creates odd feelings, tingling, burning, numbness, and a very definite feeling that something is wrong. Then, quite quickly, the virus emerges out of the body onto the surface of the skin, creating tiny blisters filled with virus particles. The pain is often excruciating and little in the pharmaceutical armamentarium can help. Occasionally there can be fever, enlarged lymph nodes, chills, malaise, loss of appetite, and stomach upset. The lesions can last up to a week or so once they emerge. There can also, rarely, be more difficult complications such as encephalitis, peripheral nerve palsies, hemiparesis, and myelitis.

The most problematic aspect of shingles is postherpetic neuropathy, i.e., pain, at the site of the eruption. It can be an unrelenting
sharp, burning, or stabbing pain that can become highly debilitating.
About half the people who get shingles also develop postherpetic neuropathy. The neuropathy is usually caused by the infection itself as it
blooms at its emergence location. The local nerves are damaged by the
inflammation and it takes them time, sometimes a very long time (7
to 10 months), to recover. The older the person, the longer they take to
heal. As long as the damage lasts, postherpetic neuropathy will remain.

The usual medical treatment is the use of antivirals such as acyclovir, valacyclovir, or famciclovir. Corticosteroids may also be used to
lessen the inflammation, especially if the complications are serious.
Over-the-counter analgesics are often used, with varying success. The
pain is sometimes so severe that opiates are necessary. Pharmaceuticals don't heal the disease but they can help reduce the length of an
episode and help with pain.

One of the better natural approaches for shingles is the use of herbs
to increase immune function to reduce outbreak frequency and herbs
that protect and restore the nerves. Specific herbs for nerve pain will
also help tremendously, especially those that affect the P2X receptors
in the brain.

Gastrointestinal Viruses (Rotaviruses and Noroviruses)

There are a number of common (and a few uncommon) viruses that
cause gastrointestinal infections in people. The two primary ones are
rotavirus and the Norwalk (norovirus) virus. Some countries now
use vaccines against rotaviruses; there is none for the Norwalk virus,
which is thought to cause 90 percent of all nonbacterial epidemic
gastroenteritis worldwide and as much as half of all U.S. gastroenteritis infections. There is also an emerging group of viruses, discovered in the 1970s, the astroviruses, that are GI tract infectives. And the
orthoreoviruses that are thought to only rarely cause human disease.

These groups of viruses are specialists in infecting human food plants and bind quite strongly to lettuce leaves, for example. They are the main cause of diarrheal outbreaks from agricultural food products. The symptoms are much the same for all: nausea, vomiting, diarrhea, abdominal pain, lethargy, weakness, muscle aches, headache, low-grade fever, dehydration. The diseases are usually self-limiting but they can be quite debilitating and a few people in the United States always die from them every year. Rotaviruses are still a major cause of child mortality throughout the world.

In essence this is what is usually called the stomach flu in the United States. It is a food-borne illness from virus-contaminated food, usually vegetables, and is commonly spread via salad bars or prepackaged spinach, bean sprouts, and so on.

The Treatment Protocols

Again, the protocols suggested in this section are *only* suggestions. There are many ways to approach treating these viruses; this is just a starting point. Comment: If encephalitis occurs from any of these viruses, the encephalitis protocol, with slight alterations for each virus, which would mean adding specific herbs to the protocol, should be used.

Cytomegalovirus (CMV)

Herbs (and supplements) that have been found active for this virus in vitro, in vivo, and in human clinical use are (in alphabetical order) *Artemisia annua* (or artemisinin), *Astragalus membranaceus* (astragalus), the berberine plants, *Bidens pilosa* (bidens), *Bupleurum kaoi, Forsythia suspensa, Geum japonicum, Glycyrrhiza glabra* (licorice), houttuynia, *Hypericum perforatum*, isatis, *Lomatium dissectum, Nigella sativa*, quercetin, *Scaevola spinescens, Syzygium aromaticum* (cloves), *Terminalia chebula, Urtica dioica* (nettles), *Zingiber officinale* (ginger).

Geum japonicum, licorice, isatis, and the berberines have been found as effective as ganciclovir in the treatment of CMV in vivo.

TREATMENT

To begin: Bidens is a potent systemic antimicrobial herb (it must be prepared from fresh leaves; for more information, see my book *Herbal Antibiotics*, second edition) and I would include it in any protocol for treating CMV. A systemic formulation that would be good is *Bidens pilosa*, houttuynia, isatis, licorice, and lomatium, equal parts of each of the tinctures, combined. Dosage: $1/4$–$1/2$ teaspoon of the tincture combination from 3–6x daily depending on severity of the infection.

Then, based on specific symptoms, add to this systemic formulation any of the following:

For GI tract symptoms: Berberine-containing plants are specific in this instance: goldenseal, phyllanthus, barberry, Oregon grape root, coptis, and so on will all work fine. My preference is for phyllanthus, barberry, or goldenseal. Dosage: $1/4$–$1/2$ teaspoon of the tincture 3–6x daily depending on severity of symptoms. The systemic tincture should also be used, with the same dosage range described above. The licorice will help any ulceration that has occurred.

For neurological symptoms: The encephalitis protocol (see page 84) plus bidens.

For pneumonia: Moderate to severe influenza protocol (see page 46) plus bidens.

Dengue Fever Virus

Some herbs and supplements effective for dengue are (in alphabetical order) *Alternanthera philoxeroides, Andrographis paniculata, Artemisia douglasiana, Azadirachta indica* (neem), the berberine (and palmatine) plants, *Cissampelos pareira, Cladogynos orientalis, Cryptocarya chartacea, Daucus maritimus, Distictella elongata, Ellipeiopsis cherrevensis, Eupatorium patens, Eupatorium perfoliatum* (boneset), *Flagellaria indica, Garcinia multiflora, Gastrodia elata, Glycyrrhiza glabra* (licorice), grape seed proanthocyanidins, *Hippophae rhamnoides* (sea buckthorn leaf), houttuynia, *Kaempferia parviflora, Lantana grisebachii, Momordica charantia, Ocimum sanctum* (mildly active), *Punica granatum* (pomegranate juice), *Quercus lusitanica* (gall oak seed), *Rhizophora apiculata, Salvia miltiorrhiza* (Chinese or red sage), *Stemona tuberosa, Tephrosia* spp., *Uncaria tomentosa.* Oligomeric procyanidins (OPCs) are also specifically antiviral for dengue. They are common in cranberry juice, pomegranate juice, grape seeds, and unripe apple peels (for example). Any source can help, but that is the reason that pomegranate is included here. In addition pomegranate is a fairly potent synergist with a wide range of antimicrobial activity.

Many of the studies did not mention the serotype of dengue tested. Most of the herbs and supplements that did specify serotype have only been tested against type 2 (out of the four serotypes). The exceptions (that I can find) are andrographis, *Momordica charantia* (type 1), *Ocimum sanctum* (type 1), and *Cissampelos pareira* (all four serotypes). It is possible that many of these herbs are active against other serotypes but no testing has yet been done.

TREATMENT

I would suggest beginning treatment with the following: *Cissampelos pareira*, sea buckthorn leaf, boneset, houttuynia, licorice, pomegranate juice, and cat's claw. *Salvia miltiorrhiza* is for hemorrhagic dengue as an adjunct.

Cissampelos pareira (in English, velvet leaf) is a widely used herb in Chinese medicine, Ayurveda, and South and Central America (where it is called *arbuta*). It is moderately findable, if you look for it. It is somewhat invasive in Florida in the United States and should be harvested for use in that region.

The herb is antipyretic, anti-inflammatory, immunomodulatory, antiplasmodial, antinociceptive, antiarthritic, antioxidant protective, antileukemic, cardioprotective, constipative, abortifacient. It should not be used if you are pregnant or wanting to become pregnant. You can use it either as a strong decoction or as a 50 percent alcohol/water tincture. It is the only herb that is considered to have strong action against all four serotypes of dengue.

Sea buckthorn leaf and boneset are both antivirals specific for dengue. The boneset, additionally, will help lower fever, reduce pains in the body, and stimulate the immune response. Houttuynia and licorice are good supportive antivirals, and both are active against dengue. (Unfortunately, all have only been tested against serotype 2.) Licorice will also act as a synergist and anti-inflammatory. Pomegranate juice constituents are antiviral for dengue and it is a good synergist and anti-inflammatory so it is perfect for keeping up fluids. Cat's claw will protect the macrophages and monocytes from dengue infection (it is very specific for this). Chinese sage should be used in cases of hemorrhagic dengue; it will lower circulating levels of von Willebrand factor in the blood. Here is a suggested protocol:

- **Strong decoction of velvet leaf:** Take 2 ounces 4x daily.
- **Tea from sea buckthorn and boneset leaves:** Add 1 ounce each of sea buckthorn leaf and boneset leaf to a quart jar (that can take heat), add boiling water, cover, and let steep 1 hour. Drink throughout the day, every day, for 2 weeks.
- **Sea buckthorn oil:** $1/2$–1 teaspoon 3x daily.
- **Cat's claw:** Tincture, 1 teaspoon 3–6x daily, or capsules, 1,200mg 3–6x daily, for 2 weeks.
- **Tincture combination** of houttuynia, licorice and Chinese skullcap, equal parts of each, 1 teaspoon 3–6x daily for 2 weeks.
- **Pomegranate juice:** Drink throughout the day.
- **Vitamin C effervescent salts:** As needed if the velvet leaf causes constipation.

For dengue encephalitis use the dengue protocol outlined in chapter 3.

Enterovirus 71

Some herbs and supplements effective for enterovirus 71 are, in alphabetical order, *Amomum villosum, Ampelopsis brevipedunculata* (porcelain berry, invasive), *Azadirachta indica* (neem), *Elaeagnus oldhamii, Euchresta formosana* (shan dou gen), *Ficus pumila, Forsythia suspensa* (lian qiao), *Glycine tomentella, Glycyrrhiza glabra* (licorice), houttuynia, *Kalanchoe gracilis, Laminaria japonica* (kombu), *Ledebouriella divaricata* (fang feng), *Lemmaphyllum microphyllum, Lonicera japonica* (Japanese honeysuckle, invasive), *Melastoma candidum* (invasive), *Melissa officinalis* (lemon balm), *Ocimum basilicum* (basil), *Origanum vulgare* (oregano), *Phragmites communis* (a.k.a. *P. australis*; invasive), *Polygonum chinense* (Chinese knotweed), *Polygonum multiflorum* (fo-ti), *Psidium guajava* (guava), *Pueraria lobata* (kudzu, invasive), *Rheum officinale* (rhubarb), *Rosmarinus officinalis* (rosemary), *Schisandra chinensis* (schisandra), *Spatholobi caulis, Thymus vulgaris* (thyme), *Toona sinensis, Zingiber officinale* (ginger).

TREATMENT

Enterovirus 71 is an emerging pathogen that has no reliable pharmaceutical treatment. Numerous invasives are specific for this disease. I would begin with these herbs as systemic antivirals (then add others specific to the symptom picture): porcelain berry, neem leaf, licorice, houttuynia, fo-ti, ginger.

Japanese knotweed (*Polygonum cuspidatum*), a.k.a. hu zhang (huchang), has not been tested for activity against enterovirus 71 to my knowledge but its constituents and actions are very similar to the two polygonums that have been tested. This is of interest to me because Japanese knotweed is an invasive and thus presents a large, easily available source of medicine.

Interestingly, a Chinese combination used for measles for several millennia has been found effective in the treatment of enterovirus 71. It is composed of black cohosh rhizome, kudzu root, red peony root, and licorice. It's a nice combination, though I don't know where you can easily find it already prepared in the West. The kudzu and the licorice are antiviral. The licorice is synergistic and immune potentiating, the kudzu and peony neuroprotective, and to some extent so is the licorice. The black cohosh is pain relieving. You can, however, buy the herbs, most of them, from 1stChineseHerbs.com (www.1stchineseherbs.com). Just because of my own preferences, I would approach my own formulation slightly differently.

In addition to the systemic antibacterials, lemon balm, especially a prepared oil infusion, is specific for the blistering that enterovirus 71 can cause on the palms and soles of the feet. If neurological complications occur, you need to add specific anti-inflammatories for the brain and neural protectors. Kudzu is a good one, and a decent choice since it is active against the virus. My general preference for anti-inflammatories in the brain these days are Japanese knotweed, Chinese skullcap, greater celandine, and lion's mane.

For simple, uncomplicated enterovirus 71, here is a suggested protocol:

- **Tincture combination** composed of equal parts of licorice, houttuynia, and porcelain berry. Dosage: From 1–5 ml, 3–6x daily, depending on the severity of the symptoms and age of child.
- **Tea** of ginger juice, neem leaf, honey, squeeze of lime, pinch of cayenne. Dosage: 3–6x daily.

For specific symptoms or complications, incorporate these additional formulations into the protocol:

For blisters: Lemon balm infused oil or cordial, applied topically to blisters, as many times daily as seems appropriate.

For diarrhea: Blackberry root infusion, consumed throughout the day as tea, with honey added as desired. Pomegranate juice is highly suggested as it is antiviral, will reduce the cytokine cascade in the body, replaces fluids, helps reduce diarrhea, and is a good synergist. A combination of pomegranate and cranberry juice is just about perfect for this.

For fever: Boneset tea, 4–6x daily. Pasque flower tincture, 5–10 drops every hour or so, can also help. It will also help reduce anxiety levels.

For encephalitis and meningitis: I would essentially use the protocol outlined in chapter 3. However, add a tincture combination of fo-ti, cordyceps, and Chinese skullcap, in equal parts, $1/4$–$1/2$ teaspoon (or more, depending on the severity of symptoms) up to 6x daily. This will reduce the cytokine cascade in the brain and CNS, protect neural structures, and reduce the symptom picture. Lion's mane tincture, at the same dosage, will help restore neural function. If neurological symptoms are very severe, add greater celandine tincture, 30–60 drops, 3–6x daily for a max of 30 days.

111

Note: When treating a child, all dosages need to be adjusted for the child's weight and age; see the appendix for specifics.

Epstein-Barr Virus

Some of the herbs and supplements effective for Epstein-Barr are *Ailanthus altissima, Alpinia galanga, Andrographis paniculata, Artemisia annua* (or artemisinin), *Azadirachta indica* (neem), *Calendula officinalis, Chrysanthemum indicum, Coix lacryma-jobi, Cochlospermum tinctorium, Curcuma longa* (turmeric), *Eucalyptus* spp., *Ganoderma lucidum* (reishi), *Glycosmis arborea, Glycyrrhiza glabra* (licorice), isatis, *Morinda citrifolia* (noni), *Opuntia streptacantha* (prickly pear cactus), *Passiflora incarnata* (passionflower), *Polygonum cuspidatum* (Japanese knotweed), *Prunus persica* (peach tree leaves), *Scutellaria baicalensis* (Chinese skullcap), *Thelypteris torresiana, Thuja* spp., *Usnea* spp., *Wolfiporia extensa* (a.k.a. *Poria cocos*, a.k.a. fu ling), *Zingiber officinale* (ginger).

Epstein-Barr acute episodes can often lead to severe chronic fatigue. Part of the fatigue comes from its impacts on mitochondrial function. It scavenges and damages mitochondria, so protecting mitochondria is important. The best herbs and supplements for this are cordyceps, *Leonurus cardiaca* (motherwort), *Passiflora* spp. (passionflower), rhodiola, schisandra, *Pueraria lobata* (kudzu), *Scutellaria baicalensis*, and N-acetylcysteine. Some of these are also very good immune herbs that will help raise immune function. Motherwort and passionflower will also help reduce anxiety and sleeplessness.

Epstein-Barr, during acute attacks, usually presents with a very severe, very painful sore throat, usually confined mainly to one pinpoint location just at the back of the throat from the mouth. I haven't found *anything* that will truly relieve it. *Echinacea angustifolia* (**not** *E. purpurea*) tincture will help a bit, if you use the tincture full strength. Keep it on the tongue a bit, let the saliva be stimulated, then let the whole mix flow *slowly* over the affected area. (But it won't do anything for the disease itself.) The root of *Artemisia absinthium* can also help if you chew a fresh root, just a bit when needed. It will really cool (almost creating a freeze sensation) the back of the throat.

TREATMENT

- **Tincture combination** of Chinese skullcap, isatis, and licorice, in equal parts, $1/2$–1 teaspoon 3–6x daily depending on the severity of the infection.
- **Ginger juice tea** (see page 44), 3–6x daily.
- **Andrographis capsules or tablets,** 1,200 mg 3x daily for 30 days. (Caution: About 1 percent of people who use andrographis get a bad case of hives; if you do, discontinue the herb, and it will clear up in a week or so.)
- **Tincture combination** of motherwort and passionflower, in equal parts, $1/4$–$1/2$ teaspoon 6x daily.
- **Tincture combination** of cordyceps and rhodiola, in equal parts, $1/4$–$1/2$ teaspoon 3x daily.

If spleen enlargement occurs, use red root (*Ceanothus* spp.). With enlarged liver, milk thistle. With meningitis use the protocols in this book for encephalitic swelling (see chapter 3).

Herpes Simplex Virus 1 and 2

There are many herbs (and supplements) useful against herpes simplex viruses; here are some of them: *Actinidia chinensis* (kiwi tree root), *Agrimonia pilosa* (hairy agrimony), *Andrographis paniculata* (andrographis), *Aristolochia debilis*, *Artemisia annua* (artemisinin), *Artemisia anomala*, *Astragalus membranaceus* (astragalus), *Azadirachta indica* (neem), the berberine plants, *Bidens pilosa* (bidens), *Boussingaultia gracilis*, *Byrsonima verbascifolia*, *Caesalpinia pulcherrima* (a strong decoction of the flower is strongest, followed by stem/leaf preparations), *Carissa edulis* (root bark), *Centella asiatica* (gotu kola), *Cordyceps sinensis* (cordyceps), *Crossostephium chinense*, *Cryptolepis sanguinolenta* (cryptolepis), *Cynanchum paniculatum*, *Distictella elongata*, *Ganoderma lucidum* (reishi), *Geum japonicum*, *Glycyrrhiza glabra* (licorice), honey, houttuynia, isatis, *Juniper* spp., *Limonium brasiliense*, *Lindera strychnifolia*, *Melia azedarach* (chinaberry leaves, invasive in the United States), *Melissa officinalis* (lemon balm), *Ocimum americanum* (hairy basil), *Ocimum basilicum* (basil),

Ocimum sanctum (holy basil, strongest of the three), *Patrinia villosa*, *Phyllanthus niruri, Pinus massoniana, Pithecellobium clypearia* (a.k.a. *Archidendron clypearia*), *Pongamia pinnata* (seeds), *Prunella vulgaris* (self-heal), *Psidium guajava, Punica granatum* (pomegranate juice), *Pyrrosia lingua, Rheum officinale* (rhubarb root), *Rhus aromatica* (fragrant sumac), *Rhus chinensis* (Chinese sumac), *Rhus javanica*, *Rosmarinus officinalis* (rosemary), *Salvia officinalis* (sage), *Sargassum fusiforme, Scutellaria baicalensis* (Chinese skullcap), *Serissa japonica* (a.k.a. *S. foetida*), *Sida acuta* (sida), *Stephania cepharantha* (stephania), *Syzygium aromaticum, Taraxacum mongolicum, Terminalia chebula, Thymus vulgaris* (thyme), *Usnea* spp., zinc, zinc sulfate cream.

Byrsonima verbascifolia is a South American herb; it is particularly antiviral for these two viruses but is hard to get in the United States. Bidens, reishi, licorice, and houttuynia are also especially strong. A combination Chinese formula, yin chen hao tang, composed of *Artemisia capillaris, Rheum officinale*, and *Gardenia jasminoides*, has shown good effect against HSV-1 and HSV-2.

Terminalia chebula, Syzygium aromaticum, Rhus javanica, and *Geum japonicum* have all been found potent against HSV serotypes. They have particularly strong actions in the brain and are synergistic with acyclovir, enhancing its actions and impacts. The use of these herbs, singly, or in combination, has been found to prevent recurrence of HSV blooms in vivo (mice). All are traditional herbs, long used in community medicine. They all have activity against a variety of viruses.

TREATMENT

- **Systemic antiviral formulation:** A combination tincture with equal parts of licorice, isatis, houttuynia, and sida, 1/2 teaspoon 3x daily. Houttuynia is particularly effective in reducing the cytokine cascade the virus starts, thus strongly inhibiting it. (In severe systemic infections, double the dose to 6x daily.)

- **Immune formulation:** A combination tincture with equal parts of astragalus, cordyceps, and reishi. (Reishi is particularly strong against these viruses.) Tonic dose: 20–60 drops 3x daily. In acute episodes: 1/2 teaspoon up to 6x daily.
- **Zinc,** internally, 25 mg daily. Double that for a few days if you feel an attack coming on.

To prevent outbreaks, try L-lysine, in a tonic dose of 1,000 mg 3x daily. (Note: If you do have an outbreak anyway, increase the dosage, up to 3,000 mg 3x daily. However, if taken regularly, the tonic dose can help prevent outbreaks from occurring.) Another helpful supplement is vitamin B_{12}, 500 mcg daily (a good B-complex is very helpful as well). Avoid L-arginine supplements and foods containing L-arginine such as nuts and chocolate. These can stimulate outbreaks.

To treat active sores, you can use zinc sulfate cream, applied 6–10x daily. This can reduce and eliminate sores within 3–5 days. The sore-relief concentrated herbal cream in the sidebar on page 117 can do the same even more quickly, within 3 days.

To reduce nerve pain, some of the things that can help are:

- **Geranium oil,** topical, applied as needed. If the pure essential oil is too strong, you can dilute it with olive oil if necessary.
- **Greater celandine (*Chelidonium majus*) tincture.** Typical American dosage is 10–30 drops 3x daily for 30 days. English dosage is higher, generally 40–80 drops 3x daily, again for 30 days. In rare instances use for longer than 30 days can cause severe inflammation of the bile ducts, so only use it for 30 days in a row.
- **Pasque flower tincture,** 10 drops every hour or so.
- **Kudzu root (*Pueraria lobata*) tincture,** 1/2 teaspoon 3 or 4x daily. This alters certain neural receptors in the brain and peripheral nervous system.
- **Theramine** can also help, sometimes a lot. It is a prescription nutriceutical that is very good for certain kinds of recalcitrant pain.

For some specific expressions of HSV, incorporate these additional formulations into the protocol:

For vaginal herpes: Prepare a douche by combining 1 ounce of a berberine plant (e.g., goldenseal, barberry) tincture and 1 ounce of
lemon balm tincture in a pint of water and use it to douche 3x daily.

For herpes eye infection: Prepare eyedrops by combining 1 ounce each
of dried licorice, houttuynia, and isatis in a heat-proof quart jar.
Bring water to a boil, then pour it over the herbs, stir well, cover,
and let sit overnight. Strain well the next day. Pour some of the
infusion into a 1-ounce brown bottle with dropper. Store the rest in
the refrigerator. Use the eyedrops throughout the day, a minimum
of 6x daily. Just 1–3 drops in each eye every hour or two until the
condition clears.

For herpetic encephalitis/meningitis: Use the protocols for viral
encephalitis delineated in depth in chapter 3. An ethanol extract
of *Cynanchum paniculatum* has been found to be very effective in
protecting the brain and neural structures in some studies and may
prove useful here.

Caution: The use of L-arginine during an *active* herpes outbreak
can sometimes exacerbate the condition excruciatingly.

Varicella Zoster Virus (Chicken Pox/Shingles)

Although chicken pox (varicella zoster virus) tends to be a self-
limiting disease a vaccine has been developed in the West; a variety
of it has also been crafted for herpes zoster (shingles). Shingles tends
to be the most problematic element of this virus; it is often extremely
painful and somewhat difficult to treat well.

I won't explore the use of herbs for chicken pox itself since, with
the vaccine, episodes in the West are becoming rare. However, modi-
fications of the protocols outlined for shingles will help with chicken
pox, especially the systemic and topical formulations. Treatment
protocols in this section are specific only for shingles.

Some of the herbs and supplements effective for herpes zoster
(shingles) are *Ampelopsis brevipedunculata*, *Astragalus membranaceus*
(astragalus), *Clinacanthus nutans*, *Ficus binjamina* (leaves), *Garcinia
multiflora*, *Glycyrrhiza glabra* (licorice), isatis, *Lonicera japonica*

(Japanese honeysuckle), *Melissa officinalis* (lemon balm), *Polygonum cuspidatum* (Japanese knotweed), *Quillaja saponaria* (Chilean soap-bark tree, inner bark infusion/decoction, low dosing), *Rhus succedanea, Ribes nigrum* (black currant).

Concentrated Sore-Relief Herbal Cream

INGREDIENTS

3 ounces licorice root

2 ounces birch bark

2 ounces lemon balm leaf

2 ounces rosemary leaf

To make:

Combine the herbs in a crock-pot with 32 ounces of water. Bring to a boil. Reduce the heat to barely under a simmer. Cook for 3 days. Turn off the heat, let cool, strain out the herbs. Return the liquid to the cleaned crock-pot, bring to a boil again, then reduce heat to just under a simmer. Let cook until the liquid is reduced to 2 ounces. (Caution: It can easily burn once it gets close, so watch it.) When reduced sufficiently, turn off the heat, let cool, and place the cream in a jar.

To use:

Apply 6–10x daily. This combination will eliminate sores, reduce pain, and promote healing very quickly, usually within 3 days or so.

TREATMENT

The basic treatment for shingles comprises 1) systemic antivirals, 2) immune formulations, 3) topical creams for skin outbreaks, and 4) treatments to reduce nerve pain and regenerate nerve cells.

  1. Systemic antivirals. I would suggest both of the following:

  • **Tincture combination** of licorice, isatis, and Chinese skullcap, in equal parts, $1/4$-$1/2$ teaspoon 3–6x daily, depending on the severity of the outbreak. This will actually help heal the nerves of the infection and prevent recurrences, if you use it over time.

  • **Lemon balm tincture** (I suggest the Herb Pharm brand), $1/4$ teaspoon 3–6x daily. This is *very* helpful over time. It is also very calming to the nerves and helps prevent recurrences.

2. **Immune formulation.** Tincture combination of astragalus, rhodiola, and cordyceps, in equal parts, $\frac{1}{2}$ teaspoon 3x daily. This will increase immune function and help reduce the incidence of future outbreaks. (Lowered immune function due to age is the main cause of shingles outbreaks after age 50.)

3. **Topical healing.** A couple of formulations can help here:

- **Lemon balm infused oil or cordial,** applied topically daily. This really does help.

- **Pine pollen cream,** applied topically daily. This really does help if you can find the cream.

4. **Nerve pain.** The herbs and supplements recommended for reducing the nerve pain of herpes simplex virus outbreaks (see page 113) will also help reduce the nerve pain that accompanies a shingles outbreak.

Herbs can also help prevent or cure the postherpetic nerve pain that comes from nerve damage after outbreaks by regenerating the damaged nerves. Two of the best regenerators (both very high in nerve growth factor) are Chinese senega root and lion's mane; vitamin B_{12} is also very helpful:

- **Chinese senega root:** 30 drops of the tincture 3x daily for 30 days, and . . .

- **Lion's mane (*Hericium erinaceus*):** 1 teaspoon of the tincture 2x daily. Note: The fresh mushroom tincture, not the dried, is preferable if you can find it. Long-term use of this herb is fine. And . . .

- **Vitamin B_{12}:** 500–2,000 mcg daily.

Supplements for both deep healing and nerve pain:

- **L-lysine:** as a tonic dose, 1,000 mg 3x daily; during a shingles outbreak, up to 3,000 mg 3x daily.

- **L-carnitine:** 500–700 mg 3x daily.

- **Alphalipoic acid:** 200 mg 3x daily.

- **Inositol:** 500–1,000 mg 3x daily.

Regular fruit intake can also be important. Low fruit intake (less than one serving per week) can lead to more frequent outbreaks.

Note: L-arginine intake can sometimes *cause* a shingles outbreak. If you have a history of shingles, I would recommend avoiding L-arginine supplementation. (Nuts and dark chocolate are fairly high in L-arginine; caution is warranted.)

Rotavirus and Norovirus

Rotaviruses are the best studied of the viral gastroenteritis diseases, in terms of herbal treatments, but for all of them, tannin-containing plants are indicated for one big reason: they inactivate the viruses. In the case of the Norwalk virus, for example, tannic acid inhibits the binding of the viral proteins to HBGA (histo-blood group antigen) receptors, thus preventing infection. There have been a number of double-blind studies using tannic-acid-containing plants in the treatment of viral gastroenteritis, and all have shown good success. Researchers have tested plants traditionally used for this kind of condition and found many of them active. The most common and strongest: *Musa* spp. (the green, unripe banana fruit, usually cooked), *Potentilla erecta* (leaves), *Potentilla tormentilla* (root), and *Psidium guajava* (guava).

The plants found effective for rotaviruses are *Aegle marmelos* (unripe fruit), *Artocarpus integrifolia* (bark), *Byrsonima verbascifolia, Eugenia dysenterica* (a.k.a. *Stenocalyx dysentericus*), *Glycyrrhiza glabra* (licorice), *Haemanthus albiflos* (bulb), *Hymenaea courbaril, Lomatium dissectum, Myracrodruon urundeuva, Myristica fragrans* (seeds), *Panax ginseng, Potentilla erecta* (leaves), *Potentilla tormentilla* (root), *Wolfiporia* (a.k.a. *Poria*) and *Polyporus* in combination (as a decoction), *Psidium guajava* (leaves), *Punica granatum* (pomegranate leaves and juice), *Quillaja saponaria, Sophora flavescens, Spondias lutea* (a.k.a. *S. mombin*; leaves and bark), *Stevia rebaudiana, Vaccinium macrocarpon* (cranberry juice).

Plants have not been tested to any extent against astroviruses though *Detarium senegalense* and *Dichrostachys glomerata* are both active against the viruses. For orthoreoviruses, the barks of both

Castanea (chestnut) and *Schinopsis* (quebracho) are active antivirals as well as tannin sources in general.

In essence, any plant that is strongly drying on the tongue is going to work: oak leaves or bark, *Krameria* (rhatany) root, pine needles (mature), acacia, agrimony, pinedrops (*Pterospora*), rose, raspberry, blackberry, and so on. Roots, leaves, and bark tend to be the most astringent parts of such plants. In my experience rhatany root, blackberry root, and pinedrops are some of the strongest, followed by quebracho, oak, and pine needles, but really, any astringent plants will do. It is just that the stronger they are, the faster they work.

Other useful plants are:

- **Berberine-containing plants.** These plants do have some antiviral properties but they also have strong actions on the GI tract membrane and help it resist any microbial infection.
- ***Bidens* spp.** These plants are strong, systemic antimicrobials and prostaglandin inhibitors and are very specific for diarrheal diseases and healing damaged mucous membrane systems.
- ***Alchornea cordifolia.*** This plant is a potent systemic antibacterial and antimicrobial that is used in traditional African medicine for a variety of conditions, including diarrhea. It has been found to reduce water and electrolyte loss during diarrheal diseases.
- ***Baccharis teindalensis, Carica papaya, Croton lechleri, Euphorbia hirta, Jatropha curcas, Jussiaea suffruticosa, Mangifera indica, Terminalia avicennoides, and Zingiber officinale.*** All have been found in a number of studies to help reduce diarrhea, limit water and electrolyte loss, and help with cramping.

TREATMENT

The treatment of these viral gastroenteritis diseases is straightforward, and while you can get fancy with this, it primarily entails the use of any plants strong in tannins, in large quantities. My preference is for their use as decoctions but even that is not necessary; unripe banana is especially useful in the regions in which it grows, for example, and is usually used as a mashed, cooked ingestible. Plants high in tannins bind the viruses while, at the same time, reducing fluid loss through firming up the stool.

Some suggestions:

- **Combination tincture** of *Alchornea cordifolia* (or any berberine-containing plant), licorice, and lomatium, in equal parts, 30 drops to 1 tsp 3–6x daily depending on the severity of the condition and age of the person.

- **Strong infusion of blackberry root:** Add 4 ounces powdered or roughly ground blackberry root to a large heat-proof jar. Add 1 quart of very hot water, cover, and let steep overnight. Drink the whole thing over the next day. Repeat daily. Increase the dosage if diarrhea is not substantially helped within 24 hours. Or . . .

- **Strong decoction of blackberry root:** 4 ounces blackberry root to 1 quart of water; boil until the water is reduced by half. Let cool and consume in equal parts throughout the day. Repeat daily.

5

HERBAL ANTIVIRALS: THE MATERIA MEDICA

A large number of structurally unique antiviral compounds from medicinal plants (herbs) have been identified. The advantages of natural compounds are fewer side effects in comparison to orthodox medical drugs, and the production of synergistic effects for a more positive treatment outcome.

— Kaio Kitazato et al., "Viral Infectious Disease and
Natural Products with Antiviral Activity"

There has been very little work in the popular press (especially in the West) on herbal antivirals — and most of what has occurred is embarrassingly poor. There are a number of reasons for this.

The field of antivirals itself, whether medical or herbal, is in relative infancy, which partly explains the problems in the literature. The general overemphasis on bacteria as disease-causing agents in the public (and medical) mind, irrespective of culture, also contributes to the problem. Then, there is the nature of viruses themselves and the difficulty of actually creating effective pharmaceutical antivirals. There are, in fact, very few pharmaceutical antivirals compared to antibiotics — generally people only hear of two: ribavirin and Tamiflu (oseltamivir). This is a much reduced pharmaceutical armamentarium compared to the scores of antibiotics that are common in most people's vocabularies; *penicillin* is, I suspect, a word known to most of the world's population.

Most of the scientific research (at least in the past and especially in the West) on viral treatment has been focused not so much on finding effective antivirals but on vaccines. And researchers have been pretty successful at this over the past 50 years — the eradication of smallpox is one of the great triumphs of technological medicine, as is the polio vaccine. So, we have vaccines now for an increasing number of viral diseases: smallpox, polio, measles, hepatitis B, influenza strains, and so on.

Thus, the focus of most medical viral research, in contrast to bacterial research, has been on vaccines. In consequence, few people ever think of *antivirals* as a specific entity that might be useful in medicine; *antibiotic* is a word that everyone has heard of, has used, and knows. The word *antiviral* is not. Nevertheless, antivirals do exist in great quantity in the world. In plants.

Viruses are an intimate part of life on this planet and every life form, including plants, has experienced viral infections during the billions of years there has been life here. Plants, the finest chemists on Earth, have created, just as they have in their dealings with infective bacteria, a wide range of compounds in response to viral infection. Similarly to plant antibiotics and bacteria, while *all* plants have created a variety of compounds to protect them from viruses, some, when used as medicines, tend to be a great deal more effective than others. The trick is to find which are the most effective, the most reliable, the most potent.

The strongest herbal antivirals are more easily revealed *if* the medicinal plant world is examined through a number of lenses and then, afterward, those findings are cross-correlated. The lenses I used for this book are:

- The history of the plants' uses in community medicine in whatever cultures have access to them — what some people call indigenous or traditional practice;
- The history of the plants' uses in developed medical systems such as traditional Chinese medicine, Ayurveda, or Western botanic practice;
- Contemporary uses of the plants among community herbalists;

- Outcome experiences among contemporary peoples who are using the plants for healing;
- Scientific study of the plants' medicinal actions as viewed through in vitro, in vivo, and human clinical study[1]; and finally
- A factor that I have found a primary indicator of strong medicinal action — the invasive status of the plant. For, interestingly enough, many of the strongest antibacterial and antiviral plants are invasives.[2]

And while I am not yet using this as a primary identifier, it is becoming evident that many of the most potent antivirals are also synergists. This is a relatively new category of herbal medicines — in the West at any rate. Synergists are plants that, when used with other medicinal substances (herbs, supplements, pharmaceuticals), through a variety of mechanisms, *increase* the potency of those substances against microbial pathogens. A number of the herbs in this book are very potent synergists.

The plants that show strong activity when viewed through a majority of these lenses end up on the list. It is then the final factor comes into play: access. There are some truly magnificent antiviral and antibacterial plants in Africa, South America, and China that simply are not to be had in the Western world, no matter how actively they are sought — unless you travel to those places. The plant medicines in this book tend to be somewhat easy to find and that is important. It's no good to know of a great antiviral if you can't find any of it to use as medicine.

Many of the antiviral herbs in this book are broad-spectrum antivirals, that is, they are active against a wide range of viruses. I tend to think of these as the most potent antivirals in a general sense (e.g., Chinese skullcap). There are others with a more narrow range but that are very antiviral for specific viruses (e.g., ginger, elder). *All* of them have shown potent activity in historical use across long timelines. *All* of them have been found effective in contemporary usage. Nevertheless, these are not the only antiviral herbs there are. These are just the ones that I have used with success, the ones that have shown up the most strongly in this examination of them, in this particular year, for these particular viruses.

Again, there are *a lot* of great herbal antivirals out there; over time, more will be understood and discussed *and* used as medicine. So, don't think these are the only ones to use; they are just the ones that I have used the most, that have the deepest historical use, that have the greatest presence in the literature, and that have the best research on them.

In this section I include the top seven antiviral herbs, five honorable mentions, one truly important supportive herb for nearly all viral infections, and two very useful antiviral supplements. Here they are.

> ## The Top Seven Antiviral Herbs
>
> Chinese skullcap
> Elder
> Ginger
> Houttuynia
> Isatis
> Licorice
> Lomatium

Chinese Skullcap

Family: Lamiaceae or is it the Labiatae, or are those synonyms? (I feel another taxonomic rant coming on.)

Species used: *Scutellaria baicalensis* is the primary species used in China and the one meant when Chinese skullcap is talked about (and the one this monograph will focus on). It most definitely does not mean the American skullcap, *Scutellaria lateriflora* — or any of the other American species. For reasons I will discuss in this monograph I strongly suggest you *not* use *S. lateriflora* as a substitute for treating viral infections. Note that *Scutellaria macrantha* is a synonym for *S. baicalensis*.

Common names: Legion for the many different skullcaps, however for *S. baicalensis*: English — Chinese skullcap, baikal skullcap, scute (really hate that one — "you are so *scute*"), golden root (really like that one). Chinese — huang qin. (Ban zhi lian is the Chinese for *S. barbata*).

Exploring *Scutellaria* Species

The Chinese do use another skullcap species, *Scutellaria barbata*, which is considered much weaker but still specific for certain conditions. There is, however, an important distinction about the medicines made from these various skullcap species. The most studied species, and the one considered the strongest, is *S. baicalensis* and with that species the Chinese use the root *only*. (See "Part Used" and "Western Botanic Practice" for more on all this.) With *S. barbata* and the various American species the aerial parts are used. This difference, aerial part versus root, makes *all* the difference in the medicinal impacts of the plants. The leaves just aren't as strong, especially for viral infections. After several millennia of use, the Chinese consider all other skullcaps to be inferior to *S. baicalensis* in their medicinal effects. And I assume (makes an ass of u and me) that they must have tried the roots of the other species and found them not as strong; nevertheless, what if they didn't . . . ? Perhaps we in the West should do a little experimenting with some roots of our own.

Now, that being said, there are 200, or 300, or 350 species in the genus *Scutellaria* . . . taxonomists are absolutely positive about those figures. Many of the various skullcaps are used similarly as medicines in the regions in which they grow; most of them contain the same constituents. However, there has been very little study on species other than *S. baicalensis*. As illustration, there are over 600 journal articles on PubMed on *S. baicalensis* (and its major constituents), but only 88 on *Scutellaria barbata*, just 24 on *Scutellaria lateriflora* (the main American species), a mere eight on *S. viscidula*, six on *S. indica*, four on *S. racemosa*, three on *S. galericulata*, and one each on *S. regeliana*, *S. incana*, *S. taiwanensis*, and *S. austrotaiwanensis*. There's even less on the others.

Some studies have shown that *S. baicalensis*, *S. barbata*, *S. lateriflora*, and *S. racemosa* have similar constituents in their roots — but then the roots of those other species are almost never used in medicine making

Part Used

The root and the root only — generally only from plants older than 3 years. There is reason to believe that the increase in pharmacological action of Chinese skullcap over the usual American species used as medicinals is due to the difference between using the root in Chinese practice and the leaf in American practice. As far as I know there has so there is no way to know if in practice they are as potent as the Chinese skullcap root. (If you try roots other than those of *S. baicalensis*, let me know how they work. Let's start something here.)

S. *lateriflora*, a.k.a blue skullcap, mad dog skullcap, Virginia skullcap, hoodwort (along with S. *galericulata*, i.e., marsh or common skullcap), is the species most commonly used in the United States. S. *racemosa* is more common in South America and S. *barbata* is the other main species used in traditional Chinese medicine. Constituent studies have found that those three varieties all contain baicalin, baicalein, scutellarin, wogonin, melatonin, and serotonin — the constituents considered to be the most active in Chinese skullcap. Other studies, on the roots of S. *viscidula* and S. *amoena*, found very similar constituents in *them*. It does seem that most of the species contain baicalein, baicalin, and wogonin at the very least — though the amounts in differing species have not been *comparatively* studied to any degree.

However, one study that did examine the constituent levels in the roots of *Scutellaria planipes* and compared them with S. *baicalensis* found that the root constituents were very similar in nature, degree, and number, and were equally active as antibacterials and antiallergics. Another study (Chinese) showed that the root of *Scutellaria rivularis* stimulated the production of monoclonal antibodies to encephalitis virus E protein, just as the root of S. *baicalensis* does.

So . . . it may turn out that many of the skullcaps can be used interchangeably with S. *baicalensis* as medicines — but *only* if the roots are used, which they generally aren't. Again, I think the roots of various skullcap species should be explored to find out if they can be used interchangeably with the Chinese variety. So, if you are using the American skullcaps, try harvesting some of the root of whatever species you are growing, and make it into medicine and find out how it works. (Then e-mail me.)

been virtually no examination of the root as a medicinal in any of the Western species.

There are, as well, no *substantive* studies on the difference between roots and leaves of any species of skullcap as regards their chemical compounds. The few I have seen that touch on it do show substantial differences between the leaf and the root and this really does need to be explored, especially if American herbalists are insisting that the American skullcaps are interchangeable with the Chinese. (And some of them are.) However, as some researchers have commented, "The results showed that the components and relative contents of the essential oils among flowers, stem, leaves, roots, and seeds have significant differences."[3] This is, of course, true of nearly all plants on Earth and one of the most basic understandings of herbal medicine.

Preparation and Dosage

Medicinals prepared from this plant are a bit hard to find in the United States, though not impossible. (I know only a few sources for Chinese skullcap root tinctures, but hundreds for the American leaf tinctures.)

TINCTURE

If making it yourself, again, use the root. After harvesting the root, cut it into easy-to-use pieces, let it dry in a cool, shaded location, then powder the root pieces and tincture them. The ratio should be 1:5 (one part herb, five parts liquid), with the liquid being 50 percent alcohol, 50 percent water. Take $1/4–1/2$ teaspoon 3x daily. In acute conditions, double that. Remember: If using for CNS damage or encephalitis, you want to flood the brain and CNS with the compounds over a long enough time period to sharply reduce the inflammation and protect and restore the neural structures of the brain. I think the tincture best for this purpose.

For sleep: The plant and root are high in melatonin, so they can help with sleep. If you are using it for that, take just before bedtime, $1/2$ teaspoon of the tincture.

Fresh leaf tincture: If you want to use the aerial parts of the plant, get or make a 1:2 tincture of the fresh leaves and stems. Tonic doses run from 10–30 drops up to 6x daily but I have taken up to $1/2$ ounce of the tincture at a time (of the American skullcaps anyway) without side effects; there apparently are none even at high doses.

POWDER

The Chinese dosages are large, as usual, generally 3–9 grams at a time. Most of the clinical studies and trials used similar dosing. If you are using capsules this is the dosage range you should be exploring, divided into three equal doses every 4 hours or so. Capsules are pretty much impossible to find but you can get the powdered herb fairly easily. I would use 1 teaspoon of the powdered root 3–6x daily.

Note: The herb reaches peak levels in the plasma and body organs in about 1 hour and only lasts in the body for about 4 hours, so you really do need to dose about every 3–4 hours.

AS A WASH

The fresh juice of the plant can be used as an eye wash for eye infections, as can the cooled infusion or decoction of the root.

Side Effects and Contraindications

Side effects from skullcap are rare, mostly gastric discomfort and diarrhea. It should not be used during pregnancy. Caution should be exercised if you are taking pharmaceuticals as it can increase the bioavailability of the drugs, thus increasing their impacts. It may interact additively with blood-pressure-lowering drugs. Type 1 diabetics should exercise strong caution with the herb as it can affect insulin and blood sugar levels.

Herb/Drug and Herb/Herb Interactions

Lots. Chinese skullcap is a synergist, perhaps as efficacious as licorice, ginger, and piperine, and should probably be added to that category of herbs. Among other things it inhibits the NorA efflux pump, which inactivates some forms of antibiotic resistance. Like the other synergists I know of, it is also a strong antiviral, which is beginning to stimulate speculation. Nevertheless, the herb strongly affects pharmaceuticals and herbs taken along with it.

Baicalein, one of the major compounds in *S. baicalensis*, is synergistic with ribavirin, albendazole, ciprofloxacin, amphotericin B.

S. baicalensis is strongly inhibitive of CYP3A4, a member of the cytochrome oxidase system. And this inhibition is dose dependent; the more you take, the more it is inhibited. CYP3A4 is a type of enzyme, strongly present in the liver, and is responsible for catalyzing reactions involved in drug metabolism. Many of the pharmaceuticals that are ingested are metabolized by the CYP3A4 system, meaning that some portion of the drug is inactivated, usually by being altered to another molecular form. With pharmaceuticals, the normal dosage range you are given is adjusted to take this metabolization into account. If you are using Chinese skullcap, then less of the pharmaceutical is going to be metabolized. In some cases this will make the impacts of the drug stronger, with the bioavailable dose higher. With other drugs it is the metabolites created by CYP3A4 that are active in the body. In this circumstance, since the herb inhibits CYP3A4, the metabolites of the pharmaceutical you are taking will be reduced in degree and have *less* effect in the body. Acetaminophen, codeine, cyclosporin, diazepam, erythromycin, and so on are all affected in one way or another. The herb does affect the amount of antibiotics that enter the system.

To make things more complicated, one of the herb's constituents, oroxylin A, is a strong P-glycoprotein inhibitor. P-glycoprotein is strongly present in the blood-brain barrier, the lining of the GI tract, renal tubular cells, capillary endothelial cells, and the blood-testes barrier. It reduces the amount of substances that cross over those barriers in order to protect what is on the other side. (This is why berberine is mostly confined to the GI tract.) P-glycoprotein inhibitors allow more of a substance to cross barriers that are high in P-glycoprotein. That means that if you are taking skullcap, any substance taken with it will end up in higher levels in the bloodstream, thus increasing its impacts in the system.

This means that Chinese skullcap will act through two different mechanisms to increase drug and herb uptake in the body.

Also, because cancer cells use P-glycoprotein as a form of efflux pump in order to eject drugs designed to kill them from the cancer cells, Chinese skullcap will increase the effectiveness of anticancer drugs by inhibiting P-glycoprotein-mediated cellular efflux. Paclitaxel uptake, for example, was increased over twofold when administered with oroxylin A.

All this applies equally to herbs and supplements that you take along with skullcap. If you are using this herb along with licorice, which is also a potent synergist, through its own mechanisms (as is ginger), everything else you take will be much more potent and pronounced in the body. (This is one reason why licorice and skullcap are considered such important medicines in Chinese practice and why they are commonly added to many herbal combinations.) *Keep this in mind.*

Habitat and Appearance

This plant likes to grow in wettish, sandy, and rocky-type seashore or creekish locations in the wild, from sea level to 6,000 feet in altitude. It is native to east Asia: China, Mongolia, Japan, Korea, Siberia, Russia. (Many of the skullcaps like it wet and tend to grow along streambeds and creeks.)

It's a perennial growing up to a foot in height (hardy to zone 5). It flowers in August, seeds are ready in September. The plants are hermaphrodites and are pollinated by insects.

And I have to admit, Chinese skullcap is beautiful, the lanceolate leaves a vibrant green, the flowers the most delicious purple. The flowers are supposedly shaped like little skullcaps — people use to wear similar, though larger, ones in the Middle Ages ... so they say. But *they* also said that the Earth was flat and that pharmaceuticals were safer than herbs and that there was no one on the grassy knoll.

I think Chinese skullcap the most beautiful of the skullcaps. Richo Cech, at Horizon Herbs, describes it like this: "The purple flowers are like schools of dolphins breaking through green waves in a summer sea." Beautifully put and very apt.

It is commonly grown in the United States as a garden plant due to its resistance to drought and cold. It can survive nearly anything. (And so can you if you use it as medicine.)

Cultivation and Collection

Sow seeds outdoors in late spring (or in a pot or cold frame in early spring). The seeds generally sprout within 10 to 20 days. Separate the sprouts when large enough to handle. Grows easily in sunny locations in ordinary garden soil that remains a bit moist. Soil needs to be well drained in sun or partial shade. It is hardy to zone 5 and survives dips as low as –23°C or about –10°F. It will survive drought pretty well once established.

You can harvest the aerial plant at flowering and make a fresh plant tincture (if that is how you are going to use it). But, again, the roots are more potent. They should be harvested after 3 years of growth (or more), cut to usable lengths, and dried carefully in the shade (though the Chinese do it in light sun). Once well dried, they should be stored in plastic bags in a plastic tub in a coolish location in the dark. Spring roots are more potent (as usual). Good-quality organic freshly dried roots should be yellowish, even a bright yellow, in color. Most of the imported Chinese roots tend to be a bit oxidized, the yellow color fading a bit. Poorly prepared or severely oxidized roots will be greenish or even black in color. Don't bother with them.

You can, if you wish, and if you are a fan of the aerial tinctures of the skullcaps, harvest the root *and* aerial parts of the plants and make a tincture from both, separately.

Properties of Chinese Skullcap

Actions

Chinese skullcap is a broad-spectrum antiviral. It inhibits hemagglu-tinin and neuraminidase, inhibits viral replication, suppresses viral gene expression, reduces viral RNA in infected cells, inhibits viral fusion with cells, protects cell membranes from virus-initiated cytokines, reduces the expression of the viral matrix protein gene, interferes with viral entry by interacting with viral envelope proteins and cellular CD4 and chemokine receptors, regulates the innate antiviral immunity of the host by modulating cytokine production at the time of viral insult, lowers host cell membrane fluidity thus inhibiting the formation of virus-induced membrane pores in host cells (which in itself stops viral entry into host cells), inhibits viral release from infected cells, inhibits viral cytokine cascades, increases apoptosis in infected cells, stimulates innate resistance to viral infection, promotes the development of monoclonal antibodies to encephalitis virus E protein, and is directly virucidal.

S. baicalensis is also:

Anodyne	Antihypertensive	Expectorant
Antianaphylactic	Anti-inflammatory	Febrifuge
Antiangiogenic	Antimetastic	Hemostatic
Antibacterial	Antioxidant	Hepatoprotective
Anticholesterolemic	Antispasmodic	Sedative (mild)
Anticonvulsant	Antitumor	Nervine
Antidiarrheal	Astringent	Neuroprotective
Antidysenteric	Cholagogue	
Antifungal	Diuretic	

Active Against

This plant is a major broad-spectrum antiviral with a wide range of activity against viruses. It is active against:

Adenovirus (3 and 7)	Hepatitis A	Human T cell
Avian infectious bronchitis virus	Hepatitis B (resistant and nonresistant)	leukemia virus
Coliphage MS2	Hepatitis C	Influenza A (H1N1, H3N2 — resistant and nonresistant)
Coxsackie B virus (3, 4, and 5)	Herpes simplex viruses	Influenza B
Epstein-Barr virus	HIV-1	Measles virus

Continued on next page

Continued from previous page

Mosaic virus
Parainfluenza viruses
  (in general)
Polio virus
Porcine reproductive
  and respiratory
  syndrome virus

Respiratory syncytial
  virus
SARS coronavirus
Sendai virus
  (parainfluenza
  type 1)

Vesicular stomatitis
virus

Chinese skullcap is synergistic with other antivirals (as is licorice, they should be used together if possible). It does have a fairly wide range of action against bacteria and some other microbes but the effects are variable; by this I mean it is not primarily a major systemic antibacterial as cryptolepis is, for example. Many of its antibacterial and antiviral effects tend to be not direct, that is, through antimicrobial actions, but sideways through the stimulation of the body's own immune responses, reduction of cytokine cascades, protection of host cells. Antibacterially, the herb does have some really potent effects against some bacteria, particularly staph organisms, resistant and nonresistant. It is also nicely active against mycoplasma and some others such as klebsiella organisms. In general, the herb can be used as a primary adjunct to any treatment of resistant bacterial disease as it is synergistic with both herbs and pharmaceuticals, will markedly reduce cytokine cascades along a rather broad range, and has its own antibacterial actions to add to the mix.

The entire list of organisms it is active against includes:

Actinomyces viscosus
*Angiostrongylus
  cantonensis*
Bacillus subtilis
*Bacteroides
  melaninogenicus*
Bordetella pertussis
Candida albicans
Chlamydia trachomatis
*Corynebacterium
  xerosis*
*Diplococcus
  pneumoniae* (a.k.a.
  *Streptococcus
  pneumoniae*)
Enterococcus faecalis

Escherichia coli
Helicobacter pylori
Klebsiella pneumoniae
*Lactobacillus
  plantarum*
*Micrococcus
  sedentarius*
  (a.k.a. *Kytococcus
  sedentarius*)
Microsporum audouinii
Microsporum canis
*Mycobacterium
  smegmatis*
*Mycobacterium
  tuberculosis*
Mycoplasma hominis

Neisseria meningitidis
Proteus vulgaris
*Pseudomonas
  fluorescens*
Salmonella spp.
Shigella dysenteriae
Shigella flexneri
Staphylococcus aureus
  (resistant and
  nonresistant strains)
*Staphylococcus
  epidermidis*
*Staphylococcus
  hominis*
*Streptococcus
  hemolyticus*

Streptococcus mutans *Toxoplasma gondii* *Ureaplasma*
Streptococcus sanguis *Trichophyton violaceum* *urealyticum*
  Vibrio cholerae

Use to Treat

Viral infections, especially pandemic influenzas and encephalitis, respiratory infections, pneumonia, infections that affect the central nervous system (essentially *any* infection that has accompanying meningitis or encephalitis such as viral encephalitis or meningitis, mycoplasma, Lyme, viral and bacterial CNS infections, and so forth), impaired brain function, fevers, intermittent fevers, GI tract disorders with accompanying inflammation, diarrhea and dysentery, hepatitis, nephritis, urinary tract infections, nervous irritability, epileptic seizures, convulsions, sleep disruptions. You can also use Chinese skullcap as supportive therapy in cancer.

Note: The root tincture of this plant is extremely specific for reducing inflammation in the brain, reducing the cytokine cascades initiated by viral and other microbial agents in the CNS, and alleviating CNS impacts of those microbes. It should be used in any treatment of viral or bacterial CNS infection.

Other Uses

Some cultures use the leaves as a steamed vegetable; the dried leaves are common as a tea.

Finding It

The best root tinctures come from Elk Mountain Herbs (www.elkmountainherbs.com) and Woodland Essence (www.woodlandessence.com). The powdered root can be purchased from 1stChineseHerbs.com (www.1stchineseherbs.com). You can get really good seed from Horizon Herbs (www.horizonherbs.com).

Plant Chemistry

More than 295 different compounds have been found in *S. baicalensis* so far. The six most important are presumed to be baicalein, wogonin, oroxylin A, baicalin, wogonoside, and oroxylin-A 7-O-glucuronide. All are strongly anti-inflammatory, antiviral, and antitumor in action. Some of the other important compounds are considered to be scutellarin, naringenin, apigenin, luteolin, melatonin, and serotonin. All are strongly biologically active. All are synergistic with each other.

Until relatively recently it was supposed that melatonin was not present in plants, only in animals. (Wrong, as such definitive pronouncements often are.) A number of plants are now known to produce melatonin (and serotonin). Chinese skullcap has some of the highest levels (7 mcg/g) so far discovered (some rice family plants have more). Studies have found that the melatonin in plants is strongly present in the plasma of animals that ingest them and that it does bind to melatonin-binding sites in the brain, creating specific effects. (One being helping with sleep cycle normalization.) Melatonin is highly active in the brain; it detoxifies hydroxyl radical, hydrogen peroxide, nitric oxide, peroxynitrite anion, peroxynitrous acid, and hypochlorous acid.

Melatonin is an upstream antioxidant; many of its metabolites, created when our bodies process it or when the plant compound detoxifies oxidants, are also potent antioxidants. It is also synergistic with a number of antioxidant enzymes and other antioxidants such as vitamin C, vitamin E, and glutathione. Melatonin is active at both the micro and macro levels, exerting antioxidative effects at the level of cells, tissues, organs, and organisms. It is a very unique substance, much different than other antioxidants — and not well understood even now. Not only does it work to repair other biomolecules but under in vivo conditions it is four times more potent than vitamin C and E in protecting tissues.

Melatonin is intimately involved in the regulation of people's circadian rhythms, including their healthy sleep cycle. Part of the reason that the sleep cycle is interrupted as people age (and during inflammatory infections in the CNS) is that the oxidative events in the brain are higher and the levels of melatonin (and its regulatory effects) are much lower. Using plants high in melatonin (which is more effective than using melatonin supplements) can normalize the circadian rhythms, including the sleep cycle, and reduce inflammation in the brain and CNS.

The constituents of Chinese skullcap do enter the plasma in substantial amounts. Baicalein is strongly concentrated in the lungs, brain, and hippocampus, wogonin in the liver, kidneys, and lungs. Baicalin concentrates in the brain, specifically in the striatum, thalamus, and hippocampus. Many of their metabolites are strongly present in those locations as well. These all provide potent CNS protection and amelioration of existing infection dynamics.

Traditional Uses

Outside traditional Chinese medicine and American Eclectic practice the uses of the skullcaps around the world are fairly uniform.

The Tibetans, for instance, use five species, including *S. barbata*, but their usages are interesting. Usually the juice of the plant or root is used for wounds, fevers, indigestion, and gastric troubles. Essentially this is showing both antiviral, antibacterial, and fever-lowering actions (and yeah, GI tract actions).

The indigenous tribes of the United States used eight different skullcaps including *S. lateriflora*. Again, the usage range is interesting. The usage range is a bit broader than the Tibetan and includes, for the aerial parts, decoctions and infusions for sore eyes, chills and fever, colds, coughs, heart troubles, and as laxatives; they used root decoction and infusion as emmenagogues and abortifacients, to expel afterbirth, as antidiarrheals, to treat the nerves and breast pain, as kidney medicine, to prevent smallpox, to prevent colds and flu, to keep the throat clean. Again, the range shows antiviral and antibacterial uses, fever-lowering actions, GI tract dynamics, female reproductive tract action, and a tiny bit of nervine action.

What is interesting about this is that the nervine use of the plants among traditional cultures is almost entirely absent. Given the historical American use of the plant, for centuries, is the leaves as a primary nervine agent and that there is pretty much no indigenous use (out of millennia of their contact with the plants) of skullcaps along that line, well, it's intriguing.

The indigenous uses, when examined in depth, do however show a difference in action between plant and root, and the root actions tend to mirror those of the Chinese skullcap.

AYURVEDA

Several skullcaps are listed in my older Ayurvedic herbals but there is nothing on use.

TRADITIONAL CHINESE MEDICINE

Skullcap is one of the 50 fundamental herbs of Chinese medicine and has been in use for over 2,000 years. It is one of the most widely used herbs in Chinese medicine.

It is considered bitter and cold and to dispel heat (fever reducer, anti-inflammatory), to expel damp heat (e.g., lung infections), to be a detoxicant, to stop bleeding, and to prevent abnormal fetal movements (which I think, in part, is an indication of its effectiveness for fetal mycoplasma infections). It is specific for fever, cough, pneumonia, hemoptysis, jaundice, hepatitis, dysentery, diarrhea, bloody stool, vexation, insomnia, headache, enteritis, acute conjunctivitis, uterine bleeding, abnormal fetal movements, hypertension, carbuncle, and furuncle. And, again, there is nothing in traditional use that emphasizes its nervine actions.

Most of the scientific studies on the plant have been conducted in China.

WESTERN BOTANIC PRACTICE

The Europeans tended to use *S. galericulata*, the American Eclectics *S. lateriflora*, and it is probably from the Europeans that the Americans got their usage range for the plant. Both were used similarly primarily as tonic, nervine, and antispasmodic herbs. The Eclectics considered their species specific for chorea (involuntary movements), convulsions, tremors, intermittent fever, neuralgia, to help sleep, and for nervous afflictions such as delirium tremens and hysteria with involuntary muscle movements. It was used in all cases of nervous excitability, restlessness, and wakefulness, especially after acute or chronic illness. It was considered to be a cerebrospinal specific. The usual dose was half an ounce of the recently dried herb in half a pint of boiling water. The herb was considered to lose its effectiveness if kept too long in the dried state.

The English use was similar with the addition of uses for nervous headaches, headaches from coughing, St. Vitus' dance (has *nothing* to do with rock and roll), hiccups, and tertian ague.

This is in fact the usage range still employed by American herbalists and very few of them, unless using the Chinese skullcap, use the root. In current American practice skullcap is considered to be a mild, soothing, and reliable nervine, less stimulating than pasque flower and without the druggy feeling that accompanies valerian if used for sleep.

Scientific Research

There are a lot of studies on Chinese skullcap: in vitro, in vivo, and human and clinical trials and studies. The compounds in the root are, not surprisingly, synergistic with each other. All that have been studied are potently antiviral, anti-inflammatory, antioxidative, and free radical scavenging. Wogonin is the most potent nitric oxide (NO) inhibitor, oroxylin is the most potent in inhibiting lipid peroxidation, baicalein appears to be the most potent antiviral compound. Together they produce effects beyond the individual constituents. (In one study the bacteriostatic effect of the root decoction was compared with that of both baicalin and debaicalin. The root decoction was the strongest.)

The root has strong cytokine impacts, reducing NO, iNOS, IL-3, IL-6, IL-17, COX-2, PGE2, NF-κB, IkappaBalpha (IκBα), IL-1α, IL-2, IL-12, TNF-α, VEGF, TGF, IFN-γ, and tends to upregulate IL-10. It inhibits the production of IgE thus suppressing the expression of histamine. It has especially strong impacts in the spleen. It attenuates the activity of c-Raf-1 kinase, MEK1 and MEK2, ERK-1 and ERK-2, p38 MAPK, and JNK.

IN VITRO STUDIES

Flavones from the root are strongly neuroprotective. Baicalein strongly inhibits the aggregation of neuronal amyloidogenic proteins and induces the dissolution of amyloid deposits. Wogonin stimulates brain tissue regeneration, including the differentiation of neuronal precursor cells. Baicalin promotes neuronal differentiation of neural stem/progenitor cells by modulating p-STAT3 and bHLH (basic helix-loop-helix) protein expression.

Wagonin is neuroprotective against cerebral ischemic insult, and at tiny micromolar concentrations completely suppresses the activity of NF-κB, and inhibits the migration of microglial cells to ischemic lesions, thus reducing inflammation at the site of injury. It inhibits the movement of the cells in response to the chemokine MCP-1.

Baicalein attenuates the induced-cell death of brain microglia in mouse microglial cells and rat primary microglia cultures by strongly inhibiting NO through the suppression of iNOS. The compound inhibits NF-κB activity in the cells as well.

Four compounds in the root inhibit prostate cancer cell proliferation.

Baicalin suppresses IL-1ß-induced RANKL (receptor activator of NF-κB ligand) and COX-2 production at a concentration of 0.01 mcg/ml. The longer the constituent is applied, the stronger the effect. Used on human periodontal ligament cells it shows highly protective effects.

Baicalein inhibits IL-1ß- and TNF-α-induced inflammatory cytokine production from human mast cells via regulation of the NF-κB pathway. It inhibits NF-κB and IκBα phosphorylation.

Baicalin promotes repair of DNA single-strand breakage caused by hydrogen peroxide in cultured fibroblasts.

The plant inhibits aromatase, thus reducing the conversion of androgens into estrogens.

There are scores of other in vitro studies such as these, all showing potent anti-inflammatory and cytokine-modulating actions of the herb and its constituents.

IN VIVO STUDIES

In rats, oroxylin A markedly enhances cognitive and mnestic function in animal models of aging brains and neurodegeneration. Baicalein is anticonvulsive, anxiolytic, and sedative in rats.

Flavonoids from the stems and leaves of *Scutellaria baicalensis* improve memory dysfunction and reduce neuronal damage and levels of abnormal free radicals induced by permanent cerebral ischemia in rats. Other studies have found that the compounds can enhance and improve learning and memory abilities and reduce neuronal pathological alterations induced by a variety of chemicals in mice.

S. baicalensis reduces symptoms associated with chronic cerebral hypoperfusion (and chronic lipopolysaccharide infusion), including spatial memory impairments, hippocampal MAPK signaling, and microglial activation.

Baicalein protects mice hippocampal neuronal cells against damage caused by thapsigargin (TG) and brefeldin A (BFA). The constituent reduces TG- and BFA-induced apoptosis of hippocampal cells, reduces the induced expression of endoplasmic reticulum stress-associated proteins, and strongly reduces the levels of MAP kinases such as p38, JNK, and ERK. It reduces ROS accumulation and levels of MMPs. It strongly protects the mitochondria from oxidative damage.

A number of in vivo studies have found baicalein to reduce both edema and intracranial hypertension during brain infection due to pertussis bacteria. It also inhibits the neurotoxic action of kainic acid in the rat brain.

Scutellaria baicalensis (in combination with bupleurum) is strongly neuroprotective against iron-reduced neurodegeneration in the nigrostriatal dopaminergic system in rat brains, showing it to be useful for treating CNS neurodegeneration.

When mice, subjected to transient global brain ischemia for 20 minutes, are treated with baicalein (200 mg/kg once daily), neuronal damage is minimal compared to controls, and MMP-9 activity in the hippocampus is inhibited. Pretreatment with baicalein prevents the damage.

Wogonin is also strongly protective in the brain. In rats damaged by either four-vessel occlusion or excitotoxic injury (systemic kainate injection), wogonin confers protection by attenuating the death of hippocampal neurons. It inhibits the inflammatory activation of the microglia by inhibiting iNOS, TNF-α, NO, IL-1ß, and NF-κB. In vitro studies have found that lipopolysaccharide-activated macrophages are protected similarly.

An ethanol extract of *S. baicalensis* has been shown to prevent oxidative damage and neuroinflammation and memory impairments in artificial senescence mice (mice that get old very fast artificially — to study aging). The hippocampus and the mitochondria are strongly protected and neuroinflammation sharply reduced. Expressions of COX-2, iNOS, NO, PGE2, Bax, cleaved caspase-3 protein are all reduced. Bcl-2 was increased. The effects are dose dependent and are most effective at 100 mg/kg (that would be 7 grams for a 150-pound person, just in the dosage range usually used in China).

Baicalin reduces the severity of relapsing-remitting experimental autoimmune encephalomyelitis induced by proteolipid protein in a mouse model of multiple sclerosis. All the histopathological findings decrease in the mice given the extract.

Baicalin has a protective effect against induced encephaledema in neonatal rats; glutamate and glutamic acid levels decrease, reducing excitotoxicity, and GABA (gamma-aminobutyric acid) increases.

Baicalin, administered to mice infected with influenza virus, increases survival time, eliminates the virus from the lungs, reduces hemagglutination titer and infectivity in the lungs, and reverses pneumonic pathological changes.

Baicalin protects rat brains from pertussis bacilli-induced brain edema. It is 20 times more potent than deferoxamine in reducing lipid peroxidation, and is markedly better at reducing edema, chelating iron, and activating SOD.

Baicalin reduces intracranial hypertension from pertussis bacilli in rabbit brains better than tetramethylpyrazine. The pathologic alterations in the brain are significantly reduced by the use of baicalin.

Baicalin, given to pregnant rats, increases the lung surfactant phospholipids in the fetus and accelerates fetal lung maturation.

Baicalein has been found to be antidepressant in animal models of depression. It reverses the reduction of extracellular ERK phosphorylation and the level of BDNF (brain-derived neurotrophic factor) expression in the hippocampus of CMS (chronic mild stress) model rats.

Oral administration of baicalein in mice infected with Sendai virus results in a significant reduction of viral titers in the lungs and a reduction in the death rate.

Oral administration of baicalein in mice infected with influenza A virus shows significant effects in preventing death, increasing life span, inhibiting lung consolidation, and reducing lung virus titer in a dose-dependent manner. Amounts as low as 1.2 mcg/ml of baicalin (the metabolite of baicalein) result in significant inhibition of the virus. (Note: Plasma levels of baicalin from the ingestion of skullcap root are significantly higher than this after dosing with 3–9 grams per day.)

Baicalein is highly synergistic with ribavarin against H1N1 influenza. The combination produces much better outcomes in mice infected with influenza A infected than ribavirin alone.

Baicalein and wogonin inhibit irradiation-induced skin damage by suppressing increases in MMP-9 and VEGF through the suppression of COX-2 and NF-κB.

In mice infected with hepatitis C virus and treated with *S. baicalensis*, the serum virus content of the mice decreases after treatment with the herb.

S. baicalensis treatment inhibits passive cutaneous anaphylaxis and reduces histamine release in rats receiving intradermal injections of anti-DNP (dinitrophenol) IgE. It is also effective in reducing IL-6 and TNF-α in mouse models of pelvic inflammatory disease. The herb is both anti-inflammatory and antinociceptive.

S. baicalensis extract stimulates the formation of red blood cells and their precursors under conditions of cyclostatic myelosuppression and sleep deprivation.

There are many more studies than these; this just gives a very good overview of the range of actions of the plant and its constituents.

HUMAN STUDIES

The root decoction has been used in a number of clinical situations in China to effectively treat scarlet fever, chronic bronchitis, and epidemic cerebrospinal meningitis. (Details are unfortunately sketchy.) The herb is almost always used in combination, so individual studies are few. But there are some here and there:

Sixty-three people with bacterial meningitis were split into two groups; 32 were treated with both an antibiotic and baicalin, 31 were treated with an antibiotic alone. The inflammatory cytokines in the CNS were markedly lower in the baicalin group, mortality was significantly reduced, and the symptom picture was markedly improved.

Sixty patients with pulmonary infection were treated with either piperacillin sodium or injection of *Scutellaria baicalensis*. Before treatment there was no difference in clinical data. Treatment outcomes were similar in both groups.

In 63 children with upper respiratory infections (51 upper acute, 11 acute bronchitis, 1 tonsillitis) 51 benefited from using the decoction of the root; temperature normalized in 3 days.

A decoction of *S. barbata* was used with 14 women with metastatic breast cancer in a trial at the Memorial Cancer Institute (Hollywood, Florida), as supportive therapy to normal chemo and radiation. The study authors commented that the herb was safe, well tolerated, and showed promising clinical evidence of anticancer activity.

A 12-week randomized trial of *Scutellaria baicalensis* and *Acacia catechu* in Alabama in the dietary management of knee osteoarthritis found that the placebo group had a much higher incidence of respiratory infections than the herbal group. (No mention is made in the study abstract of the herbal compound's effects on osteoarthritis.) However, another study in Arizona, in a randomized, short-term, double-blind event, found that the same mixture (code-named flavocoxid) was as effective as naproxen in controlling signs and symptoms of osteoarthritis of the knee. There was, again, a higher incidence of other effects in the nonherbal group, including more edema and musculoskeletal discomfort.

Russian studies with the root found that it increased the relative number of T lymphocytes in lung cancer patients receiving antineoplastic chemotherapy. Another Russian study with 88 lung cancer patients found that ingestion of a powdered extract of *S. baicalensis* root was accompanied by increased hemopoesis and an increase in immune markers.

There have been a number of combination therapies using *S. baicalensis* in China in the treatment of minimal brain dysfunction, bacillary dysentery, eye infections, and leptospirosis. All showed good outcomes.

Baicalin has been used effectively in treating meningitis, infectious hepatitis, hepatitis B, and acute biliary tract infections. In one study, baicalin was used in the treatment of bacterial meningitis. Sixty-two people with the condition were separated into two groups; one received an antibiotic, the other baicalin. The levels of TNF-α, NO, IL-1 in both plasma and cerebrospinal fluid were monitored. The cytokines were significantly lower in the baicalin group, and mortality was significantly reduced as well.

S. baicalensis has also been found to ameliorate irinotecan-induced gastrointestinal toxicity in cancer patients.

The tincture of *S. baicalensis* was used effectively in treating 51 cases of hypertension. Blood pressure levels dropped with accompanying symptom improvement.

Elder

Family: Caprifoliaceae or maybe Adoxaceae, the literature isn't clear.

Species used: There are five or maybe 30 species of elders. Taxonomists are not sure . . . again. They used to be in the Caprifoliaceae or honeysuckle family (the taxonomists, not the elders) but DNA scientists got involved again and decided that, no, *this* is not a honeysuckle, as anyone looking at a taxonomist can plainly see. It is an Adoxaceae. The suffix -*aceae*, by the way, indicates the members of a plant family, and the prefix *adox-* is the descriptive of that family. *Adox* comes from the ancient Greek and means "not according to right reason, absurd, opposed to common sense." The taxonomists are, however, pretty sure that the elders are in the genus *Sambucus*.

Roughly, there are two forms of elder, the red and the blue. (The red are smaller, conservative, and somewhat toxic, the blue are larger, more progressive, and people friendly.) Some people (i.e., taxonomists) say, inevitably, that there are really *only* two species of elders: *Sambucus nigra* (the blue/black berry group) and *Sambucus racemosa* (the red berry group). So, *Sambucus canadensis* is not really *Sambucus canadensis* anymore but *Sambucus nigra* ssp. *canadensis*. Because of the (reputed) higher toxicity of the *S. racemosa* group, the blue species are the ones usually used for medicine. (Though, to be clear, indigenous peoples use every species irrespective of berry color for both medicine and food. And the medicinal uses are very similar, irrespective of color. Please see the preparation section for more on this.)

And just to make it more complicated, there are two species that have white berries (red, white, *and* blue — they are a patriotic genus): *S. australasica* (okay, okay, the berries on this one *are* kind of yellow, hence the name *yellow* elderberry) and *S. gaudichaudiana*, the Australian white elder.

The most commonly used medicinal species is *Sambucus nigra*, which grows throughout North America, Europe (into the Scandinavian countries), western Asia, northern Africa, New Zealand,

Australia, many Pacific islands, and so on. It's an invasive, making it dear to my heart.

Even though the other blue-fruited species are not quite as widely established, being, I guess, less invasive, most, if not all, of them can be used as medicine: *S. australis* (southern elder, found in South America and Australasia), *S. canadensis* (American elder, found in eastern North and Central America to Panama), *S. cerulea* (blue elderberry, found in western North America), *S. ebulis* (European dwarf elder, found in central and southern Europe, northwest Africa, southwest Asia), *S. javanica* (Chinese elder, found in southeast Asia, Malaysia, the Philippines), *S. lanceolata* (Madeira elder, found on Madeira island), *S. melanocarpa* (found from the western United States into Canada), *S. mexicana* (Mexican elder, found in the Sonoran desert), *S. neomexicana* (New Mexico elder, found from the western United States up into Canada), *S. palmensis* (Canary Island elder), *S. peruviana* (Peruvian elder, found in South America), *S. simpsonii* (Florida elder, found in the southeastern United States), *S. velutina* (velvet elder, found in southwestern North America). The only blue/black berry species I know personally are *S. nigra, S. cerulea, S. mexicana,* and *S. canadensis.* I've used them all for medicine at one time or another. They seem pretty interchangeable to me.

No matter where you live, you will probably be able to find an elder someplace near that you can use as medicine. However . . . I will talk mostly about *Sambucus nigra* with a bit on the others here and there.

Synonyms: The genus and its various species are in flux due to taxonomitis and synonym accusations are flying everywhere. For sure, *S. cerulea* and *S. caerula* are probably the same plant, but then again, maybe they are really *S. mexicana,* or maybe *S. nigra,* or something.

Common names: Legion. Everyplace the plant grows, it has a local name. The plants have been used in food, medicine, and crafts since people have been. In the West, elder — reputedly from the fact that if you use the plant as medicine you will become one. Some say that the plant itself is an elder to the plant communities around it, a gateway to the depths of the plant world.

Parts Used

Most commonly the berries and flowers but the leaves, bark, and root all have a long tradition of medicinal use. You will often see warnings not to use the inner bark, leaves, or root of this plant but that is a rather recent phenomenon (since 1910 or so). Historically, they have all been used with good effect. (The secret is in the preparation.)

This particular genus, like some others such as comfrey, is suffering from a certain, unfortunately common, form of phytohysteria known as "this-plant-will-poison-you-because-someone-got-sick-from-it-once." So, *don't use herbs!* Most of us who are members of the neo-herbal renaissance have suffered its effects in one form or another. Nevertheless, I have used most parts of this plant for medicine and found them all beneficial. It just depends on what you are needing, why, how you prepare it, and the dose.

More on this next. Kind of a rant actually.

Preparation and Dosage

Most people these days are working with the berries only (a very few American herbalists use the flowers medicinally, but not normally as a primary treatment approach). Usually what is used, especially in Germany — and probably because of German approaches everyplace else — is a standardized liquid extract (or standardized lozenge) or some other variation of the berry juice: expressed juice, syrups, a tea, or a juice decoction. Dosage usually being a cup of the tea or a glass of the juice or a couple tablespoons of the syrup for influenzal infections for reducing fever. I don't agree with this limitation on the medicinal use of the plant but then I tend to be grumpy.

Rant: In reading articles about elder it is common to continually be exposed to the phytohysterical pronouncement that the plant is poisonous. Well, it is not. The various parts of the plant are emetic (and purgative if you take enough) *if used fresh*. That simply means that you will feel nauseous and possibly vomit if you take too much. The flowers are the least likely to cause any nausea or vomiting and thus are considered safe by most phytohysterians everywhere. The berries may cause some degree of vomiting and nausea if you take too much at once (see the discussion of side effects on page 152 for an amusing anecdote) or if you are especially susceptible to the compounds in the plant. But they are fairly safe in that respect, so the hysteria alert level is only Orange with the berries. The rest of the plant, however, is in the Red alert level range and from reading about it, I am pretty sure the plant could kill off most of the Western hemisphere with just a few drops of the leaf tincture.

Here is a sampling. This first one is from *HerbalGram* and runs mild on the Panic Index:

> Improperly prepared elder preparations can induce toxic effects in humans through poisonous alkaloid and cyanogenic glycosides that are found in the roots, stems, leaves, bark, and unripe berries. Effects of cyanide, also known as hydrocyanic acid (NCN [sic, this should be HCN])), on humans include nausea, vomiting and diarrhea, as well as central nervous system and respiratory depression, and general lethargy.[4]

Here's one, however, that tips the needle into the Red, and it is not uncommon: "One word of caution: don't eat raw elderberries. They are poisonous! In the raw form, they produce cyanide."[5] I can just hear the exclamation points on that last word, can't you? There's about eight of them! Then there is this one: "Elderberries must never be eaten raw. All parts of the plant contain the toxin hydrocyanic acid which is destroyed by cooking."[6] (That last bit is the important part and I will get back to it in a minute.)

The hysteria about the red berry varieties is even more pronounced because the HCN in them is in higher quantities. Nevertheless, they can be used as well . . . if you treat them just as the black berry varieties, discussed below, are. Essentially you *heat* them.

The cyanogenic compounds in elder, which are also strongly present in cherries and apples, for example, *can* poison you . . . if you take them as isolated compounds. But the "poisoning" they are talking about here merely consists of nausea, weakness, dizziness, and vomiting — the usual things that happen when you eat something that disagrees with you. The plant is *not* a poisonous plant the way hemlock is (see Socrates for more on this); it's an emetic (vomit) and in large doses a purgative (poop) and the word "poisonous" really should not be used to describe it.

The plant uses these compounds to protect itself from predators, especially vegetarians. When plant-eating animals forage too much from elder, they get dizzy and weak and if that does not stop them and they keep at it, they eventually wander away to vomit. At that point, they pretty much forget about eating altogether, which is the point. If the plant were poisonous, it would just kill the animals, but it doesn't. In fact, it likes to be foraged a bit; it helps the growth and health of the plant (and the health of the animal). However, the compounds in the plant that cause vomiting occur in just the right amounts to stop foraging when the limit of the plant's tolerance is reached. The cyanide compounds in plants such as elder are normally held separately in different parts of the plant. When the animal chews the leaves, the crushing of the leaves, bark, and so on frees the compounds and combines them, making, in the case of cherry, cyanide gas. Both this and HCN slow (or even paralyze) respiration by inhibiting an enzyme in the mitochondria of cells, cytochrome c oxidase. This is what makes the eater dizzy and a bit breathless. It is also why cherry bark is such a good herb for coughs, or why it has antitussive actions (this is basically what *antitussive* means). In essence, it paralyzes the lungs, which is how it stops hacking coughs. If understood properly, elder can also be used as a potent antitussive herb for unremitting coughs.

Raw kidney beans (and a few other beans) are also considered poisonous unless they are cooked sufficiently by briskly boiling for at least 10 minutes — after having been soaked for 5 hours. (Crock-pots that never reach high temperatures can increase the toxicity fivefold.) But you never see the same kind of phytohysteria about kidney beans as you do with elder. People are simply told to cook them sufficiently to avoid the problem. So, let's stop it all right here and begin talking about what is true for this plant.

Boiling the plant (that is, the leaves, berries, bark, or root), beginning with cold water and raising the heat, for 30 minutes will reduce the cyanide (or HCN) content to nearly nothing. (With cassava, for instance, the fresh leaves contain 68.6 mg/kg of HCN. Boiling them, beginning with cold water, for 30 minutes reduces this to 1.2 mg/kg, making them safe for use. If you start with hot water, the reduction is only to 37 mg/kg.) The longer the boil, the lower the cyanide compound content.

This is why, in the Asian traditions, they use the stems, leaves, and roots (of the *red* species no less) with impunity. To treat broken bones ½ to 1 ounce of the leaves is boiled in 3 cups of water until reduced to 1 cup, which is then consumed. And this is continued for 2 weeks. The root is used similarly for arthritic conditions. The boil time on this is long, much longer than 30 minutes. They are producing what is called a concentrated decoction.

The many chemical compounds contained in the plant are much stronger in the leaves, stems, and roots and by this I am talking about not just the HCN content but the antiviral compounds, the antibacterial compounds, the anti-inflammatory compounds, and so on. The best medicines are going to come from a much more sophisticated preparation process of the plant than any I have so far read of. To elucidate . . .

The leaves, like peach leaves, are a very reliable nervine. That is, they relax the nervous system. That is why the herb was used for epileptic fits and various dementias and uncontrollable movements by both European and American herbalists for centuries. Dosage of the fresh leaf tincture runs from 5 to 10 drops, taken no more than each hour (though some people can take much higher doses — in fact up to 1 teaspoonful every hour).

Because the fresh stem, leaf, and root can cause nausea, they also cause sweating. This helps lower fevers and is very useful during viral infections. A tincture of the stem can be used to initiate sweating if you take just enough to cause that and not enough to start vomiting. This varies for each person but in general, the dosage range is similar to that of the fresh leaf tincture. (I haven't yet worked with the root and so can't comment on it. However, the Asians use it, as a concentrated decoction, for arthritic inflammation and, given its constituents, it would be very good for that.)

The flowers are best if they are prepared as a hot infusion, covered. That is, put 1 ounce of the flowers, dried or fresh, in a quart of hot water, cover, and let sit until cool. This retains the essential oil compounds of the flowers in the liquid and they have unique antiviral qualities themselves. You can drink as much as you wish of it.

The berries are fine, but the seeds possess HCN and this is what makes some people vomit. So nearly all sources recommend cooking them first. Below is a very good recipe.

Elderberry Syrup for Colds and Flu

INGREDIENTS

1 cup dried elderberries (or 2 cups fresh)

2 quarts water

20 cups sugar (yes, yes, I know)

To make:

If you are using dried elderberries, soak them overnight in the refrigerator in the water. In the morning, put the pot on the stove and bring the contents to a boil. Once boiling, reduce the heat to a simmer, and cook until the liquid is reduced by half. (Hours). Do *not* skim the surface of the liquid; this keeps the resins in the syrup, which you want to do. When the liquid is reduced by half, remove from the heat, let cool, then strain through a wire strainer, mashing the remaining liquid out of the berries with a strong spoon. Throw the berries away, return the liquid to the pot, set it over medium heat, and add the sugar, stirring until it is completely dissolved. Let cool.

The amount of sugar in the syrup will stop it from spoiling. Bacteria cannot live in high-sugar-content solutions such as honey. If you don't want this much sugar, you can use half as much but you should add 20 percent alcohol to keep the mix from going bad.

To use:

Dosage for adults is 2–4 tablespoons every 2–4 hours during the early stages of a cold or flu infection. This is what is called a concentrated decoction and it is pretty good, if used at the first signs of infection.

If the flu gets established, use this syrup along with the influenza protocol in chapter 2 or, at the very least, the fresh ginger juice tea on page 44. If you'd prefer an elderberry-only treatment, you can add the syrup to 8 ounces of an infusion of the leaves and drink every 3 hours or so. I would also use 8 ounces of the flower infusion and 5–10 drops of the leaf tincture on the same time schedule.

If you are using the fresh juice, which many do, it will be less strong than the syrup, so you will need more. Just test it to make sure you are not easily nauseated.

It is possible, with practice, to create a mixture based on this type of formulation that would be a powerful treatment for respiratory viral infections, one much more sophisticated than just the syrup. It would be strongly antiviral, strongly anti-inflammatory, and potently analgesic. For example:

Antiviral Elder Recipe

INGREDIENTS:

1 cup dried elder leaves

$^1/_2$ cup dried elder stems

$2^1/_2$ quarts water

1 ounce elderberry syrup (see recipe at left)

1 ounce fresh elder leaf tincture

1 ounce elder stem bark tincture

To make:

Powder the dried leaves and stems as finely as possible in a blender or grinder. Place in a pot with the water and bring to a boil. Reduce the heat to a simmer and cook until the liquid is reduced by two-thirds. Remove from the heat and let cool. Press the decoction through a cloth to remove the plant matter. Add the elderberry syrup and tinctures to the liquid and stir well.

To preserve this, you may need to add sugar to the stem/leaf decoction after you press it. If so, reheat, add enough sugar to bring the sugar content up to 65 percent or so, and let cool before adding the rest of the ingredients. However, you can also refrigerate it, or add enough alcohol to bring the alcohol content up to 20 percent, in order to preserve it.

To use:

Take 2–4 tablespoons every 2–4 hours, less if you feel nauseous. Start slow and work up.

Caution

I have seen people eat handfuls of ripe elderberries or drink copious amounts of the fresh-juiced berries without nausea *and* I have seen one person eat a small handful of ripe elderberries or drink a small amount of the juice and vomit explosively. *There seems to be a wide range of sensitivity to the HCN in the plant.* And there is HCN in the fresh tinctures that has not been removed by heating. If you are going to use the antiviral elder recipe above — or any of the fresh leaf and stem tinctures — I recommend that you test your sensitivity by beginning with small doses and working up until you find your nausea level. The majority of people appear able to take the herb with impunity.

Also note that the fresh juice of the leaves, the stems, and the roots are potently emetic. If you need to vomit, for whatever reason, they can be used in small doses for this purpose.

Plants harvested near roadways and industrial sites have been found to have much higher levels of heavy metals than those in other locations. Careful where you harvest.

Side Effects and Contraindications

Sometimes . . . diarrhea, nausea, vomiting, depending on the dose, what part of the plant you are using, how it is prepared, and your individual biological response to the medicinal. There are few reports of side effects from these plants except for that.

From individual reports, *S. mexicana* berry appears to be a bit more nausea-inducing than the other varieties of blue/black berry species.

Eating Fresh Berries

Because the fruits contain potently active antioxidants, if you juice the berries in the presence of oxygen (essentially in your kitchen or herb room) many of the constituents will combine with oxygen as the cell walls are broken, reducing the potency of the compounds. Eating the berries fresh eliminates this problem.

There is one report of a group of people drinking juice pressed from "the berries, leaves, and stems" (Juice from the leaves and stems? Are these crack babies?) and 11 of them, within 15 minutes, experienced weakness, abdominal cramps, nausea, and vomiting. Eight of them were taken (by helicopter for god's sake!) to the hospital, where the physicians remarked on the dangerousness of self-medicating and the natural world in general (especially the intersection of the two). "All recovered quickly." Well, I guess so. Look, it will just make you vomit and only then if: 1) you take too much, or 2) you have an individual reaction to the plant, or 3) you take too much of the fresh or raw leaves, stem, root, or, sometimes, the uncooked berries. Once the stuff is out of your system, that's it. No more trouble.

Because the individual response to the herb varies so widely, you should start with low doses and work up. Some people can take large amounts — that is, handfuls of raw (or dry) berries all day long, or large doses of the leaf tincture, while with others, 10 ripe, raw or dried, berries will cause nearly immediate vomiting.

Herb/Drug and Herb/Herb Interactions

None have been noted but speculation abounds that elder may exert additive actions when combined with laxatives or diuretics or decongestants or various jams and jellies (producing sugar overload, just an FYI on that one). A couple of reports say that, in rats, the herb interferes with the impacts of phenobarbital and morphine, reducing their effects.

Alternatives: Poke root, *Phytolacca americana*, has a number of similarities to elder including its medicinal actions and the hysteria about being poisonous. The plant (all parts: leaves, roots, berries) contains a tremendously potent antiviral compound, pokeweed antiviral protein (PAP), that is broad-spectrum against a wide range of viruses (and other antiviral compounds as well). Used in its purified form it has inactivated the HIV virus in mice, making them HIV free. The poke plant itself could very well be a potent broad-spectrum antiviral and it should be examined in some depth for this use. As well, the root is a very strong lymph system herb, one of the few that I know of besides red root, so it also helps clear the lymph system of viral and bacterial debris and potentiates the actions of the nodes, spleen, and so on. I suspect that poke, as a medicinal plant, can be prepared identically to elder in order to use the plant as a reliable antiviral. Because the plant also has major impacts on the spleen and lymph system, that would make it a primary plant to use for viral encephalitis.

Habitat and Appearance

Most people describing elder say it is a largish shrub, occasionally a small tree. But all the elders I have known look like trees to me and pretty much to everyone I know who has seen a live one. (Well, okay, *S. canadensis* is more bush-like; it does stay pretty small. And, well, *S. neomexicana* is pretty bush-like, too, I guess.) I have seen *S. cerulea* up to 40 feet tall and sources say others in this genus can reach 50 feet. I just can't get the descriptive "small" from that. But I guess when they were young . . .

The branches of the tree/bushes have leaves that are pinnate, meaning for every leaf on one side of the stem, there is another opposite, and in spite of the fact that everyone I know calls these leaves they are really leaflets, I guess; the whole stalk that has leaves on it is a pinnate leaf, or something. Anyway, once seen never forgotten. The leaflets usually are a bit serrated along the edge. However . . . one species, black lace elder, a developed species, has leaves a bit more "lace-like." It's an ornamental, if you like that sort of thing, but not really a member of the medicinal group, historically speaking. I don't know if it is usable medicinally.

The flowers form an umbel (flattish umbrella-like cluster), often the size of an adult hand or larger. They produce black or blue or purplish or black/blue/purplish berries when ripe (except for the red/white/yellow berry species, which I am not going to go into here). In some species, the flowers are usually white (occasionally pink) and possess a marvelous smell. All the ones I use usually smell heavenly. But in some species they reputedly smell fetid. The flowers are upright on the stems in very prolific clusters. The berries, when ripe, are heavy and hang down from the weight.

The bark is very rough and corrugated when older. I've never harvested the root, so don't know what it looks like (yet). It is reported to be a potent emetic, so, if you need to vomit . . . and we all need to sometime or another . . . that's the ticket.

S. nigra grows in pretty much any kind of terrain: from floodplains to forest gaps to suburbs to industrial wasteland. The only limit seems to be highly shaded areas; it needs some sun to be happy. I have seen various *Sambucus* species growing from sea level to over 9,000 feet in altitude, in wet locations, in dry locations, in hot, rarely cold climates, in extremely cold climates (in Canada, for example), in wilderness, and in cities. It's a great invasive medicinal.

Cultivation and Collection

Richo Cech, of Horizon Herbs, my go-to guy for reliable information on growing medicinals, recommends that you take the dried berries, soak them overnight, "smash them, and remove the seeds. Sow in outdoor conditions, in pots or flats, and expect germination in the spring. . . . The best conditions for germination are cool, moist shade. . . . Elderberries will not grow properly in sterile soil. Sow seeds in very rich and composty soil medium. . . . Once germinated, the seedling grows very rapidly into a handsome bush or small tree. Grow out in a shaded place in pots for a year before transplanting to final location." The flowers appear in about 3 years and are normally pollinated by beetles and flies of various sorts with a few bees thrown in for good luck.

The flowers are collected in full bloom (June/July), the berries when ripe (August/September), and either dried out of the sun and stored in plastic or glass containers in coolish, dark locations or used fresh in tinctures, cordials, cough syrups, and so on. The leaves can be picked at any time and tinctured fresh or dried for use later, with the same storage conditions. The inner bark is treated similarly.

Properties of Elder

Actions

In my opinion this herb is a narrow-spectrum antiviral but a fairly good one in its range. (I am starting to suspect its range is much greater than any of us realize, however.) Currently, I think it the least strong of the herbs listed in this section but I suspect that is because of the failure to commonly use the leaves and bark as antivirals. The flowers and berries are most commonly used and they appear to be the weakest parts of the plant. Nevertheless, the berries do possess some good activity against, primarily, influenza viruses (and some other enveloped viruses, especially respiratory) *and* the plant is a moderate invasive and broadly available throughout the world. If you have nothing else handy for a severe respiratory infection, use it. For some people it works very well, especially if you use the herb *right at the beginning of an influenza infection*, just when that tingle in the bones begins.

As an antiviral, elder inhibits viral replication, inhibits neuraminidase, reduces hemagglutination, binds influenza viruses thus inhibiting them from infecting host cells, contains nontoxic type 2 ribosome-inactivating proteins, is directly virucidal, inhibits maturation of viruses, is a depurinating agent — with depurinating activity against both viral nucleic acids and infected host cell ribosomes — and protects against viral infection if taken prophylactically.

It is also antibacterial (directly and through anti-quorum-sensing activity), antifungal, analgesic, anti-inflammatory, antinociceptive, anticancer, antiangiogenic, antiteratogenic, diaphoretic, diuretic, prostaglandin synthesis inhibitor, antipyretic, antioxidant (the berries have more antioxidant strength than vitamins C and E), moderate immune stimulant.

Active Against

As an antiviral, elder is primarily active against enveloped viruses (see "Plant Chemistry" for more). The flowers, berries, leaves, and bark all have a range of activity against microbial pathogens; however, the berries have been the most exhaustively tested. Still, in spite of the hysteria about using the bark and leaves, they are also potently antimicrobial though more needs to be done in looking at just *what* range of microbes they are active against and *how* they are to be prepared for use. I suspect the antimicrobial actions are consistent among the different parts of the plant but no one has really explored that to any extent. However, a look at the plant chemistry reveals that all parts of the plant contain compounds specifically active against enveloped viruses; these are not just confined to the berries and flowers. And *the compounds are much stronger in the leaves, bark, and roots.* Given the historical importance of the plant and its common use as a medicinal throughout the world, there is just too little research on it. This section contains *only* those microorganisms that some part of the elder plant has been tested against:

Elderberries: influenza A (H1N1 — various strains; H5N1 — KAN-1; H3N2 — various strains), influenza B (three different strains), animal influenza (three different turkey and swine strains), HIV (four serotypes), feline immunodeficiency virus (FIV), herpes simplex viruses, tobacco mosaic virus, various mycoviruses, *Haemophilus influenzae*, *Staphylococcus aureus* (resistant and nonresistant), *Streptococcus pyogenes*, group C and G streptococci, *Branhamella catarrhalis*, *Helicobacter pylori*, *Bacillus cereus*, *Pseudomonas aeruginosa*, *E. coli*, *Salmonella poona*, *Shigella* spp., *Mycobacterium phlei*

Elder flowers: influenza A and B, *Staphylococcus aureus* (resistant and non-resistant), *Bacillus cereus*, *Salmonella poona*, *Pseudomonas aeruginosa*, *Mycobacterum phlei*

Elder leaves: tobacco mosaic virus, lymphocytic choriomeningitis virus, Columbia SK virus, *Bacillus cereus*, *Serratia marcescens*, *E. coli*, *Epidermophyton floccosum*, *Microsporum canis*, *Microsporum gypseum*, *Trichophyton mentagrophytes*, *Trichophyton rubrum*

Elder stem bark: respiratory syncytial virus, lymphocytic choriomeningitis virus, Columbia SK virus, *Candida albicans*, *Trichosporon beigelii*, *Malassezia furfur*, tobacco mosaic virus

A combination formula made from *Sambucus nigra*, *Gentiana lutea*, *Primula veris*, *Verbena officinalis*, and *Rumex* spp. (called Sinupret in Europe) was found to be broadly antiviral, showing activity against influenza A, parainfluenza, human rhinovirus B, Coxsackie virus, adenovirus C, and respiratory syncytial virus.

Use to Treat

Influenza and other respiratory infections. Most commonly this usage includes only the berries as a concentrated decoction or syrup (or, more weakly, an infusion of the flowers). However, a concentrated decoction of berries, stem bark, and leaves gives the most potent antiviral combination of all.

The leaves, root, and stem bark, decocted, for internal inflammations, broken bones, and arthritic complaints. The leaves, decocted, for liver disease and inflammation. But again, see the preparation section for more on this.

Continued on next page

Continued from previous page

The leaves and bark for topical fungal infections. All parts topically for herpes sores and skin inflammations.

The leaf tincture in small doses as a nervine relaxant, an internal anti-inflammatory, and an analgesic for pain.

The root tincture if you really, really need to vomit explosively. (Really, it's much better than ipecac.)

A number of cultures use elders (e.g., *Sambucus ebulis*) as a primary, first-use anti-inflammatory, feeling that it is especially useful when compared to pharmaceutical anti-inflammatories. A brief look at the Iranian usage range gives a good overview of the plant's capacities.

In Iran the root is particularly valued as an anti-inflammatory (the leaves as well) and is used topically to reduce swellings from bites, stings, infected wounds. There is also judicious use of the root and leaf internally as nonsteroidal anti-inflammatories for rheumatoid complaints along with the topical use. (Normally they are decocted prior to internal use; see the preparation section.) The leaves are widely used in Iranian herbal practice to reduce swellings in the liver and kidneys, as a diuretic, and as a liver protectant. The undecocted root (tincture or infusion) is commonly used, in tiny doses, as a tea for dropsy (essentially reducing leg edema through diuresis). Larger amounts are used as a purgative, to induce vomiting in case of poisoning or to realign the stomach mucous membranes (similarly to the American physiobotanical uses of lobelia in the nineteenth century).

Other Uses

The flowers as fritters or as adjuncts in wine and beer, the bark for dye, the berries for wine, beer, jellies, jams, and pies (black *and* red varieties), and the odd whistle here and there from the stems.

Finding It

Not hard. Decent tinctures that have moved outside the elder*berry* box are rare though.

Plant Chemistry

The elders contain several hundred identified compounds including fairly high levels of phosphorus, vitamins A, B_6, and C, and most if not all the amino acids. They are also heavy in polyphenols and anthocyanins. The main anthocyanins are cyanidin 3-glucoside (Cy3G), cyanidin 3-sambubioside, cyanidin 3,5-diglucoside (Cy3,5dG), and cyanidin 3-sambubioside-5-glucoside. These have a wide range of effects; cyanidin-3-glucoside, for example, is a rather potent anticancer agent. They are all highly antioxidant. Fruits of the plants contain from 360 to 1,300 mg/100 g and from 270 to 660 mg/100 g of CY3G and Cy3,5dG, respectively.

As with all plants, there are variations in chemical profiles even among different plants of the same species. Nevertheless, all elders (red and black berry types) contain very similar chemical profiles. All elders are particularly high in compounds with a wide range of antiviral activity. To elucidate further . . .

They contain a unique group of compounds called ribosome-inactivating proteins (RIPs). There are two known types of these proteins, types 1 and 2. Until recently the main ones known were type 2 RIPs such as ricin and abrin. All are extremely toxic. In contrast, those in elder are *not* toxic, putting them in a unique chemical class of their own.

S. nigra bark contains a complex grouping of type 2 RIPs such as nigrin b, basic nigrin b, SNA, SNA 1′, and SNLRP. The berries contain nigrin f and nigrin s. Leaves of the dwarf elder, *S. ebulis*, contain type 2 RIPs ebulin 1 and ebulin r1 and r2 as well as type 1 RIPs called ebulitins. The fruits contain a type 2 RIP called ebulin f. These ebulins are strongly antiviral with low toxicity and represent a novel antiviral mechanism in plants — they essentially use these compounds to protect themselves from plant viruses. As researchers have noted, "Biochemical and molecular studies have shown that the elderberry tree expresses a complex mixture of type-2 RIPs and/or lectins in virtually all tissues . . . [and] the antiviral activity of RIPs against plant viruses is well-documented."[7] But these compounds also have activity against a wider range of viruses such as HIV and influenza.

The plants are also very high in flavonoids that have been found to bind to H1N1 virions, inactivating them. Once the viruses are bound, they can't infect host cells. Elder flavonoids have a very strong affinity for influenza viruses, somewhat like a magnet and iron filings. The degree of inhibition of these flavonoids is similar to that of Tamiflu.

Specific compounds such as apigenin, beta-sitosterol, betulin, caffeic acid, chlorogenic acid, cyanin, ferulic acid, glycyrrhetic acid (present in some species), isoquercetrin, kaempferol, linoleic acid, linolenic acid, lupeol, malic acid, oleanolic acid, oleic acid, palmitic acid, quercetin, rutin, sambucine, shikimic acid, stigmasterol, tannic acid, tyrosine, undecylenic acid, and ursolic acid are also antiviral, some strongly so.

These compounds are active across a range: herpes simplex viruses, Coxsackie B1 and 3, enterovirus 71, HIV (and SIV), influenza, chikungunya virus, Epstein-Barr, hepatitis B, hepatitis C, hepatitis E, Japanese encephalitis, West Nile encephalitis, vesicular stomatitis virus, poliovirus, adenovirus-3, porcine circovirus, porcine epidemic diarrhea virus, rhinoviruses, Junin virus, cytomegalovirus, respiratory syncytial virus, tobacco mosaic virus, SARS and other coronaviruses, dengue, fowlpox, rotavirus, canine distemper virus, murine norovirus, feline calicivirus, and Ebola.

The compounds in elder are particularly active against enveloped viruses. These include the influenza viruses, herpesviruses, pox viruses (shingles/chicken pox), hepatitis B and D, the flaviviruses (West Nile, dengue, tick-borne encephalitis, yellow fever, Japanese encephalitis, and so on), coronaviruses (upper respiratory and GI tract infections and SARS), paramyxoviruses (mumps, measles, respiratory syncytial virus, parainfluenza), rhabdoviruses (vesicular stomatitis virus), bunyaviruses (hantavirus), filoviruses (Ebola, Marburg), and retroviruses (HIV). Various parts of the plant *have* been tested against some of the viruses in these groups and have been found active against them. Further, historical use in a number of cultures includes some of these disease categories. It seems as if the plant may in fact be a broad-spectrum antiviral for all enveloped viruses.

Many of these compounds act synergistically. The result is a fairly potent grouping of compounds that deeply affect influenzal and other enveloped organisms. As only one example . . .

Palmitic acid is a rather novel CD4 fusion inhibitor that blocks HIV entry and multiplication while a number of other compounds are directly virucidal against the virus and still other compounds such as astragalin stimulate immune function and response. Palmitic acid also stimulates viral clearing responses against influenza viruses. But it, at the same time, induces a long-term memory (up to several years) in the body's CD8 T cells of that response against influenza viruses *and* inhibits the production of mature viral particles while, again, numerous other compounds in elder are directly virucidal for the organisms, and others inhibit viral binding to host cells, and others stimulate specific immune responses.

The elders also contain cyanogenic glycosides such as sambunigrin and ebuloside — and these compounds are higher in leaves, stems, and roots, respectively, which is why people rather frantically say you should not use those parts of the plant for medicine. These are the compounds that raise the phytohysteria levels among those who understand medicinal plants . . . not.

The particular compounds that cause these effects have very specific medicinal actions as well and very useful ones at that. As usual the dose is the thing (eat 5 pounds of sugar and tell me how you do) *and* the preparation. Again, please see some details on this in the "Preparation and Dosage" section. There is more to this than meets the stomach lining.

Traditional Uses

This plant has been used by people as medicine since people have been on every continent on which it grows.

The genus name, *Sambucus*, comes from ancient Latin, Greek, and Aramaic roots and is the name of an ancient musical instrument, a.k.a. panpipes, made from the hollow stems of the plant. The plants used to be (or maybe still are) in the Caprifoliaceae family. *Caprifolia* itself is from the ancient Greek as well and means "goat leaf." It was the ancient name for a honeysuckle. But the meaning goes deeper than that as the ancient god of wild woods, fields, and music, Pan, possesses, in part, a goat shape. The elders were felt to be a primary plant of the god Pan. The plant was felt to cure nearly all the ills of humankind (thus allowing one to *become* an elder). That is, it is a *pan*acea.

The word *pan* is also from the ancient Greek, meaning "all, wholly, entire, altogether, by all, of all" — and yes, I have read philological treatises on the topic, so tear thy hair not oh ye reasonless reductionists.

AYURVEDA

Sambucus nigra and *S. ebulis* both exist in Ayurvedic practice but not in any depth. *S. ebulis* has a minor role, the roots used in dropsy.

S. nigra use is more extensive; the flowers, berries, roots, leaves, and stem bark are used, the flowers and leaves used fresh. The inner bark is a hydrogogue, cathartic, and antiepileptic. The flowers are diaphoretic, sudorific, and laxative. The berries increase renal function, the root is an aperient.

TRADITIONAL CHINESE MEDICINE

I don't find anything on this genus in my research library, which is extensive in some respects, though it seems as if there should be something since the plant grows in that region. But, after way too much searching of journals on the Internet, I did begin to find some information here and there. Still, it took a bit of serendipity and some cleverness to find it. Despite this, the genus doesn't seem to be considered a major medicinal in any sense of the word. The usage range is odd as well. It doesn't overlap well with the genus use in the Americas or in Europe, in spite of the fact that constituent studies find very similar compounds in the Chinese species.

Three members of the genus, all red berry species, have been used in China for millennia (they just don't seem very excited about it).

Sambucus formosana (one site lists the Chinese name as mao gu xiao) appears to be the least used member of the genus and I can find little on it. It, like *S. chinensis*, has been used to treat liver disease. One site lists this species name as a synonym of *S. chinensis*, another site as a synonym for *S. javanica*. (There are apparently taxonomists *everywhere*.)

I do find a bit more on *Sambucus chinensis* (in traditional Chinese medicine known as lu-ying, in English as Chinese elder) but it did take some searching. (At least one site lists this plant name as a synonym for *S. javanica*.) Syrups of the berries *and* the leaves are used (decoctions again). The herb is considered to be warm and bitter and is used for dispelling blood stasis and dispelling wind rolling. Lu-ying's primary uses seem to be for the treatment of hepatitis and liver injury, for inflammations, and as an analgesic. It is also used to induce sweating, as a diuretic, for bruises, rheumatism, dislocations, nephritis, edema, beriberi, and urticaria.

Assuming this species name *is* a synonym, then the use data expands a bit (but . . . the plant under the name *Sambucus javanica* is listed by a number of sources as *not* growing in China even though it is called Chinese elder — are taxonomists even human? Have they no mercy?). The whole plant would be then anodyne, antiphlogistic, depurative, diuretic, emetic, and purgative. The leaves and root are used for pain and numbness, bone diseases, and rheumatic problems. The fruit is used as a depurative and purgative. A decoction of the berries is used to treat injuries, for skin diseases, and for swellings. A decoction of the leaves is used as a diuretic and an anodyne (pain reliever).

In Indonesia *S. javanica*'s leaves are primarily used for pain relief. One-half to 1 ounce of leaves is boiled in 3 cups of water and reduced to 1 cup, and the decoction consumed for 14 days. (Note: No emetic warnings are shouted.) For beriberi 1 to 2 ounces of fresh root, stems, and leaves is treated similarly, the cooled decoction consumed for 14 days. (Again, no emetic warnings occur.) For jaundice, the roots only are used, as a concentrated decoction. (Another site lists multiple synonyms for this plant, including *Ebulis chinensis*, though, upon examination, that also seems to be the name of an Argentine mussel. So, no, taxonomists have no mercy.)

Sambucus williamsii is also listed as a species long in use in traditional Chinese medicine. On that I do find a bit more usage, over centuries, for inflammation, broken bones, and joint diseases. There are actually some good studies on the actions of the plant leaves in healing broken bones and osteoporosis (see the "Scientific Research" section). This use for broken bones and bone loss is interesting and potentially opens up a whole new range of action for this genus. *S. javanica* is also used for this; it makes sense to explore it further. The action appears specific to the leaves (concentrated decoction).

Sambucus williamsii is also considered anodyne, carminative, diaphoretic, diuretic, and emetic. The leaf is also used to treat (and alleviate, i.e., break) ague fits (essentially intermittent fevers with sharp swings into both extremely hot and cold states, i.e., fits). The flowers are diaphoretic and diuretic. The juice of the stem is used as an emetic. A decoction of the root for arthritis inflammations.

Still, there is so little on the genus compared to so many others; it doesn't appear to have a major place in traditional Chinese medicine.

WESTERN BOTANIC PRACTICE

Elders have been used in European medical practice for over 2,500 years for inflammatory conditions, for sore throats, as a purgative, as an emetic, and for wounds. The leaves were a major ingredient in salves for the treatment of wounds, bruises, and sprains. Used internally, they are expectorant, diaphoretic, and diuretic. The berries were used for rheumatism, erysipelas, colic, diarrhea, epilepsy, and dropsy.

The use of the various *Sambucus* species by the indigenous peoples of the Americas was extensive, for both red and blue berry species. *S. canadensis* bark was used as an emetic, laxative, blood purifier, for wounds to prevent infection, for skin inflammations, for jaundice, as a wash for pain, as a poultice for headaches, as a laxative for children, to treat measles, diphtheria, and mumps. The leaves were used in ointments for wounds and burns, and a leaf infusion to wash skin sores to prevent infection, as a diuretic, for dropsy, and for jaundice. The berries for rheumatism, as a wine as a tonic, and for fevers. The flowers to sweat out fevers, for colds and pulmonary troubles, and to treat colic in infants. The root as an emetic, for liver troubles, as a poultice for swollen breasts, and as a poultice for a baby's unhealed navel.

And so on and on and on.

The various species (*S. cerulea, S. mexicana, S. neomexicana, S. nigra, S. velutina*, and so on) were all used pretty similarly. In essence: for fevers and colds, as an emetic, as a purgative, for skin inflammations, for rheumatism (arthritic complaints) and sore joints, to treat wounds, as a diuretic, and for liver troubles.

The American Eclectic botanical physicians had a similar range of use.

There has been very little new exploration of this plant as a primary medicinal by contemporary American herbalists, probably due to phytohysteria contamination.

Scientific Research

There hasn't been nearly enough study on this plant. However, the pharmacokinetics of this plant, at least of the anthocyanins, are good.

Anthocyanins are a group of water-soluble pigment compounds that exist in plants, in all their tissues, but we notice them primarily in the fruits. They create the various colors of the fruits: red, purple, or blue. They are a kind of flavonoid. Closely related compounds called anthoxanthins are what are contained in the white and yellow berry species of elder. These kinds of compounds have been extensively studied as medicinals and they do have a wide range of actions: anticancer, antiaging, neuroprotective, anti-inflammatory, antioxidant, antibiotic, analgesic, and blood sugar regulating. The anthocyanins in elder are particularly potent and are the compounds in elder that have been most extensively studied.

They reach peak presence in the body within 30 to 60 minutes after ingestion. They are high in the urine and GI tract mucosa, and in the liver and bloodstream to a lesser extent. The half-life is about 2 hours. They are absorbed in the small intestine and can be found in the body (and urine) as intact glycosides, methylated forms, and glucuronidated derivatives.

There have also been some studies of the pharmacokinetics of ursolic acid, which is present in fairly high quantities in the plant. Ursolic acid has anticancer properties, is potently anti-inflammatory through its down-regulation of MMP-9 and inhibition of COX-2, stimulates anabolism (increasing muscle mass and decreasing fat accumulation), thus reducing muscle atrophy, and is cardioprotective, analgesic, antibacterial, antiviral, antidiabetic, and antioxidant. Once ingested, it is widely present in blood plasma, reaches peak concentration in 1 hour, and reaches its half-life in 4 hours.

Elder is a potent COX-2 inhibitor and inducer of quinone reductase. (*S. racemosa* inhibits ornithine decarboxylase.) It also tends to act in the body as a cytokine modulator; it increases the body's production of IL-10 if it is taken during an infection, downregulating the levels of other cytokines as necessary, but if taken early in the disease process, it inhibits viral upregulation of IL-10 and increases antiviral cytokine production and activity. One study found that ethanol leaf extracts of *S. ebulis* reduce TNF-α and its associated induction of VCAM-1 (vascular cell adhesion molecule-1). Intracellular adhesion molecule-1 (ICAM-1) levels were also reduced in that study. Elder modulates the production of interferon gamma (stimulating it if necessary, lowering it if it is too high) and hematopoietic growth factor GM-CSF by monocytes and lymphocytes. In vivo studies with mice have found that elderberry extracts enhance the immune system through increased levels of T cells, B cells, interferon, and IL-2. (There are some reports that show that Sambucol, a proprietary elderberry extract, stimulates TNF-α production. This perplexes scientists but in fact the herb tends to modulate cytokine production, raising it if necessary, lowering it if it is too high.)

Normally, when herbs or their compounds are tested by scientists in their labs, they do it in vitro (lab/test tube), in vivo (animal), or with human clinical study or trial. Unknown to most people there is a fourth category, in planta (i.e., in plants). This will, I suspect, be a growing category for research as time goes by. Most of the studies on elder and its constituents have been in vitro, and many of those findings have already been scattered throughout this monograph. Here are a few from the other categories.

IN PLANTA

Elder has been found to be directly virucidal against tobacco leaf virus, to inactivate the virus through depurination, and to be host protective if later challenged by viruses.

IN VIVO

Sambucus ebulis protects mice from the teratogenic effects of albendazole. TheraMax, a proprietary blend of green tea and elderberry (*Sambucus nigra*), is effective against seven of eight strains of influenza A and B (in vitro); when used on mice infected with mortal doses of influenza viruses, it significantly slowed the arrival of death, curtailed weight loss, and improved lung hemorrhage scores. *Sambucus ebulis* leaves were found to possess potent wound healing activity when used as an ointment on mice. *Sambucus williamsii* extracts (part of plant not stated but it was apparently the leaves or stems) exerted protective effects on ovariectomy-induced bone loss in rats. It improved trabecular bone mass and cortical bone strength, decreased urinary calcium excretion, increased serum calcium levels, increased tibial bone mineral density, and exerted beneficial effects on the microarchitecture of the trabecular bone. A methanolic extract of the stems of *Sambucus sieboldiana* (*S. racemosa* subtype) was found to possess antiosteoporotic activity. It inhibits bone resorption in ovariectomized rats.

In a particularly interesting study, mice were given Sambucol, an extract of elderberry. It caused a shift in immune response in the face of microbial challenge. In mice then infected with leishmania parasites, Sambucol delayed the onset of the disease by upregulating Th1 cytokines. However, when given to mice challenged with malarial parasites, the incidence of cerebral malaria increased substantially. In essence it exacerbated the Th1 dominant cytokine cascade during malarial infection, leading to a worsening of symptoms. The berries appear to *possibly* act as a Th1 activator, while the leaves act as a Th1/Th2 modulator. (So, don't take the berry syrup if you have malaria.)

HUMAN STUDY

Sixty patients, aged 18 to 54, suffering from influenza symptoms for 48 hours or less, were enrolled in a randomized, double-blind, placebo-controlled study of the effectiveness of elderberry syrup. Participants received 15 ml ($^1/_2$ ounce) of an elderberry syrup or placebo for 5 days. Symptoms were relieved on average 4 days earlier in the elderberry group.

Sambucol, in a placebo-controlled, double-blind study, was used to treat a group of individuals in Panama during an influenza epidemic. Those using the elderberry extract experienced a significant improvement in symptoms, including fever, in 2 days. A complete cure was recorded for most within 2 to 3 days. Serum examination showed high hemagglutination inhibition titers to influenza B.

Ginger

Ginger is a decent antiviral *only* if you are using the fresh rhizome, not the dried root. Specifically: the juice of the fresh root (though an alcohol tincture of the fresh root *will* work, it's just not as good). In Chinese medicine the dried root and the fresh root are considered different medicines with *very* different actions — because they are. The plant's constituents alter considerably with drying as many of the volatile oils are lost; other constituents morph as they dry.

Family: Zingiberaceae. There are about 1,400 members of the family, ordered in four subfamilies, five tribes, and 52 genuses, genii, or genera (whatever). The *Zingiber* genus is usually referred to as the *true* gingers and is the one most people have heard of though nearly everyone knows *only* the main culinary variety, *Z. officinale*.

Members of the *Alpinia* genus (whose members are known as the galangals — and I actually know a person with that last name) are probably the other most commonly used medicinals (and culinary additives) in the family. Some of them do have a similar range of actions. (Cardamom and turmeric are both gingers but they belong to other genera — or perhaps genuses, maybe genii.)

Species used: There are 85 or maybe 100 species of plants in the genus *Zingiber*. (Why have taxonomy anyway?) *Z. officinale*, the common food ginger, is the most famous and the one generally used for medicine. Many of the species in this family contain similar constituents and can be used medicinally. Some are similar in their antiviral actions, some are very different. This short monograph explores only the culinary ginger, *Z. officinale*.

Common names: Ginger in English and about a billion other names depending on which culture and language you are using.

Part Used

The root (yes, I know it's really a rhizome, but no one cares).

Preparation and Dosage

If you are using ginger as an antiviral, the fresh juice cannot be surpassed in its effectiveness. It takes about 30 minutes after drinking the fresh juice as a hot tea for ginger's compounds to enter the bloodstream; they reach peak concentration in about 60 minutes and then begin to decline. The fresh juice tea should be consumed every 2 to 3 hours in acute conditions or at the onset of colds or flu to keep the constituents at high levels in the blood.

FRESH GINGER JUICE TEA

Juice one or more pieces of ginger, in total about the size of a medium to large carrot, or four pieces the size of your thumb. *Save the plant matter that is left over* after juicing (for making an infusion; see below) or else squeeze it as dry as you can to extract all the juice still in it — there's a lot.

Combine ¼ cup of the fresh juice with 12 ounces hot water, 1 tablespoon wildflower honey, one-quarter of a lime (squozen), and ⅛ teaspoon cayenne. Drink 4–6 cups per day.

INFUSION

Method one: The leftover plant matter from juicing the root can be put into 1–2 cups hot water, depending on how much you have left, and allowed to steep for 4–8 hours, covered. Strain, and use the infused liquid as you would ginger juice in making fresh ginger juice tea (above). It will be almost as useful as the fresh juice but not quite.

Method two: This is the method to use if you don't have a juicer for juicing the ginger root. Grate or chop the ginger (a piece about the size of your thumb) as finely as you can. Steep in 8–12 ounces hot water for 2–3 hours, *covered* in order to preserve the essential oils in the tea. Drink 4–6 cups daily.

In acute conditions: 6 cups of the infusion per day minimum.

TOPICALLY

Ginger juice is exceptionally good (sometimes) in relieving the pain of burns and speeding up healing. Apply the fresh juice topically to the affected area with a cotton ball. It is also a good antibacterial and antifungal when applied to skin infections.

AS TINCTURE

Fresh root, 1:2 (1 part ginger to 2 parts liquid), in 95% alcohol. Dosage: 10–20 drops up to 4x daily. (I do not prefer this approach, as the fresh juice is much, much better — nevertheless it is a million . . . well, okay, a billion . . . times better than using the dried root.)

AS FOOD

In everything and anything, often.

Side Effects and Contraindications

Large doses should be avoided in pregnancy due to the plant's emmen-agogue effect, though the dried root can be used to help morning sickness in moderate doses. May aggravate gallstones, so caution is advised. Rarely: bloating, gas, heartburn, nausea — usually when using the dried, powdered root.

Herb/Drug Interactions

The root is synergistic with a number of antibiotics, especially the aminoglycosides, increasing their potency, especially against resistant organisms.

Alternatives: *Alpinia galanga*, also known as galangal, is a close relative of culinary ginger and is also used in cooking, primarily in Asia (it is common in Thai food, for example). It has a similar range of anti-viral action. Again, the fresh juice and the ethanol extract of the fresh root are the strongest antiviral forms of the medicine to use. Other edible gingers, such as *Zingiber zerumbet*, another Southeast Asian culinary ginger, are also very high in antiviral activity.

Habitat and Appearance

The exact geographical location of the original ginger plant is unknown — most likely someplace in Asia. It has been cultivated for 4,000 or more years in China and India and reached the West around 2,000 years ago. The genus name *Zingiber* is of ancient Hindu extrac-tion; it means "horn-shaped." ("They" say it's from the shape of the root, but I don't believe it; I've seen ginger roots. But perhaps it came from a double-blind study . . . that's where they blind *both* the taxono-mist's eyes and . . .) The roots form dense clumps as they grow and that is what everyone harvests.

The plant is a perennial and likes warm, humid climates from sea level up to about 5,000 feet (1,500 m) in altitude. It is rarely found wild; it's a cultivated medicinal.

The plant grows 2 to 3 feet (up to 1 m) in height and looks like sort of a shortish bamboo with a thin central stalk. *Zingiber* plants look much alike and are often confused with the alpinias, another genus in the family.

Cultivation and Collection

Again, the root of ginger is really a rhizome but nobody cares about the distinction except for phytogrammarians, so I will just call it a root as nearly all people who use language do.

Ginger is almost always cultivated from pieces of the living root, like potatoes. Simply allowing some ginger root to begin budding, then cutting it into pieces, each with a bud, and planting them is usually how it is done. Most ginger plants on Earth are rootstock clones (kind of a Stepford Wives sort of thing). It is one of the most heavily cultivated plants on Earth. *Everybody* loves it (well, almost everybody). The plant is considered a perennial but it generally depletes the soil in which it is grown so it's usually rotated every other year. Unless it is in the exact right location it won't last once the soil is depleted.

Ginger is a tropical plant. It likes sheltered locations, filtered sunlight, warmth, humidity, rich soil. It hates direct sun and so on; basically it wants to be pampered and protected from the elements. It can't take freezing.

The root cuttings should be planted in late fall or early spring. No direct sun locations. Plant the cuttings 2 to 3 inches deep (5 to 10 cm) with the bud upward.

The plants need a lot of water, so don't let the soil dry out. Mulch them thickly. They hate dry air. The leaves die back in 8 to 10 months, and that is when the roots should be harvested. The roots will last a long time before they dry out; they should be used fresh if you are using them as antivirals.

Properties of Ginger

Actions

As an antiviral, ginger inhibits the attachment of viruses to the cell, inhibits hemagglutinin, inhibits viral proteases, inhibits neuraminidase, stimulates antiviral macrophage activity, is virucidal. It is also:

Analgesic	Antifungal	Diaphoretic
Anthelmintic	Anti-inflammatory	Elastase inhibitor
Antiarthritic	Antispasmodic	Hypotensive
Antibacterial	Antitussive	Immune stimulant
Antidiarrheal	Carminative	Synergist
Antiemetic	Circulatory stimulant	

Active Against

Ginger has been used across the world for treating a large range of viral infections including colds, influenza, hepatitis, herpes, yellow fever, measles, chicken pox, and enterovirus. Note: The list that follows contains *only* those viruses (and other microbes) that it has been found effective for in medical research studies; it has been used against a wider range in historical practice.

Given the test range, ginger should be thought of as a narrow-spectrum antiviral — primarily specific for respiratory viral infections, though its range of actions makes it a very good supportive herb for most viral infections. It is active against influenza A, rhinovirus (especially 1B), human cytomegalovirus, hepatitis C, HIV-1, Epstein-Barr, HSV-1 and HSV-2 (resistant or otherwise), Newcastle virus (Ranikhet strain), vaccinia virus, tobacco mosaic virus, and poliovirus (type 3 — mildly so).

The herb has a decent range of antimicrobial actions as well, against:

Acinetobacter baumanii	*Dirofilaria immitis*	*Porphyromonas*
Angiostrongylus	*Escherichia coli*	*endodontalis*
cantonensis	*Fusarium moniliforme*	*Porphyromonas*
Anisakis simplex	*Haemonchus contortus*	*gingivalis*
Aspergillus niger	*Haemophilus*	*Prevotella intermedia*
Bacillus subtilis	*influenzae*	*Proteus vulgaris*
Campylobacter jejuni	*Helicobacter pylori*	*Pseudomonas*
Candida albicans	(cagA+ strains)	*aeruginosa*
Candida glabrata	*Klebsiella pneumoniae*	*Salmonella*
Coliform bacilli	*Listeria* spp.	*typhimurium*

Shigella dysenteriae *Staphylococcus* *Toxoplasma gondii*
Shigella flexneri *epidermidis* *Trypanosoma evansi*
Staphylococcus aureus *Streptococcus viridans*

Use to Treat

Ginger is best thought of in the following way: as a respiratory antiviral circulatory stimulant that will calm nausea, reduce diarrhea and stomach cramping, reduce fever (by stimulating sweating), reduce cold chills, reduce inflammation in bronchial passageways, thin mucus and help it move out of the system, reduce coughing (as much as codeine cough syrups), ameliorate anxiety, and provide analgesic relief equal to or better than ibuprofen. It is a synergist, increasing the actions of other herbs and boosting their effectiveness by relaxing blood vessels and increasing circulation, thus carrying the active constituents of the other herbs more efficiently throughout the body.

If used at the onset of a cold or flu, i.e., *the very day you sense it coming on*, it can cut down sick time to 3 days or less and the episode will often be mild. If used once the flu or cold is fully blown it will help ameliorate the symptoms considerably and shorten the illness. How much depends on your general immune health. If you've been burning the candle at both ends and putting off resting for too long . . . well, get some soup and settle in for some time off.

The herb can also be used in some bacterial diarrheal conditions, especially where there is cramping (cholera, dysentery, *E. coli*, etc.), for reduced circulation with coldness in the extremities, for migraine headache if accompanied by cold hands or feet, and for a sluggish constitution.

Finding It

Grocery stores everywhere.

Plant Chemistry

There are over 400 constituents in the root, including gingerols, zingiberol, zingiberene, zerumbone, shogaols, 3-dihydroshogaols, gingerdiols, mono- and diacetyl derivatives of gingerdiols, dyhydrogingerdiones, labdadiene, and so on. The volatile oils such as the gingerols are very potent but much reduced in the dried roots. They are present at levels 6 to 15 times higher in fresh roots. Many constituents convert to shogaols as the root dries. The volatile constituents are the most antiviral.

Traditional Uses

Ginger has been used every place it is grown as a medicine. *Everyone* not trapped in a technological culture uses it for healing (colds and flu, nausea, poor circulation), for food preservation, and so on. In general, the methods of preparation are the same and they entail the use of the fresh root, *not* the dried.

In Burma, fresh ginger root is boiled in water (with palm sap to sweeten it) to get a hot infusion for treating colds and flu. In Congo, ginger is crushed and mixed with mango tree sap for colds and flu. In the Philippines fresh chopped ginger is boiled with water, and sugar added, for sore throats. It is used similarly in China and India. (There is a reason it is done this way.)

Ginger has a long historical tradition in warm climates as a food additive. Like many culinary spices it possesses strong antibacterial activity against a number of food-borne pathogens — especially against three of those now plaguing commercial foods: *Shigella, E. coli,* and *Salmonella.*

Two of the best ways to take ginger as food are the pickled ginger often served along with sushi in Japanese restaurants or candied ginger root slices. Both make great snacks, can be eaten in large quantities, and are a healthy stimulant for the system.

AYURVEDA

Ginger has a very long history in Ayurveda, which calls it srangavera and about 50 other names depending on where you go. It is used for dyspepsia, flatulence, colic, vomiting, spasms of the stomach and bowels attended by fever, cold, cough, asthma, indigestion, lack of appetite, diarrhea, fever. The fresh juice (ahh!), mixed with sugar and water, is a common form of preparation.

TRADITIONAL CHINESE MEDICINE

Fresh root: sheng jiang. (The dried root is termed gan jiang — a very different medicine.) Considered pungent and warm in traditional Chinese medicine, it is used as a diaphoretic, antiemetic, mucolytic, antitussive, detoxicant, anti-inflammatory. It is considered specific to warm the lungs, for pathogenic wind-cold conditions (i.e., severe intolerance to cold), slight and for fever, headache, general ache, nasal congestion, runny nose, cough, vomiting. It is usually prepared by decoction in water or pounded and the juice added to warm water (ahh! once more). Ginger is generally combined with other herbs in traditional Chinese medicine as it is considered to be a "guide" drug that carries the other herbs where they need to go. Ginger is also considered to be specific for ameliorating the toxic effects of other drugs or herbs. Estimates are that up to half of all Chinese herbal formulas contain it.

WESTERN BOTANIC PRACTICE

Everyone in the West has used ginger in much the same ways though, historically, most of them tended to focus on its use for stomach and bowel complaints.

Scientific Research

The research on ginger has been problematic in that distinctions haven't been made (or looked for) between the actions of the fresh root and the dried root. (Common among scientists.) Nor has there been clarity about *how* the herb is prepared or what effect that might make on outcomes. (Common among scientists.) It is very rare that fresh preparations have been tested. (Ridiculous since that is the *primary* form of the medicine the world over.) Water extracts of the dried roots show very little antimicrobial activity — though they remain potently anti-inflammatory.

If you don't understand the problems inherent in the journal papers, the outcomes — which vary all over the place — are hard to understand. Sigh. Plants possess very different medicinal actions depending on when they are harvested, how they are harvested, if they are dried or fresh, how they are prepared as medicines, how often they are taken, how much is taken, and if they are taken in isolation or in combination. Scientists coming from a reductionist orientation have a hard time understanding all that; they don't understand that herbal medicine really *is* rocket surgery.

In the case of ginger, a further irritant is that there has been no clinical work on its use for viral diseases in spite of the fact that everyone on Earth uses the herb for colds and flu. (And if there were studies, they would probably have used the dried root and found it, unsurprisingly, to be useless.)

As an overview: There have been some 30 clinical trials with 2,300 people using ginger root. Following is just a sampling of a few of those and of a few in vivo and in vitro studies. There are about 1,400 journal listings at PubMed for studies on the plant.

OTHER ACTIONS

Anti-inflammatory actions. Gingerol and its related compounds are potent inhibitors of lipopolysaccharide-induced PGE2 production in vitro. They are also very strong inhibitors of NF-κB expression and TNF-α. In vivo, through such inhibition, the herb reduces the incidence of liver neoplasms in mice and blocks the development of liver cancer.

Ginger inhibits both COX-1 and COX-2 in vitro through inhibiting several genes involved in the inflammatory response (acting on cytokines, chemokines, 5-lipoxygenase, and COX-2). In a trial with 56 people (28 with rheumatoid arthritis, 18 with osteoarthritis, 10 with muscular discomfort) who took dried ginger, 75 percent reported relief from pain and swelling. In a double-blind, randomized, placebo-controlled clinical trial with 102 people with osteoarthritis, ginger was found to be as effective as ibuprofen in relieving pain and swelling. Numerous other in vivo studies have shown that ginger root has both anti-inflammatory and analgesic actions; some used the essential oil massaged into the affected area — it works really well.

Antiemetic/antinausea actions. Various clinical studies have found that ginger root is especially effective for treating severe morning sickness in pregnant women. The dried root was used, of course, and was found more effective in severe cases. (The fresh root is better for nausea.)

Antiadhesion actions. In vivo, ginger root interferes with the adhesion of enterobacterial disease organisms to the intestinal wall. This, in essence, reduces entero-infection of the GI tract, short-circuiting the disease process. Ginger is also an elastase inhibitor. Many bacteria use elastase to break down cellular tissue, helping their penetration of the body. (Ginger also reduces spasms in the intestinal tract, relaxing the intestinal wall, at the same time.)

Antidiarrheal actions. Ginger root interferes with the colonization of cells by enterogenic bacteria, thus reducing diarrhea and reducing bacterial load. The root alters bacterial and host cell metabolism through a unique-to-ginger mechanism.

Cerebroprotective actions. In vivo studies found that ginger root protects rats from brain damage and memory impairment.

Immunostimulant actions. In vivo studies with ginger root have found that it increases immune markers across the board, pre- and post-infection.

Detoxification actions. In vivo rat studies found that ginger reduced cadmium levels and toxicity in rats, acting as a heavy metal detoxifier. And ginger root in vivo reduces the effects of organophosphate insecticides.

Anthelmintic actions. Ginger was found to be effective in the treatment of endoparasites and stomach problems in ethnoveterinary practice in Pakistan, killing all red stomach worms (*Haemonchus contortus*) in test animals. It has been found active against a number of other endoparasites in other trials.

Synergist actions. Compounds from ginger have been found to be not only antibacterial but to modify bacterial resistance in *Acinetobacter baumanii* and to help potentiate the action of tetracycline. Ginger also potentiates the activity of aminoglycoside antibiotics (arbekacin, gentamicin, tobramycin, streptomycin) and other antibiotics such as bacitracin and polymyxin B against vancomycin-resistant enterococci.

Other studies have found antiulcer, antitumor, gastric antisecretory, antifungal, antispasmodic, anticonvulsant, and antiallergenic actions in the plant.

Houttuynia

Family: Saururaceae.

Species used: *Houttuynia cordata* almost always. There are two species in this genus but the most recent one, *Houttuynia emeiensis*, was only discovered in 2001. Some taxonomists consider this second species identical with *Houttuynia cordata*, the species used for millennia in the East and first identified by the West in 1783. Some insist it is different. There has been some intense name-calling as a result. (Taxonomists are like our children.) The two species are used interchangeably but the newest one grows in a very limited range and is not widely available.

There is reportedly a wide range in the taste of *Houttuynia cordata*, which a number of sources attribute to chemical variations in the species depending on where it is grown. The Chinese/Vietnamese chemotype is reported to possess a taste/smell similar to coriander; the Japanese chemotype, according to one anonymous reporter, has "a strange lemon or orange odour that is often compared with ginger." To those who hate the taste every species apparently tastes like rotten fish. To those who like it, heaven itself has become food, and, they insist, the plant never has smelled or tasted like fish.

One of the plant's closer relatives is yerba mansa (*Anemopsis californica*), which grows in similar terrain, has a very similar flower, and has a somewhat similar range of medicinal actions. Yerba mansa was once named *Houttuynia californica* in the nineteenth century, which does lead, occasionally, to some confusion.

Synonyms: *Houttuynia foetida, Polypara cochinchinensis, Polypara cordata, Gymnotheca chinensis,* and, sometimes, if one group of taxonomists wants to make the other group really mad: *Houttuynia emeiensis.*

Common names: It's pronounced "hoo-TY-nee-ah" big fella, and, yes, you may yell that loudly at square dances, hootenannies, and cattle roundups. Other names: heart-leaved houttuynia, lizard tail, Chinese lizard tail, chameleon plant (as opposed to the specific variety called 'Chameleon'), heartleaf, fishwort, fishmint, bishop's weed, doku-dami (Japan), and yu xing cao (China). The Chinese name literally means "fishy-smell herb" because, well, it smells like fish.

Parts Used

The aerial parts are used for medicine, the roots and leaves as pot herbs everywhere they grow (well, except in the United States).

Preparation and Dosage

The fresh plant is much more antibacterial/antiviral (as is the tincture) and is traditionally pounded to make juice for oral administration internally, on wounds, or as eyedrops. The remaining mashed plant can be used as a paste applied topically to wounds and bites; the decoction (allowed to cool) can be used for an external wash. The

Japanese use a tea, taken regularly, as a tonic medicine. I prefer a tincture of the fresh plant leaves.

FRESH PLANT TINCTURE

The tincture should preferably be made 1:2, that is, one part herb to two parts liquid. The liquid should be pure grain alcohol if you can get it. So, if you have 16 ounces of plant leaves, you would add 32 ounces of alcohol, let it macerate for 2 weeks, decant, and press out the liquid.

Contrariwise, you can make it 1:5 from the dried leaves. That is, one part dried leaves, five parts liquid. In this instance the liquid should be half pure grain alcohol and half water, essentially a 50 percent alcohol liquid. So, if you have 1 ounce of leaves you would use 5 ounces of liquid and then continue as above.

As for dosage:

For viral infections: $1/4$–$1/2$ teaspoon up to 6x daily, depending on how acute the condition is.

For mycoplasma and bartonella: $1/2$ teaspoon 3x daily.

The tincture can taste nasty, very fishy to some, so put it in something with a strong taste to cover it (fish soup?). Otherwise it can be hard to get it down — for some. I don't find it all that bad myself. It is not great but is only mildly fishy to my incredibly sensitive ("Hey! Are you looking at me?") taste buds.

There are a few companies selling the tincture for absurd prices, which, given that the plant is an invasive and very easy to grow, I find obscene.

DECOCTION

Traditionally the herb (sometimes the root) is used, either dried or fresh, to make a decoction. For dried, 15 to 30 grams (about $1/2$ to 1 ounce) of the dried plant is decocted (that is, briefly boiled), allowed to cool, then consumed. Fresh, 30 to 50 grams of the fresh herb is decocted similarly. Examination of the decocted herb has, however, revealed that it loses much of its antibacterial/antiviral actions upon being boiled (which is why the Chinese tend to boil it really, really briefly). If decocted intensively, the plant works well to stop diarrhea but is relatively inactive antimicrobially.

POWDERS AND CAPSULES

You can also find the powder, sometimes concentrated at 5:1, sometimes just the regular old powdered herb, from some Chinese herb companies. You can encapsulate the powder if you cannot take the taste of the tincture. I have been unable to locate any pre-encapsulated forms on the market. The herb really isn't that popular in the West at this point.

If you do encapsulate it yourself, use 00 capsules. I would begin with two capsules 3x daily and see how it goes, adjusting the dose depending on how it works for you. Contrariwise, you can work with the powder directly. I would begin with 1/2 teaspoon 3–6x daily and see how it works. (I normally only use the tincture.)

I have never been sure of how to dose the 5:1 concentrated powders that the Chinese often make; presumably you would take one-fifth the dose of the nonconcentrated form but that is just a guess.

Side Effects and Contraindications

Fishy-smelling breath (according to several former spouses). The taste can be terrible to the point of gagging (some say). Other than the nausea from the taste there are no reported side effects in the literature from oral ingestion of the plant.

It does have emmenagogue actions (though oddly enough the herb is not traditionally used for starting menstruation) so it should not be used in pregnancy. However, a few individual reports from China say it can, very rarely, cause congestion in the vagina (but I am not really sure what that means unless it is an overproduction of mucus, as in "congested" lungs or nasal passages; it certainly can't be congestion as in "traffic congestion," as in "traffic on I-80 is backed up to the State Street Parkway so take an alternate route").

The Chinese sometimes use it as an injectable and there have been some severe anaphylactic reactions to that. So . . . don't inject it.

Herb/Drug and Herb/Herb Interactions

None have been noted in the literature or in any anecdotal reports that I can find.

Habitat and Appearance

Houttuynia is a creeping perennial. The stem is a sort-of trailing viney thing that creeps along the ground and from which sub-stems sprout vertically to about 14 inches in height at most. When thickly growing, it can look a bit like a small bush. The leaves are heart-shaped, alternate, from 1 to 3 inches wide, and 1 to 3 inches long. The (original, noncultivar) plant leaves actually look quite a lot like those of the common violet. The noncultivar flowers are pretty, four-petaled, greenish-white with an upraised spike sort of like a tiny cattail (a.k.a. the terminal spike).

There are a number of cultivated varieties that have been mucked about with to give color variations. They may be mottled green and red, green and yellow, green-leaved with a rim of red, magenta and green, and orange or even mixes of all of those. There is even a nearly black-leaved variety. And of course the flowers have been altered as well, with some of the varieties sporting red blooms. These varieties have the usual ridiculous names associated with them: Chameleon, Flame, Joker's Gold, Sunshine, Variegata, and so on. They are common in gardens throughout the world.

The roots are more correctly creeping rhizomes that run just under the soil in a tangled mat something like a writhing mass of spaghetti noodles. They are sort of golden in color.

The original native range of the plant was wide, from Nepal and India through China and Indochina into Japan, and south into Vietnam, Thailand, and Java. But it's a good hitchhiker and spread, in its original form, throughout the Pacific islands, Australia, and New Zealand as ships sailed here and there over the centuries. Once it was introduced as an ornamental it went everywhere and is now common throughout Europe and North America. It has an especially strong presence in eastern Europe, the U.K., and Russia.

The plant will grow from sea level to 2,500 meters (7,500 feet) and it likes it wet, that is, if it is growing wild. Its standard terrain is ravines, streamsides, forests, wet meadows, slopes, thicket and field margins, trailsides, roadsides, and ditch banks.

It tends to prefer moist loamy soils, shallow water, and low light conditions (dappled sun/shade) either in forests or not. It is particularly fond of growing on the margins of ponds and waterways — really any type of wettish to boggy location that is coolish and shaded. It is highly tolerant of cold and is hardy to about 0°Fahrenheit (–18°C) but can tolerate dips to –30° F (–34° C). (Horizon Herbs grew it in unheated greenhouses in February in the state of Oregon just fine.) It is hardy in zones 4 through 11, essentially most of the United States. In spite of its natural preferences, the plant can tolerate full sun (though it may scorch — it really does like a bit of shade) and is drought resistant. Few animals will eat it; rabbits (reportedly) detest it (they have the second kind of taste buds — *bunny* buds).

Cultivation and Collection

Houttuynia is an invasive, which makes it of particular interest to me. Like many invasives it is potently medicinal and a decent edible, if you like the flavor. I consider it another plant that should be planted by everyone who wants healing independence and wide availability of potent medicinal plants for themselves and their families. Once it's planted you will have both food and medicine forever. Just don't let your neighbors catch you — practice the confused look you developed in high school for the time someone brings up the fact the plant is killing off the *real* American plants and that you, yes *you*, have a duty to stop it.

The plant is banned from importation in New Zealand (too late) and a number of other places (still too late). The plant is reportedly invasive in Texas, Louisiana, Alabama, Florida, North Carolina, and Pennsylvania.

Houttuynia is a hermaphrodite — another reason many Americans are uncomfortable with the plant. Thus, it can self-seed — there doesn't have to be a mommy *and* a daddy. There are some 1,000 seeds per 0.04 gram of seed weight and every plant produces a lot of seed. Any and all portions of the root will grow as well. It is just reproductively irritating no matter how you look at it.

Once established it just doesn't let go. There are numerous humorous reports on the Internet of people planting it as a ground cover and having it take over their gardens, yards, and lives. Digging it out is difficult as every piece of overlooked root, no matter how small, will, well, root and produce a new plant, something every eradofanatic discovers the next spring. From one killed plant, a thousand rise to take its place. Often the Internet stories end with the writers adding rather glumly that their houses are for sale.

Plant sex, destroying American suburbs everywhere.

Reportedly the growing condition that will produce the strongest growth is a clay, loam soil, 5.9 pH, with 78 percent moisture content. Still, houttuynia can be grown in much drier conditions than it normally likes as long as you keep it watered. It will tolerate sandy, loamy, and clay soils. It can even grow in water up to 2 inches deep. It flowers in June (usually). It grows extremely quickly.

Houttuynia is reportedly very hard to grow from seed but those who have done it say that you should sow the seeds in a greenhouse in spring, keeping the soil moist, then separate them into individual pots when they are big enough. Transplantation can occur any time after that.

The more variegated the plant, the less hardy, the less medicinal, the less invasive. Most of the variegated species will tend to relapse into the more basic unvariegated state if you let them. Gardeners are warned to pick off and dispose of any green leaves that show up to keep this from happening. I would suggest the opposite approach.

In China, the plant is traditionally harvested after flowering and then dried in the sun. It is usually used as a decoction, 15 to 30 grams of the dried plant or 30 to 50 of the fresh. It is usually not decocted for long in order to prevent the heat loss of volatile oils. The more it is heated, the worse its antimicrobial actions become. The primary reason it is heated is to get rid of the fishy smell — about 1 minute does it, so they say. However, in spite of all that, the Chinese consider the fresh plant the strongest form of the herb.

If you are making tinctures use the fresh plant picked just at flowering. If you want to dry the plant, bundle and hang it, and when it is completely dry store it in plastic bags out of the sun, preferably in plastic tubs, well sealed.

Note: Houttuynia hyperaccumulates lead and arsenic, so don't harvest it from around mines.

Finding It

If you are going to grow it for medicine, try to get the original, unmucked-about-with plant if you can, not the highly variegated varieties ('Chameleon' is the worst to use for medicine). Horizon Herbs sells the plants and they are pretty good ones — www.horizonherbs.com. You can get the seeds from suppliers here and there but the plants are reportedly hard to grow from seed; the easiest way to grow the herb is from divided rootstock. If you want a very good fresh tincture at a decent price try Woodland Essence (www.woodlandessence.com). The dried herb (in both powder and cut form) is available from 1stChineseHerbs.com (www.1stchineseherbs.com).

Properties of Houttuynia

Actions

As an antiviral, houttuynia inhibits viral replication, interferes with the function of the viral envelope, is directly virucidal, stops virion release from infected cells, prevents viral infection if taken prophylactically. It is also:

Analgesic	Antimicrobial	Febrifuge
Anthelmintic	Antioxidant	Hemostatic
Antibacterial	Antitussive	Hypoglycemic
Anticancer	Astringent	Immunomodulatory
Antifungal	Diuretic	Larvacidal
Anti-inflammatory	Depurative	Laxative
Antileukemic	Emmenagogue	Ophthalmic

Active Against

Moderately broad-spectrum antiviral. It is active against influenza virus A (H1N1 strains), SARS-related coronavirus (FFM-1, FFM-2), dengue virus serotype 2, avian infectious bronchitis virus (a coronavirus), enterovirus 71, enteric cytopathic human orphan (ECHO) virus, herpes simplex virus 1, herpes simplex virus 2, HIV-1, cytomegalovirus, porcine epidemic diarrhea virus, and pseudorabies herpesvirus. Studies have found it ineffective against polio and Coxsackie viruses.

The herb also has a good range of action against bacteria and other microbes. It is active against:

Aedes aegypti larvae	Fusarium oxysporum	Neisseria catarrhalis (a.k.a. Moraxella catarrhalis)
Aspergillus spp.	Haemophilus influenzae	
Candida albicans		Proteus vulgaris
chromomycosis fungus	Hymenolepis diminuta	Salmonella choleraesuis (a.k.a. S. enterica)
Colletotrichum capsici	Leptospira spp.	
Corynebacterium diphtheriae	Malassezia pachydermatis	Salmonella enteritidis
Cryptococcus neoformans	Microsporum ferrugineum	Sarcina ureae
Diplococcus pneumoniae (a.k.a. Streptococcus pneumoniae)	Microsporum gypseum	Shigella flexneri
	Mycobacterium tuberculosis	Shigella schmitzii (a.k.a. S. dysenteriae)
Epidermophyton rubrum	Mycoplasma hominis (30 strains)	Shigella shigae (a.k.a. S. dysenteriae)

Continued on next page

185

Continued from previous page

Shigella sonnei	Staphylococcus aureus	Tinea imbricata
Sporotrichum spp.	Streptococcus	Vibrio cholerae
Staphylococcus albus	hemolyticus	

There are a number of Internet sites insisting that the herb is active against trichophyton and gonococci but intensive searching has failed to turn up any relevant documents supporting it. Every site I can find simply repeats the same thing — all apparently from the same initial site, wherever that is. It is reported that James Schaller, M.D., found the herb effective, in vitro and in vivo, against bartonella species but I can't find any actual data on that to support it.

Use to Treat

Respiratory viral infections — especially SARS and influenza, ECHO infection, neurological enterovirus infections, neurological encephalitis infections, and dengue fever.

The herb is also excellent for mycoplasma infections, any serious infections in the lungs especially with abscesses, infections in the urinary passages and kidneys, genital infections, dysentery and any bacterial diarrheal conditions, various diseases of the eye (fresh juice or tea applied

Plant Chemistry

Houttuynoside A, various houttuynoids (A through E), houttuynin, lauryl aldehyde, caprylic aldehyde, quercetin 3-rhamnoside, quercetin 7-rhamnoside, n-capric acid, cordarine, quercitrin, isoquercitrin, decanoyl acetaldehyde, alpha-pinene, beta-pinene, linalool, camphene, myricene, limonene, caryophyllene, afzerin, hyperin, chlorogenic acid, beta-sitosterol, stearic acid, oleic acid, linoleic acid, myrcene, 2-undecanone, hyperoside, p-cymene, eucalyptol, beta-ocimene, nonanal, fenchyl alcohol, menth-2-cn-l-ol, trans-pinocarveol, verbenol, topically), skin infections with pus or boils. It is especially indicated if any of these conditions are accompanied by foul-smelling discharge.

Other Uses

As food. The young shoots and leaves are very tender (later in the year the leaves become somewhat bitter) and are a major food source in all the plant's native regions. There are varying reports on the taste and smell. Some say that the leaves have a slight orange smell and taste, others that it is reminiscent of coriander, others insist it is actually a slight fishy smell and taste, and still others report that it is more akin to rotten fish. From all accounts this is another of those plants like cilantro — you either love it or hate it. If you hate it, the taste is rank (in varying degrees of rankness depending on your level of hate). However, if you love it, it is wonderful with delicate shadings of flavor. (Taxonomists are now arguing that there are two species of taste buds, one that . . .)

The leaves, for those who like it, are used in salads or are steamed as a pot herb or even blended with rice as a main dish. The rhizomes are washed and cut in 3- to 4-inch lengths and added to stir-fry. Both are sometimes used as a main ingredient in meat and other dishes. The leaf tea (dokudami cha) is common in Japan as a medicinal drink.

camphor, beta-terpineol, pinocarvone, isoborneol, pelargol, terpinen-4-ol, myrtenal, alpha-terpineol, verbenone, trans-carveol, piperitone, isopulegol acetate, bornyl acetate, isobornyl acetate, benzyl isobutyrate, undecanal, alpha-terpinyl formate, dihydrocarvyl acetate, neryl acetate, undecyl alcohol, geranyl acetate, 4-acetamido-1-hexanol, beta-caryophyllene, beta-farnesene, lauryl alcohol, beta-chamigrene, valencene, methyl undecyl ketone, alpha-bulnesene, dodecanoic acid, nerolidol, spathulenol, caryophyllene oxide, viridiflorol, juniper camphor, methyl tridecyl ketone, phytone, heptadecanol, phytol, phytol acetate, a variety of aristolactams, piperolactam, aporphines, splendidine, lysicamine, 4,5-dioxoaporphines, norcepharadione B, noraritolodione, various amides, and so on. The herb is reportedly high in potassium, magnesium, and sodium.

A significant number of these compounds possess antiviral and/or antibacterial actions. The whole herb was found to be more effective than any of the isolated constituents, showing a profound synergism in its chemical actions. One study found *Houttuynia emeiensis* to be more potent in its antibacterial effects than *H. cordata*. (Several taxonomists were found fighting in the parking lot just afterward.)

Traditional Uses

There is a lot of indigenous and local use of the plant throughout its native range, both for food and medicine. The tribes of the Kameng district of Arunachal Pradesh (which is in northeast India) use 1½ ounces of the fresh root, boiled as a decoction until reduced by half. The dose is half a glass of the decoction twice daily for a week in the treatment of dysentery, diarrhea, and cholera.

In Nepal the fresh juice of the root is used for indigestion, topically for skin diseases, as eyedrops for eye infections. The juice of the leaf is dripped into wounds to prevent infection, to kill maggots in the wounds, and to accelerate healing.

In Thailand the herb is used to treat venereal and skin diseases and as a diuretic and urogenital antiseptic.

It is used in Japan as a tonic tea, for chronic earache, as a lotion, and as a liquor. Its name in Japanese, dokudami, literally means poison-blocking. It is considered to be an herb for detoxification of the blood to increase overall health of the body. Usually 4 to 12 grams (¹/₇ to a bit less than ¹/₂ ounce) are used to make the tea. The lotion is made by soaking the dried plant in shochu liquor (about 25 percent alcohol) for 10 days, straining it, then adding glycerin. It is then used on the skin for healing. The liquor is made by putting the dried plant in a bottle, adding shochu to about three-quarters the level of the bottle, then adding honey to top it off. After 3 months, the herb is filtered out and the liquor stored in the refrigerator. It is drunk as a tonic. Essentially this is what we herbalists in the United States would call a cordial.

The greatest depth of use has been in traditional Chinese medicine.

AYURVEDA

In spite of tribal use, I can't find much on the plant as a part of formal Ayurvedic practice. It is apparently used in combination formulas for the treatment of AIDS (as an antiviral adjuvant) throughout the country but that is about all I can find.

TRADITIONAL CHINESE MEDICINE

In traditional Chinese medicine yu xing cao is considered to be slightly cold, pungent, and specific for the lung channel. It has traditionally been used for removing toxic heat, eliminating toxins, reducing swelling, discharging pus, and relieving stagnation. It is specific for promoting drainage of pus, lung abscess with purulent expectoration, heat in the lung with cough, lung abscesses, cough with thick sputum, dyspnea, edema, carbuncles and sores, dysuria, leukorrhea, acute dysentery, and acute urinary infections. It is considered latent-heat clearing, antipyretic, detoxicant, anti-inflammatory, and diuretic. The fresh juice is used for snakebite and skin infections. Common medicinal use in China is for chronic nephritis, inflamed pelvis or cervix (pelvic inflammatory disease), gonorrhea, rheumatism, anal prolapse, hemorrhoids, inflamed respiratory tract (including pneumonia and bronchitis with or without edema), prevention of postoperative infections, inflammation and pus in the middle ear, measles, tonsillitis, chronic sinusitis, nasal polyps, inhibiting anaphylactic reactions, and various cancers.

Again, the fresh leaf is considered to be more efficacious than the dried.

WESTERN BOTANIC PRACTICE

Very little use in the West until recently. Few American herbalists use it. Most understand it not at all. It has achieved some prominence from those treating Lyme and its coinfections, usually bartonella.

Scientific Research

Most of the scientific studies have occurred in China, often with injectable forms of the herb. Numerous others have been conducted in India and Thailand. Few have occurred in the United States. (The herb tastes funny.) In general, the studies found that the effects were dose dependent, in other words, the more they gave, the better the outcome. Since the herb has shown no toxicity from oral ingestion (up to 16 grams per kilogram in mice, a huge dose), that would indicate that largish doses can be used very effectively.

In vitro studies found that the herb (water extract) significantly increases IL-2 and IL-10 cytokines. IL-10 is also known as cytokine synthesis inhibitory factor; it is an anti-inflammatory cytokine. It essentially downregulates other cytokines and blocks NF-κB activity. It is specific for counteracting the effects of mast-cell-initiated allergic reactions, which is why the herb is good for stings and bites and anaphylactic reactions. The herb also stimulates the production of CD4+ lymphocytes. It is especially active in the spleen.

Herpes simplex virus (HSV) 1 and 2 depend on NF-κB activation for replication. In vitro studies found that houttuynia suppresses HSV infection by inhibiting NF-κB activation. The herb's inhibition of NF-κB has also been found to significantly reduce chemotaxis during infection, reducing cellular migration. The herb also inhibits hydrogen peroxide impacts on cells and lipid peroxidation by 80 percent.

In vitro research found that the herb is active against 21 staph aureus strains (but is not very active in

stopping biofilm formation in that organism).

In vitro study found that while the herb is strongly active against enterovirus 71, its activity is much higher in cells pretreated with the herb than if it is administered postinfection.

In vitro the herb inhibits the production lipopolysaccharide-induced COX-2 and PGE2 in mouse macrophages. The herb reduces Th2 cytokines, specifically IL-4 and IL-5. It inhibits HMC-1 cell migration. It also inhibits DNA topoisomerase 1 activity.

Houttuynia liquid extract protected and restored white blood cell counts in mice X-rayed and administered cyclophosphamide. It normalized connective tissue growth factor and increased levels of adiponectin in streptozotocin-induced diabetes in rats.

Eight hundred mg/kg of the herb reduced the numbers of *Hymenolepis diminuta* flatworms in rats by nearly 75 percent and the egg count by nearly 60 percent. In comparison the drug praziquantel showed 87.5 and 80 percent effectiveness.

Water extracts of the herb significantly reduced NO levels in *Salmonella*-infected macrophages and extended life spans of *Salmonella*-infected mice given a lethal dose of the bacteria from 7 days (no herb) to 23 days. The effects were dose dependent.

The herb is strongly inhibitive of avian infectious bronchitis in vitro and was found to protect chicken embryos from infection by the virus and to protect 50 percent of mature chickens from infection.

The herb, as a water extract, was used to treat bleomycin-induced pulmonary fibrosis in rats. The herb significantly decreased SOD, malondialhehyde, hydroxyproline, interferon-gamma, and TNF-α. The morphological appearance of the lung was markedly improved.

A number of studies found that the herb strongly inhibited induced-oxidation events in rats. It specifically inhibited NF-κB, TNF-α, NO, COX-2, and PGE2. It also inhibited passive cutaneous anaphylaxis (PCA) in mice, inhibited IgE-mediated systemic PCA, reduced antigen-induced release IL-4 and TNF-α, inhibited degradation of IkappaBalpha. It specifically inhibited antigen-induced phosphorylation of Syk, Lyn, LAT, Gab2, and PLC gamma-2. Further downstream it also inhibited Akt and MAP kinases ERK-1, ERK-2, JNK-1, and JNK-2 but not p38.

Extracts of the herb protected rat kidneys when rats were injected with streptozotocin. TGF-ß1 and collagen type 1 levels in renal tissues decreased, and BMP-7 increased.

Water extracts of the herb showed antiobesity effects in mice by inhibiting glycerol absorption and corn-oil-induced increases in triglyceride levels. The herb inhibited oleic acid increases in blood plasma.

Cows with bovine mastitis were treated with a form of houttuynin, a compound from houttuynia. In acute mastitis 88 percent were cured and 53 percent showed microbiological clearance. In cows treated with combination penicillin/streptomycin the rates were 90 and 55 percent respectively. In subacute conditions the houttuynin results were 94 and 48 percent. In the pharmaceutical group they were 94 and 44 percent. (This finding is significant because of the degree of mycoplasmal infection in dairy herds, a major cause of bovine mastitis.)

A modified form of houttuynin both protected mice from and corrected induced membranous glomerulone-phritis in mice. It inhibited the expression of NF-κB and MCP-1.

A water extract of the herb protected rat primary cortical cells from beta-amyloid-induced neurotoxicity, specifically through modulating calcium influx and protection of mitochondria.

Researchers in Korea are interested in a class of food herbs they are calling phytobiotics, among which is houttuynia. In one study, researchers found that adding it to chicken feed instead of antibiotics found that it has similar effects on weight, disease reduction, and health as pharmaceuticals without the negative side effects, including antibiotic resistance. Lipid oxidation in the meat was significantly reduced. In another study, the mortality of chicks challenged by *Salmonella* was significantly reduced when the herb was included in their feed. PGE2 synthesis decreased, CD4+ increased, the CD4+:CD8+ ratio balanced, immune function in all chicks was enhanced.

Many of the human studies with the herb used an injectable form and found it highly effective for treating bronchopulmonary complaints including pneumonia. Oral dosing of a compound formula that included *Platycodon grandiflorum* was also effective. Both oral and injectable forms were found prophylactic for leptospira infections. Used alone or in combination with *Artemisia annua* the herb was an effective treatment for leptospirosis.

Cotton impregnated with the water extract (or oral tablets) was used in treating chronic cervicitis with lesions.

Applied once every day for 5 days (243 people participating) the cure rate was 81 percent.

Of 100 cases of chronic suppurative otitis media treated with ear drops of the distillate of the herb, 95 were cured. Thirty-one of 33 cases of atrophic rhinitis benefited from nose drops of the solution. Irrigation with the extract was effective in treating chronic maxillary sinusitis. And in other studies houttuynia (water extract) was used to irrigate nasal passages after endoscopic sinus surgery for those with chronic sinusitis and/or nasal polyps. The herbal extract was found to be more effective than two other irrigants used.

A clinical trial in China in the treatment of chronic-relapsing ulcerative colitis found that herb cured 20 of 21 and gave improvement in the other. Stool normalization, cessation of diarrhea, reduction of blood in stool, and abdominal pain disappearance all were faster in the herbal group than in those being treated with pharmaceuticals. (Again this is an important study as this kind of condition is relatively common in chronic mycoplasma infection.)

The herb's constituents move fairly rapidly into the bloodstream and maintain a high presence. The absorption half-life after oral ingestion is 3.5 hours. The herb's constituents are present in the highest amounts in the lungs, heart, liver, kidneys, and serum in that order. Elimination of constituents, metabolized or not, in the urine and feces is very low; the main route of excretion is the lungs (breath). Radioactively labeled houttuynine was found in rat tissues for up to 48 hours. The highest levels were in the bronchi (especially at 1 and 4 hours postinjection) and in descending order in the gallbladder, liver, ovaries, intestine, spleen, kidneys, and lungs. Oral dosing found the highest levels in the bronchi after 24 hours.

Isatis

Family: Brassicaceae. (This family is the home of all cruciferous vegetables such as cabbages, broccoli, and brussels sprouts and the reason why the tincture of this plant tastes kind of like spoiled broccoli/cabbage. So, if you combine it with houttuynia . . . well, let's just say you are in for a treat.)

Species used: There are somewhere between 30 and 80 species in this genus. Well-degreed taxonomists speak authoritatively, and rather insistently, of just how many species really are in this genus — few of them cite the same figures, or the same plants. As yet, I cannot find a definitive work on the genus. So, there's 30, or 48, or 79 — a bunch of plants anyway. (Taxonomist: a person who is taxing, that is, someone "not easily borne, wearing, burdensome, onerous.")

The most commonly used species is *Isatis tinctoria* (worldwide) but *Isatis indigotica* is fairly prominently used in China (as is *tinctoria*), *Isatis costa* is used in Pakistan, *Isatis cappadocica* in Iran, and still others here and there. All the species seem to contain similar chemistry; all (at least all the sources I have read say so) have been used to produce the indigo dye that the genus is known for.

Synonyms: Some taxonomic compulsivists list *Isatis indigotica* as a synonym for *tinctoria* but chemical examination of the two continually reveals significant differences (not that *that* will deter them).

Common names: Isatis, woad, dyer's woad.

Parts Used

Root and leaves.

Preparation and Dosage

Isatis has traditionally been used as a decoction in China, where the longest history of use has occurred. The use of isatis tinctures is fairly new although the Chinese and Japanese have been testing the activity of alcohol extracts for several decades. The plant is rarely used as a single tincture but is normally combined with other herbs. If you are going to use it as a single you might consider using it as a decoction as the Chinese have traditionally done. (I do not think that capsules or tablets are an effective form for the herb; there is no clinical data on them and I have not seen good effects in practice from their use.)

In traditional Chinese medicine the roots and leaves are considered to be different medicines and are used for slightly different things (see the section on traditional Chinese medicine; pages 204–205). Most people in the United States who do make tinctures are using the root; nevertheless, the leaves are exceptionally potent and are considered to be more specific for upper respiratory infections than the root — they are the most antiviral part of the plant.

I agree with a number of practitioners who have found the leaf better for acute conditions, and the root for chronic. The root seems to be better at modulating immune dynamics, increasing immune response, and moderating inflammation — just helping to tone down and even out everything while increasing immune potency. It, as well, does have a number of the potent antiviral compounds in it, so I like to include it, with the leaves, in formulations. It is also the most antibacterial part of the plant. The best tincture formulation, in my opinion, comes from a mixture of the root and leaves: one part root, two part leaves. The roots are sometimes hard to dig if you are wildcrafting them, however the aerial parts can easily be wildcrafted and both root and leaves can be bought online.

The leaves need to be dried before tincturing; do not use them fresh unless you are making dye. In addition, they need to be heated (as does the root) to better extract the polysaccharides. (The Chinese do things for thousands of years for a reason.) Also: You need soft water, that is, acidic, anywhere from a pH of 1 to 6, in order to more effectively extract the bioactive alkaloids from the plant. Most of the constituents are soluble in water, so you won't need much alcohol, mostly just enough to bring out a few alcohol-soluble constituents and to stabilize the tincture so it won't go bad when stored. Studies have found that high-alcohol-content extractions are not as effective as water extracts for treating virus infections; alcohol/water combinations are better than pure alcohol or pure water for extracting the constituents needed to treat bacterial infections.

TINCTURE

Use an herb:liquid ratio of 1:5, with the liquid being 25 percent alcohol. Use two parts leaves, one part root. (Tastes terrible.)

Take (for example) 5 ounces dried root (grind it well) and 10 ounces dried leaves (also ground well). That makes 15 ounces of herb. You will need five times that of liquid, that is, 75 ounces. Of that liquid, 25 percent (one-quarter of it) will be alcohol, the rest will be water. You will need, then, 56 ounces of water, 19 of alcohol.

Add the ground-up herbs to a cooking pot, mix in the 56 ounces of water, bring to a boil. *If you do not have soft water, or if you do not know, you will need to add 1 tablespoon of vinegar as well to help extract the alkaloids.* Cover the pot and boil for 30 minutes. Then let it cool to room temperature. You can put the covered pot in the sink with cold water to speed this up. (Don't let it tip over; just an FYI on that one.)

When the mix is cool, pour it all into a large jar with a lid, and add the 19 ounces (liquid measurement) of alcohol. Put the lid on and let it sit for 2 weeks. Shake it every once in a while.

When done, pour off the liquid, and squeeze the marc (the herbs) to extract as much liquid as you can. Then throw the pressed herbs away (in the compost or garden of course). Bottle and label. As for dosage:

As a preventive: 30 drops up to 6x daily.

In acute conditions: 1 teaspoon up to 10 times daily.

Note: Again, I would not normally use this herb as a single, but only in combination with other herbs such as lomatium or licorice.

DECOCTION

The Chinese dosage is quite high, as usual, compared to Western approaches. Root decoctions: 10–30 grams ($1/3$–1 ounce) of the root boiled for 30 minutes; 1 cup drunk 3x daily for a max of 3 weeks. Leaf decoctions: 9–15 grams; 1 cup drunk 3x daily (in acute conditions 60–120 grams).

CAPSULES OR TABLETS

Again, I am not convinced this is a useful way to take this herb; all indications from the research are that the herb is most effective if heated in water and a decoction made. Nevertheless, if you must: 200 mg 3x daily. In acute conditions: 2 grams daily. Again, the leaves are better for viral influenzas.

Side Effects and Contraindications

Leaf: Occasionally nausea, rarely vomiting. Root: Rarely allergic reactions, urticaria, cyanosis of the face, dyspnea — but these were from intramuscular injections; there is no evidence of this from oral ingestion.

However caution should be exercised in long-term use. Normally, you would not take isatis for longer than 3 weeks. This should be sufficient to deal with anything you have, especially if you have combined the herb with other antivirals. You should avoid using the herb as a single medicinal if you are presenting with a subjective feeling of cold without fever. The herb *may* induce a deep chill with overuse (longer than 3 weeks). Under some circumstances, longer use can lead to feelings of weakness, light dizziness, and an odd feeling in the bones. Stopping the herb will correct the condition within a few days. Isatis should not be used by people on dialysis or those experiencing renal failure — high doses or long-term use may negatively affect the kidneys.

Herb/Drug Interactions

Synergist with antibiotics and viral vaccines, increasing the activity of both. The herb may interfere with tests for measuring total bilirubin content.

Habitat and Appearance

Isatis is native to southeastern Russia and China but has hitchhiked widely with people and is now common throughout Europe, northern Africa, Japan, the United States, and Canada. Isatis is mainly a northern hemisphere plant. It was a major agricultural crop a great many places, planted widely for several thousand years, due to its use as an indigo dye for cloth — but it escaped. (Italy has now begun growing it again as an important agricultural crop — a source of natural, nonpolluting indigo dye.)

Isatis is invasive nearly everyplace it gets transplanted — yet another potent invasive medicinal for emerging infections. The plant is especially invasive in the western United States, up into Canada, and around the Great Lakes region. It can be found wild in California, Colorado, D.C., Idaho, Illinois, Montana, Nevada, New Jersey, New Mexico, New York, Oregon, Utah, Virginia, Washington, West Virginia, Wyoming, British Columbia, Ontario, Quebec. It is considered invasive in Canada and at least eight western states. A few isatis plants even traveled as passengers on the first Chinese space mission — one giant leap for plantkind.[8]

Like many of the potent antimicrobials that we need for resistant infections, this one is growing all around us, insisting we notice it. Nevertheless, as an invasive, it has been targeted as a plant to be terminated with extreme prejudice. Plant purists (phytoaryans) of various stripes exist in many locations and spend a great deal of their time working to eradicate isatis. They tend to exhibit phytohysteria at the simplest provocation and will speak badly of the plant if you bring it up in conversation — forgive them, for they know not what they do.

Isatis is a biennial (usually) though it can annualize if the climate forces it to or even straggle on as a perennial for a while. The plant begins as a basal rosette and looks something like a cross between the dandelion rosette and that of broccoli. It does have some small, rounded teeth on the first-year leaves that the second-year leaves don't have, but there isn't the same kind of toothiness as that belonging to dandelion leaves. The leaves in first-year rosettes are up to 7 inches in length with a cream-colored midrib. They are broadest at the tip and taper to a point at the base. I think the plant looks more broccoli-like in color and texture the second year; the stalk it sends up reminds me quite a lot of that pile of semi-edible stuff you have left after you take the broccoli heads off for cooking, or at least a well-watered plant does. (Unfortunately, to my tongue, the tincture tastes not like broccoli but a bit like spoiled cabbage or broccoli — interfering with my enjoyment in taking it . . . a lot — and I work to mask it with other herbs such as yerba santa. It helps. A little.) Isatis growing in more semiarid locations tends to get a bit woody and darker in color as it ages, the stem being, like the ripe seeds, a bit purplish/brown in color. The second-year leaves clasp the stem rather than having a slender stem (petiole) attachment.

The flowering stalk that it sends up the second year, to my eye, looks a bit like broccoli when it has gone to seed — the agriculturally grown isatis more so. The flowering stalk can be from 1 to 4 feet in height; it puts out clusters of yellow flowers that look to my eye a great deal like those of St. John's wort. They are bright yellow. It flowers in May/June and begins to set seed immediately. The flowers continue growing up compounded racemes, the seeds following closely behind, developing from the earlier flowers that have already matured. It takes about 8 weeks from the beginning of flower-stem growth to the setting of the first seeds.

If environmental conditions don't support seed production the second year, the plant can continue as a rosette for several years until they do. That plant, not surprisingly, tends to be bigger, both roots and rosette.

The seed pods (each containing one seed) are flattish and remind me of rolled oats, in spite of their green color when young. They turn a dark purplish-brown when ripe. The pods hang off the flowering stalk in their thousands, lined up like paratroopers about to exit a plane over enemy-controlled territory. Each plant can put out as many as 500 seeds a season; later generations tend to spread out from that first plant in a sort of expanding zone of conquest, extending from a common center. It doesn't take long to dominate the landscape. The seeds can remain viable for years in the soil. Once freed from the seed pod, *every* seed will germinate. (It can't be bargained with. It can't be reasoned with. And it absolutely will not stop. Ever.)

The plant loves alkaline, semiarid soils and it does very well in them. It spreads rapidly in such soils, and doesn't need disturbed soils to extend into a new locale; it crowds out normal vegetation just fine. The plant seeds produce potent chemicals that inhibit competing plants; even its own seeds won't germinate until the chemicals are leached out of the soil after the parent plant dies the second winter.

Isatis is especially invasive in ecologically disturbed areas (even if they appear sound to the eye), especially where there has been overgrazing by cattle. The rate of spread is intense, one site in Montana reporting an increase from infestation in 2 acres to over 100 in 2 years. It reduces cattle grazing capacity by about 40 percent on infested range

— part of its ecological function. Even sheep and goats don't like to eat it and that is saying something. It is intensely bitter the older it gets.

Radishes are also a member of the Brassicaceae family and the root of isatis is indeed sort of radish-like, a bit like a cross between a daikon radish and a carrot, except for the color. The first-year root tends to be a bit fuller, more plump, and the root bark (tannish-brownish with a hint of gold) a bit lighter in color. The plants send out lateral roots in the upper foot of soil to tap surface water as well as sending down a taproot to drink from deeper sources. The second-year roots go much deeper, up to 5 feet (3 feet is more common). The root bark the second year is a bit darker. When sliced the inner bark is a light cream, the core darker, the same color as the outer bark. The roots are fleshy, generally 1 to 3 inches in diameter and, unless garden-grown, hard to dig up except for the top layers. They like tough soil.

Finding It

Plant it, you won't regret it (though antiphytoimmigrants probably will if they find out). It will supply potent medicine for you and your family indefinitely as it reseeds easily once established. Or if you live in the right region you can wildcraft it; the invasive plant societies will love you for it. Seeds are available from Horizon Herbs (www.horizonherbs.com).

You can get bulk isatis root, powder, cut and sifted, or concentrated from 1stChineseHerbs.com (www.1stchineseherbs.com). They carry the leaf as well. You can also get a very nice tincture of the root from Sage Woman Herbs (www.sagewomanherbs.com).

Properties of Isatis

Actions

As a broad-spectrum antiviral, isatis is directly virucidal, inhibits viral replication, inhibits virus attachment to cells, inhibits hemagglutination, inhibits viral neuraminidase (equivalent to Tamiflu in potency), inhibits RANTES. It potentiates the effectiveness of viral vaccines and is an immune stimulant, anti-inflammatory, antipyretic, antinociceptive, antiallergenic, tyrosinase inhibitor, antioxidant, antifungal, antibacterial, antiparasitic, antileukemic, antitumor, potent urease inhibitor, potent cross-class serine protease inhibitor, butyrycholinesterase inhibitor, lipoxygenase inhibitor, antiendotoxin, dioxin antagonist (including against TCDD or 2,3,7,8-tetrachlorodibenzodioxin, the most potent).

Active Against

Isatis is a very broad antiviral herb. It is active against influenza viruses A and B (various strains of H1N1 as well as H6N2, H7N3, H9N2), SARS coronavirus, Coxsackie virus (B2, B3, B4), rubella virus, avian infectious bronchitis virus, respiratory syncytial virus, human adenovirus type 3, measles, mumps, varicella virus (chicken pox/shingles), Epstein-Barr, hepatitis B, herpes simplex virus 1, cytomegalovirus, hemorrhagic fever with renal syndrome (HFRS) virus, porcine reproductive and respiratory syndrome virus, swine pseudorabies virus, Newcastle disease virus, goose parvovirus, and porcine parvovirus.

It has some antimicrobial actions as well, against *Staphylococcus aureus, Toxoplasma gondii, Plasmodium falciparum, Leishmania* spp., *Pseudomonas aeruginosa, Trichophyton schoenleinii, Aspergillus niger, Candida albicans, Trichophyton simii, Macrophomina phaseolina, Bacillus pasteurii* (a.k.a. *Sporosarcina pasteurii*), leukemic and liver cancer cells, and possibly other cancers. Alcohol/water extracts of *Isatis microcarpa* (dried) leaves are active (in vitro) against *Bacillus subtilis, B. sphaericus, Staphylococcus aureus, Pseudomonas* spp., *E. coli, Salmonella* spp., *Aspergillus niger, A. flavus, Fusarium oxysporum, Alternaria tenuis, Microsporum fulvum.* Water extracts of the root are active against *Staphylococcus* spp., *Bacillus subtilis, E. coli, Salmonella typhi, Streptococcus* spp., and *Haemophilus influenzae.*

The isothiocyanates in the plant, especially phenethyl isothiocyanate, are potently inhibitory of *Clostridium difficile.* (Some monographs on isatis list a number of other organisms against which the herb is supposedly effective, e.g., *Neisseria* spp. The data they cite comes from Chinese texts that don't identify which plants were tested — see the section on traditional Chinese medicine.)

Use to Treat

The herb is strongly specific for influenza (all strains irrespective of source), SARS, all primary respiratory virus infections, viral pneumonia, meningitis, pseudomonas lung infections, scarlet fever, sore throat, laryngitis, tonsillitis, Epstein-Barr (especially with acute-onset sore throat), gastroenteritis, hepatitis, bacterial conjunctivitis (as eyedrops), leukemia, chicken pox, shingles — generally, any viral infection including encephalitis.

Isatis is strongly active against paramyxoviruses, which include respiratory syncytial virus, mumps, measles, and Newcastle disease. Although not tested against other members of this group (rinderpest, canine distemper, metapneumovirus, Hendra virus, Nipah virus, morbillivirus) it is being used in veterinary practice with good effect for canine distemper, rinderpest (before eradication), and Newcastle disease. It seems to be broadly active against this group. The herb is widely used in China for viral hepatitis but I have located only two tiny studies on its activity in this regard.

The herb is also widely used for encephalitis in China with apparently good results. I can find nothing testing the antiviral activity of the herb against any encephalitis viruses. However, the herb is strongly active against the rubella virus, which is a member of the Togaviridae family of viruses, which also includes a number of encephalitis viruses. There are some clinical studies of the herb being used for encephalitis B (Japanese encephalitis virus) in China with very good outcomes (see the "Scientific Research" section for more). And the herb is high in kaempferol, common in many plants, that is specifically, and strongly, active against the Japanese encephalitis virus. Its history of use in China for these viral diseases strongly supports the herb's use in these conditions. I would use it as an adjunct for *any* encephalopathy of viral origin.

Other Uses

The plant has a very long history as a dye plant for making an indigo dye for cloth. There is a very good description of how to make the dye from fresh plants at www.woad.org.uk/html/extraction.html ("How to Extract Woad Dye in 10 Easy Stages," by Teresinha Roberts, June 5, 2012), though by googling the Internet you will get a number of good sites. The same dye was sometimes used for tattooing and also body paint by the Picts and the Brittanni (Mel Gibson in that movie).

Cultivation and Collection

Isatis *loves* semiarid, alkaline, average-to-poor soils with enough water to ease its thirst but not to overhydrate it. However, if you garden-raise it and water it well, it will grow fleshy and fat and look much more like a broccoli plant than otherwise. The plant has very low nitrogen requirements. It propagates easily from seeds sown in sunny locations. Sow in fall or spring. It seeds itself readily once established. Survives to –30°F (–34° C). Doesn't like the shade; needs sun. Will grow from sea level to 7,000 feet or so (2500 m). Tolerates salty air and soil. *Isatis tinctoria* is often one of the earliest plants to emerge in spring (self-motivated, early riser).

Usually, *only* the leaves and roots are used medicinally. The stems are discarded, the flowers ignored, the seeds overlooked. The seeds are most likely highly medicinal but for some reason no one has explored their medicinal uses. (They contain a large amount of diverse fatty acids and are very high in the anticancer compounds glucobrassicin, neoglucobrassicin, and glucobrassicin-l-sulfonate. They also contain the glucosinolate precursors to the anti-inflammatory compound tryptanthrin.) The leaves and roots have somewhat different actions, so harvest and store them separately. (See the "Preparation and Dosage" section for more.)

The root should be harvested in the fall of the first year or the spring of the second. Clean and slice the roots while they are still fresh, as you would carrots. Layer them on a tray and dry out of sunlight in a warm location.

Harvest the leaves from the first-season and second-season plants prior to flowering (if possible). The plant will releaf as it is harvested. When the plant is cut or the leaves damaged, later leaves can produce up to 65 times as much glucobrassicin. The leaves contain a number of important chemical precursors when they are harvested fresh; *they need to be dried at heat* for the chemicals to convert to their final form. The most important end-product chemicals are tryptanthrin and indirubin. Tryptanthrin is a potent anti-inflammatory compound that strongly inhibits prostaglandin and leukotriene synthesis — it is also potently antiparasitic against toxoplasmal, malarial, and leishmanial parasites. It is found in much higher levels in dried leaves than in fresh. Indirubin is potently anti-inflammatory as well, although in different ways. It is strongly cytotoxic to leukemia cells and is very virucidal. Indirubin is three to five times higher in the dried leaf than in the fresh.

Traditionally, the leaves are harvested, then allowed to dry in the sun for several days, then brought inside to finish drying. The most tryptanthrin is produced when the plants are dried at around 100°F (40°C).

Bag both leaves and roots, separately, in plastic when completely dry. Store in plastic tubs out of the sun. Leaves will last several years, roots much longer. If you can't store this way, replace the leaves yearly, the roots every other year.

A Eurasion rust fungus has been imported by the phytopolice to try to kill the plants off. Check any plants you harvest and skip those with the rust fungus present. You will know it when you see it: The leaves look sick, turning brown, spotted, shriveling.

Plant Chemistry

More than 65 nonvolatile plant compounds have been identified in the leaves of isatis: alkaloids, flavonoids, fatty acids, porphyrins, lignans, carotenoids, glucosinolates, and cyclohexenones. And another 70 volatile compounds as well: aliphatic hydrocarbons, acids, alcohols, aldehydes, esters, aromatic aldehydes, ethers, furans, isothiocyanates, thiocyanates, sulfurated compounds, nitriles, terpenes, sesquiterpenes — the usual suspects. The isothiocyanates account for about 40 percent of the total volatile fraction.

Isatis also contains indican, isatin, isatisine A, indirubin, bisindigotin, kaempferol, indigotin, epigoitrin, isatinones A and B, trisindoline, salicylic acid, syringic acid, benzoic acid, gamma-linolenic acid, indolin-2-one, anthranilic acid, 3'-hydroxyepiglucoisatisin, epiglucoisatisin, various flavone C-glucosides, various sphingolipids, mannitol, various glucopyranosides, indolinone, indigo, alpha-linolenic acid, cytidine, hypoxanthine, uridine, xanthine, guanosine, L-pyroglutamic acid, sinigrin, uracil, beta-sterol, daucosterol, o-aminobenzoic acid, glucobrassicin, neoglucobrassicin, glucobrassicin-l-sulfonate, along with several hydroxycinnamic acids and, as usual, a whole bunch of other stuff. There is 20 times more of the cancer-preventing gluco-brassicin in isatis than its relative broccoli.

Traditional Uses

Isatis has been used for millennia in Asia as a medicinal and has been cultivated since neolithic times elsewhere for its use in textiles, body paints, inks, and medicine. It was widely cultivated throughout Europe until the early twentieth century when chemical dyes replaced the need for natural indigo sources. The name of Glastonbury, a town in Somerset, England, is thought to mean "place where woad grows." Many archaeological sites from the neolithic contain isatis remnants, including the French cave of l'Audoste, in Bouches du Rhône, and the Iron Age settlement of Heuneburg in Germany. Isatis seed impressions have been found on many examples of ancient pottery. Egyptian mummy wrappings were sometimes dyed with the plant. Dye shops with the remains of isatis plants have been found in ancient Viking settlements. The author of the Lindisfarne Gospels used a woad-based pigment (isatis) for his blues. Deep blue dye plants were very rare in the ancient world and the color was highly prized.

Since woad is biodegradable and renewable it is beginning to be commercially grown again to make both ink and dye (for inkjet printers and small craft dyers).

AYURVEDA

Isatis is traditionally used in Ayurvedic practice but I can find little on it. Used as a digestive tonic and for GI tract problems.

TRADITIONAL CHINESE MEDICINE

Isatis has been used for millennia in China. The leaves of the plant are referred to as daqingye, the root as banlan'gen; they are considered to be close but somewhat different medicinals with slightly different actions. However there is a problem in extrapolating from Chinese studies of the herb (a point rarely made when citing the Chinese studies). The problem is that four different plants (all from different genera) are referred to as daqingye in Chinese medicine, and two different ones as banlan'gen. While the plants are used interchangeably with each other, the problem is that the early Chinese clinical trials with the plants did not differentiate species in a number of instances. Later studies are much better.

The leaves (daqingye) are used as a bitter, cold herb, anti-inflammatory, detoxicant, for reducing fever, and for removing heat from the blood. It is considered specific for fever, colds and flu, maculae, papulae, pharyngolaryngitis, parotitis, encephalomeningitis, encephalitis B, erysipelas, carbuncle. It is considered good for headache and sore throat. The root is considered to be bitter, cold, with latent-heat-clearing properties, antipyretic, detoxicant, and anti-inflammatory, and for clearing heat from the blood. It is used for erysipelas, macular eruption due to pathogenic heat, loss of consciousness, hemoptysis, pharyngitis, mumps, conjunctivitis.

The Chinese used the leaf decoction to good effectiveness in treating the SARS outbreak there several years ago. It is now widely used for influenza and viral pneumonia, hepatitis, mumps, encephalitis, and gastroenteritis.

WESTERN BOTANIC PRACTICE

Isatis has a long history of use in Europe, at least as far back as the fifth century BCE. Hippocrates recommended the plant for treating wounds, ulcers, and hemorrhoids. Galen and Pliny recommended it as well. In the late Middle Ages it was used for snakebites, wounds, and inflammation. The American Eclectics didn't use it much, mostly as a vulnerary and styptic. It has only just recently emerged into Western awareness as a medicinal, mostly for its antiviral properties. As yet, it is still little understood by American herbalists in spite of its being an invasive in the United States, and those who do use the plant generally use it the wrong way. They use the root as the main medicinal instead of the leaf, which is more active, especially against viral infections. Most use the plant as tablets or capsules even though it is not very active in those forms — water extracts, for example, are significantly more effective in stimulating immune responses than both high-concentrate alcohol extracts and the herb in solid form.

Many American herbalists, regrettably, don't know the plant at all.

Scientific Research

There have been a number of good clinical trials in China on the use of the herb for various things; I am not going into any depth on the ones that don't make a distinction as to which plant was used. Trials where the plant (leaf) is not clearly identified were conducted with upper respiratory infections, influenza, mumps, measles, infectious hepatitis, and infectious lymphocytosis. Trials where the root is not identified occurred with chicken pox, encephalitis B, hepatitis, mumps, influenza, infectious mononucleosis, herpes simplex, herpes zoster, pityriasis rosea, verruca plana, cerebral meningitis, diphtheria, and fulminant conjunctivitis.

Given the many later studies (in vitro, in vivo, human) that show that isatis is active against many of these organisms and/or conditions, there is good reason to believe that it was isatis that was used in some or all of the studies.

Isatis tinctoria leaf was used to treat patients with encephalitis B (Japanese viral encephalitis). Headache and other symptoms were sharply reduced, and the mortality rate was decreased in both mild and serious cases — in critical patients, Western intervention was needed along with the herb in order to prevent death.

Sixty people with rubella were randomly assigned to two groups. One received a combination formula of isatis root, milkvetch root, and basket fern, while the control group received ribavirin — both for 20 days. The isatis formula and ribavirin were effective for both groups; the isatis group responded more quickly to treatment.

Twenty healthy people experienced induced contact dermatitis; they were then treated with a variety of isatis extracts as well as pure tryptanthrin. The isatis extracts were more effective than the tryptanthrin in resolving the dermatitis.

A randomized, double-blind, parallel study was conducted with 200 people suffering from bacterial conjunctivitis. Isatis root eyedrops were used (versus levofloxacin) to treat them. The drops were administered six times daily; 90 percent were cured.

Twenty patients with head or neck cancer were split into two groups in order to test isatis root for the treatment of radiation-induced mucositis. The first group received normal saline, the second gargled, then swallowed an isatis root decoction. Those receiving the decoction had significantly reduced severity of mucositis and anorexia and less swallowing difficulty. This study echoes other reports that the root decoction heals ulceration in and regenerates mucous membranes.

Purified extracts from isatis — indirubin and meisoindigo (an indirubin metabolite) — were used to successfully treat chronic myelogenous leukemia.

In vivo trials with isatis leaf in rats found that the herb was highly effective in treating chronic pseudomonas lung infection (similar in its dynamics to cystic fibrosis). The herb reduced the incidence of lung abscesses, decreased the severity of macroscopic pathology in lung tissue, and altered the inflammatory response in the lungs from an acute inflammation dominated by polymorphonuclear leukocytes to a less-intense chronic type inflammation dominated by mononuclear leukocytes.

In vivo trials with mice found that isatis enhanced the protectiveness of viral vaccines (foot and mouth disease). In other trials, extracts of isatis leaf reduced induced inflammation in mice. Both topical and oral ingestion were effective; purified tryptanthrin extracts were not effective. (Unusual extracts were tested: supercritical CO_2 and dichloromethane.) An in vivo study with mice found that dichloromethane extracts of isatis leaf were effective as an anti-inflammatory in the treatment of arthritis. And extracts of isatis leaf were found to inhibit allergen-induced airway inflammation and hyperreactivity in mice.

Isatis root extracts were found to be highly protective of mice after total-body irradiation, modulating inflammation and reducing tissue damage. And when endotoxins from Gram-negative bacteria were injected into rabbits, administration of an extract from isatis root (o-aminobenzoic acid) reduced fever and destroyed 84 percent of the endotoxins. Deaths dropped from 70 percent to 20 percent.

Isolated fatty acids (compound K) from *Isatis tinctoria* leaf prolonged survival of cardiac allografts in alloantigen-primed mice. Compound K, when combined with tacrolimus, significantly inhibited heart transplant rejection in mice.

An isolated constituent of isatis, indirubin, and an indirubin metabolite, meisoindigo, are used as a combination therapy in the treatment of myelogenous leukemia in China. They have been found to be antiproliferative and cytotoxic to cancer cells, and in clinical use they have extended survival times considerably, inducing hematologic remission.

Scores of studies have been conducted on the antiviral, antibacterial, antifungal, and cytoinhibitory actions of both the leaf and root. Crude extracts of isatis (and various isolated constituents) have been found more effective than ribavirin in their antiviral actions on Coxsackie viruses. They are as effective as Tamiflu (in vitro) in inhibiting viral neuraminidase. (Neuraminidases are enzymes that are essential for viral entry into the host cells.) Tamiflu acts as it does because it inhibits the enzyme that allows influenza viruses to enter cells to replicate.

Several compounds in the plant have been found to be potent urease inhibitors. Urease is an enzyme found in many bacteria, yeast, and fungi. A urease inhibitor is, in essence, an antimicrobial against microbes that need that enzyme to function (such as some of the mycoplasmas).

Tryptanthrin (especially), gamma-linolenic acid, and an indolin-2-one derivative are highly anti-inflammatory, inhibiting COX-2, 5-lipoxygenase (5-LOX), the expression of inducible nitric oxide synthase (iNOS), human neutrophil elastase, and the release of histamine from mast cells. Indirubin is a potent inhibitor of cyclin-dependent kinase 5 (CDK5), glycogen synthase kinase 3ß, and inflammatory reactions in delayed-type hypersensitivity.

Licorice

Licorice is an unusual medicinal. It is potently antiviral, moderately antibacterial (but fairly strong against a few bacterial species such as *Staphylococcus* and *Bacillus* spp.), moderately immune potentiating, and a very potent synergist. So, where to put it? (Throws dart.) Ahhh, the antivirals.

Licorice should also be considered a primary synergist plant. *It should rarely be used alone or in large doses for extended periods.*

Family: Leguminosae.

Species used: Primarily *Glycyrrhiza glabra*. There are 18 or 20 or 30 species in the *Glycyrrhiza* genus. (So, you're saying taxonomy is a *science*?) They are native to Europe, North Africa, Asia, Australia, North and South America. All species have been used medicinally but the two most common are *Glycyrrhiza glabra* — the European licorice — and *Glycyrrhiza uralensis* — the Chinese. (Though the Chinese primarily use *G. glabra* now, and grow it extensively, because it generally contains the most glycyrrhizin.)

The Russian licorice *G. echinata* is often used in that region and other sweet licorices such as *G. inflata* and *G. eurycarpa* are used wherever they grow. The American licorice *G. lepidota* is rarely used these days in spite of its wide native range but was frequently used as a medicinal by the indigenous peoples in the Americas. (And, yeah, they used it just the same way.)

In this section I will talk mostly about *G. glabra* as it is the most commonly used medicinal species, referring to it as "the plant" or "licorice," sometimes as "it." If I talk about another species' actions, I will usually list it by name.

Common names: Licorice in the West, gan cao in China, mulathi in India, kanzou in Japan where it is a prominent herb in Japanese kampo (traditional) medicinal practice.

Part Used

The root. The leaves have similar but much milder actions than the root.

Preparation and Dosage

Used as tincture, as tea, in capsules. Again: This herb is best used with other herbs in a combination formula.

One of the primary things to keep in mind when using licorice is that the higher the glycyrrhizin content, the more antiviral the herb will be. If using the herb as an antiviral you *should not* use deglycyrrhized licorice.

There is a lot of variety in the glycyrrhizin content of licorice roots. It varies depending on species as well. In the Japanese pharmacopoeia the glycyrrhizin content of the root has to be at least 2.5 percent, i.e., 25 mg per gram of root. In the Chinese (as well as under WHO guidelines) it has to be 4 percent, that is, 40 mg per gram of root. Unfortunately, in the United States growers don't test the glycyrrhizin (a.k.a. glycyrrhizic or glycyrrhizinic acid) content of their harvested roots. So there is no way to know how much is in there. I rarely am a fan of such testing but in this case I think it warranted for two reasons: 1) It will be easier to create proper dosages of the herb in practice and 2) it makes it easier to determine the likelihood of side effects and how to dose the additives that, if taken with the herb, will reduce or eliminate the chance of those side effects.

Glycyrrhiza uralensis generally has less glycyrrhizin than *G. glabra* though tests have shown that Mongolian varieties of *G. uralensis* run higher, from 27 to 58 mg/g though the low end is more common. I would not use *G. uralensis* for treating viruses unless that was all you had; in fact, most species roots run under 25 mg/g. *G. glabra* really is the way to go on this one.

Because the Chinese actually have to create 4 percent product by law, I would tend to buy imported roots if you really want to make sure you have at least that level of glycyrrhizin. They do sometimes import bad product into the United States but assuming that they have not in this case, if you buy from a Chinese herb supplier such as 1stChinese Herbs.com you would theoretically be getting around a 4 percent root.

To begin, the roots you use must be 3 years or older (4 years if you are using *G. uralensis*). The glycyrrhizin content of younger roots is very low compared to the older roots.

There are a number of beliefs about how the root should be prepared. Some people feel that an infusion or decoction, or even a concentrated decoction, of the root (with the later addition of 20 percent alcohol to stabilize it) produces the best extract. I am not so sure. Studies in China and Japan have found that the glycyrrhizin is best extracted in a water and alcohol blend, not in water. In fact a mix of 50 percent alcohol and 50 percent water produced the most efficient extraction in all the studies I have read. So, I am going to take a wild guess and go with that here.

TINCTURE

Use the dried root, in a 1:5 herb:liquid ratio, with the liquid being 50 percent alcohol and 50 percent water. In general, the glycyrrhizin extracts better in lower-pH water (somewhat acidic), so you might want to add a tablespoon of vinegar to your water.

Dosage: 30–60 drops up to 3x daily. In acute conditions: 1/2 teaspoon (2.5 ml) 3–6x daily, blended with other herbs, and generally for a maximum of 6 weeks at this dose and only if you take the additional supplements described under contraindications (page 212).

A company called Standard Process makes a standardized tincture, 1:1. Average dosage is 2.5 ml daily, which will give 75 mg glycyrrhizin. Dosage for acute viral infections would be 2.5–5 ml 3x daily (see the discussion of WHO, EU, Japanese guidelines below). Note: This brand is not easily found but you can find it if you google "licorice high grade 1:1." Some sources sell it by the 500 ml bottle, that is, about 16 ounces.

It will last awhile; the pricing is actually reasonable on that size. If you actually do want a reliable product as regards glycyrrhizin content, I would suggest this one.

INFUSION

Combine 1/2 to 1 teaspoon of powdered root with 8 ounces water, simmer for 15 minutes, uncovered, then strain. Drink up to 3 cups a day. In acute conditions, drink 1 cup every 2 hours.

DECOCTION

The traditional preparation in Japan (standard now in the Japanese pharmacopoeia) is as follows: 6 grams powdered root in 500 ml (about 16 ounces) water; bring to a boil, uncovered, and let boil moderately until the liquid is reduced to 250 ml. (This will be fairly mucilaginous.) Then add enough water to bring the volume up to 1,000 ml. Drink throughout the day. Tests in Japan found that this preparation will have about 50 mg/g of glycyrrhizin. (I assume here that the powdered root they used conformed to the Japanese standard of 2.5 percent glycyrrhizin.)

CAPSULES OR POWDER

Take 4,000 mg (i.e., 4 grams) daily in three divided doses. Note: 1/4 teaspoon of the powder is about 2,000 mg. *However* . . . Chinese doses run high, as they tend to do, up to 9 grams daily. Oddly, the WHO monograph lists the dosage range as 5–15 grams daily, somewhat higher. Assuming that you are getting a 4 percent glycyrrhizin content in the root, that will give you 200–600 mg of glycyrrhizin daily, which is the WHO suggested limit. The European Union standards suggest that people not consume any more than 100 mg of glycyrrhizic acid per day. In Japan glycyrrhizin intake is suggested to be kept to 200 mg per day. So, as usual, you have a range to choose from. *If* you are struggling with a severe viral infection for which this herb is specific, especially if it is severe encephalitis, there is no reason, keeping the contraindications in mind, to not use the higher WHO dose during limited treatment of 4 to 6 weeks' duration. Again, please keep in mind the side effects and contraindications.

Note: You can get licorice root standardized to either glycyrrhizin or glycyrrhic acid content if you look for it. Douglas Labs makes a 500 mg capsule standardized to contain 12 percent glycyrrhizin per capsule. This will give you 60 mg glycyrrhizin per capsule. For acute viral infections, if you are using this brand, take 1 or 2 capsules 3x daily. Note: Make *sure* you don't accidentally buy the deglycyrrhized stuff by accident; they make both kinds. It is a fairly easy brand to find online.

There are a number of different brands that have licorice root standardized for anywhere from 12 to 25 percent glycyrrhizic acid. I would take these similarly during acute viral infections, looking to get up to 600 mg daily of glycyrrhizic acid.

Side Effects and Contraindications

Generally, licorice is nontoxic, even in high doses. However, long-term use, especially if you use the herb as a single (rather than in combination), and most especially if you use large doses, can cause a number of rather serious side effects. Even the use of a tea over several years will do it and every now and then, due to the rather good range of effects the herb has, someone does. (This makes antiherb proponents *very* excited.)

Note: *This herb should rarely be used in isolation or in large doses or for long time periods* — that is, longer than 4 to 6 weeks. (However, see the comments in the next paragraph.) The side effects can be severe: edema, weak limbs (or loss of limb control entirely), spastic numbness, dizziness, headache, hypertension, hypokalemia (severe potassium depletion) — especially in the elderly. Additional problems are decreases in plasma renin and aldosterone levels, and at very large doses decreased body and thymus weight and blood cell counts. Essentially, this complex of symptoms is a condition called pseudoaldosteronism, which licorice can and indeed does cause if you take too much of it for too long. However . . .

Taking licorice along with some other supplements *can* reduce or even eliminate the tendency of the herb to produce pseudoaldosteronism. There is an intravenous form of glycyrrhizin commonly used in China that contains 40 mg aminoacetic acid (glycine), 2 mg

L-cysteine, 1.6 mg sodium sulfite, and 4 mg monoammonium glycyrrhizinate (glycyrrhizin) per 2 ml vial. Normal dosing is 40–60 ml IV
and up to 100 ml. The oral therapeutic dose is as high as 200 mg daily.
This combination eliminates pseudoaldosteronism as a side effect.
You can add both glycine and L-cysteine to your protocol to limit
the potential for pseudoaldosteronism if you are taking large doses
of licorice for extended periods. (Glycine, minimum 2,000 mg daily;
L-cysteine, minimum 500 mg daily.) The addition of potassium (5,000
mg daily) will also help prevent the hypokalemia. Again: Licorice
should be taken in combination with other herbs — this reduces the
tendency for side effects by itself. And, if you do need to take largish
doses of licorice, even with other herbs, for severe viral infections,
please add these supplements to your regimen and carefully monitor
for side effects.

Because of licorice's strong estrogenic activity it will also cause
breast growth in men, especially when combined with other estrogenic herbs. Luckily all these conditions tend to abate within 2 to 4
weeks after licorice intake ceases. Caution should be used, however, in
length and strength of dosages.

A number of studies have found that large doses of licorice taken
long term during pregnancy have detrimental effects on the unborn
children. Low doses are apparently safe. Again, this plant should not
be used in large doses or for lengthy periods of time *especially if you
are pregnant.*

The herb is contraindicated in hypertension, hypokalemia, pregnancy, hypernatremia, and low testosterone levels. However, for short-
term use in those conditions (10 days or less), in low doses combined
with other herbs, it is very safe.

Herb/Drug Interactions

The plant is highly synergistic. It is also additive. It should not be used
along with estrogenic pharmaceuticals, hypertensive drugs, cardiac
glycosides, diuretics such as thiazides, loop diuretics, spironolactone,
amiloride, corticosteroids, hydrocortisone.

Alternatives: *Taverniera cuneifolia,* endemic to northeastern Africa and southwestern Asia, has a very similar chemical profile, also contains a large amount of glycyrrhizin, and can be used similarly to commercial licorice.

Habitat and Appearance

The *Glycyrrhiza* genus is a member of the pea family with the usual pea-type leaves — a bunch of oval leaflets running along a central stem. The plants are perennials, can grow to 6 feet (2 m) in height, and bush out to 3 feet (1 m). The plants produce spikes of the usual pea-family flowers during the summer. They range in color from yellowish to blue to purple in the various species. The plant sends out both roots and rhizomes, the roots thick and fleshy, up to 4 inches in diameter, going as deep as 3 feet (1 m). The creeping rhizomes spread out from the pri-mary root, up to 26 feet (8 m) in length, often sending up shoots of new plants far from the original. The roots and rhizomes of the cultivated species are light in color, the wild species darker. The inside of most of the species is yellowish, and, in the commercial species at least, quite sweet. The native American species is not very sweet, though a lot of sources say it is (I first tasted it in 1987, still waiting for that sweet taste to emerge on my tongue). The American species, though low in sweet-ness, possesses many of the same medicinal actions, according to most sources, as the more prominent medicinal species. (Though, since glyc-yrrhizin is considered to be the primary active constituent *and* is the source of the sweet taste in licorice, I am confused by that assertion.) I've not encountered any of the other, less common species in practice.

The licorice flowers mature into clusters of spiky brown seed cap-sules about the size of a grape (at least in the American species — the only one I have seen).

The genus ranges from semiarid desert to lush, wet climes such as Yorkshire, England, and from sea level to 8,500 or so feet (2,500 m) in altitude. When wild, the plants often like growing along waterways in sandyish soil. The American species is endemic throughout Canada and most of the United States excluding the Southeast. *G. glabra* is cultivated in many places in the Americas but has escaped and can be found here and there in California, Nevada, and Utah. I can't find a record of any wild species in mid- to southern Africa (though it is most likely grown there) but the genus seems to have spread pretty much everywhere else. If you look around you will probably find a licorice native in your ecorange someplace.

Cultivation and Collection

The plants grow fairly easily from root cuttings; the seeds are more demanding. The seeds need to be stratified for several weeks, then scarified and soaked for 2 hours in warm water before sowing if you want an easy germination. Treated seeds will germinate at about an 80 percent rate, untreated at around 20 percent. Once started, the plants are pretty intent on remaining and spreading wherever they want to. Make sure you want it where you plant it — you won't be able to get rid of it if you change your mind. A few places here and there consider it an invasive because, well, it is.

Both the European and Chinese varieties warrant planting in the wild and letting them go; they are well able to look after themselves if released from captivity. As they are a major medicinal, the more they spread, the better off we will be.

The plants like a free-draining friable soil with a pH between 6 and 7 but they can take on a greater range than that and do quite well. They are drought tolerant and like the sun but do need a bit of water; they often grow wild along streambeds, where they are very tenacious.

It takes a few years for the plants to establish themselves (3 years is a good minimum period of time; earlier than that and the glycyrrhizin content in the roots is too low) but once they do, you will be able to harvest from them pretty much forever. You will rarely, if ever, be able to dig the entire root system of an established plant, so it will continue to grow and spread from what is left. Commercial growers generally achieve somewhere between 15 and 50 tons per hectare (2.5 acres) of roots once the plants have matured. The older the plants and the deeper the dig, the bigger the yield. The plants produce a lot of root mass. You can get enough medicine for an entire family from just one established plant, pretty much forever.

If you are growing *Glycyrrhiza glabra* harvest the roots after 3 years. The glycyrrhizin content is highest in August/September. The larger the roots, the higher the content. (The greatest concentration of glycyrrhizin in this species' roots, when it was grown hydroponically, was produced by the use of a quarter unit of Hoagland solution.)

If you are growing *Glycyrrhiza uralensis* (the other major species used as medicine), harvest the roots of 4-year-old plants and older in mid-July, which is when the glycyrrhizin content is highest for this species. The glycyrrhizin content begins to fall in early August, becoming very low by November. It begins to rise again in March, reaching its peak between late June and mid-July.

Once you've harvested them, dry the roots out of the sun. The larger roots should be cut into smaller sections before being dried. The larger the root diameter, the higher the glycyrrhizin content.

In general, studies have found that wild plants are higher in glycyrrhizin than domesticated plants. *Glycyrrhiza uralensis* tends to have much less glycyrrhizin than *G. glabra*. Normally it runs 1 to 4 mg/g but some studies have shown it to be as low as 0.52 percent by weight of the root.

Finding It

You can buy very good-quality organic licorice root from Pacific Botanicals (www.pacificbotanicals.com), my preferred source for high-quality grown herbs. Regrettably there is no way to determine the glycyrrhizin content of their product. (I still like it though; it *feels* good.) 1stChineseHerbs.com (www.1stchineseherbs.com) has the Chinese-grown *G. glabra*, which, while not organic, is definitely supposed to be at least 4 percent glycyrrhizin by weight. Seeds can be had from Horizon Herbs in Oregon (www.horizonherbs.com) or from Richters (www.richters.com), an international seed merchant.

Note: Some of the licorice in commerce comes from eastern Europe (which possesses some of the highest levels of soil and air pollution in the world). It makes no sense to buy potentially contaminated herbs to use for their broad-spectrum immune and liver actions.

Properties of Licorice

Actions

As a major broad-spectrum antiviral, licorice prevents viral replication across a wide range of viruses and inhibits viral growth, viral uptake, neuraminidase in numerous influenza strains, virion-associated RNA-dependent DNA polymerase, casein-kinase-II-mediated activation of HIV-1 enzymes (including HIV-1 protease and reverse transcriptase), viral antigen expression of human cytomegalovirus, and protein-kinase-A- and casein-kinase-II-mediated phosphorylation of the ICP27 regulatory protein of HSV-1. It inactivates virus particles, strongly inhibits viral cytokine cascades, stops the ballooning degeneration of fused cells, modifies the intracellular transport and suppresses sialylation of hepatitis B virus surface antigen, inhibits RANTES secretion, lowers lipid bilayer membrane fluidity, thus stopping the virus-induced development of membrane pores through which the viruses can enter host cells. It is strongly virustatic, somewhat virucidal.

The herb has other actions as well:

Adrenal cortex stimulant
Adrenal tonic
Analgesic
Antibacterial
Anticancer/tumor inhibitor
Antihemolytic
Antihyperglycemic
Anti-inflammatory
Antioxidative
Antispasmodic
Antistressor

Antitussive
Antiulcer
Cardioprotective
Demulcent
Estrogenic
Expectorant
Gastric secretion inhibitor
Hepatoprotective
Immunomodulant
Immunostimulant
Laxative (gentle)
Mucoprotective

Prevents biofilm formation
Protects from effects of radiation exposure
Smooth muscle relaxant
Stimulates pancreatic secretions
Synergist (potent)
Thymus stimulant
Tyrosinase inhibitor
Xanthine oxidase inhibitor

As an immunostimulant, it stimulates interferon production, enhances antibody formation, stimulates phagocytosis. As an immunomodulant, it will reduce interferon-gamma levels if they are high and upregulate them if they are low.

Licorice is a fairly potent synergist. It has been found to potentiate the action of antituberculosis drugs, increasing positive outcomes in treatment. It potentiates the action of oseltamivir against resistant influenza

Continued on next page

Continued from previous page

strains. It reduces toxicity and potentiates other medications in the treatment of rheumatoid arthritis. Licorice potentiates the effect of the neuromuscular blocking agent paeoniflorin, enhances the solubility of compounds from other plants (during tincturing) by a factor of up to 570 (e.g., the sapogenin isoliquiritigenin and the saikosaponins from ginseng), and increases the immune-stimulating action of other herbs such as *Echinacea purpurea* significantly.

It takes 4 to 8 hours (depending on what and how it is taken) for the glycyrrhizin to reach maximum serum concentration after oral ingestion; then it is slowly excreted and eventually eliminated entirely about 72 hours after ingestion. (Most of it is gone after 24 hours.) It stays in the body a long time.

Active Against

Licorice is broadly antiviral. It is active against a wide range of viruses through multiple mechanisms. It strongly inhibits the ability of many viruses to create the membrane pores through which the viruses then enter cells. This slows or even ends the viral infection right there. For other viruses, it is directly virucidal, and for others it stimulates the host immune system specifically to attack the invading virus. Licorice, and its constituent glycyrrhizin, are especially effective against enveloped viruses, and this covers a wide range: herpesviruses, poxviruses, hepadnaviruses, flaviviruses, togaviruses, coronaviruses, hepatitis D, orthomyxoviruses, paramyxoviruses, rhabdoviruses, bunyaviruses, filoviruses, and retroviruses. It is not active against all viruses in these groups but it is against many of them. Chinese skullcap and licorice in combination should be considered the main antivirals to use for any viral infection.

The viruses that licorice has been found effective for, irrespective of mechanism, are influenza A (various strains, H1N1, H2N2, H5N1, H9N2, novel H1N1, oseltamivir-resistant novel H1N1, and so on), SARS-related coronavirus (FFM-1, FFM-2 — multiple isolates), respiratory syncytial virus, parainfluenza virus 3, Japanese encephalitis virus (multiple strains), tick-borne encephalitis, West Nile encephalitis, yellow fever, dengue, viral pneumonia, avian infectious bronchitis virus, enterovirus 71, rotavirus, adenovirus type 3, Coxsackie B3, Newcastle disease virus, vaccinia virus, vesicular stomatitis virus, HIV-1, cytomegalovirus, herpes simplex 1 and 2, hepatitis (A, B, C, E, and most likely D), varicella zoster, Epstein-Barr, poliovirus (wild and vaccine types 1, 2, 3), measles, Chandipura virus, pseudorabies virus, vovine immunodeficiency virus, murine retrovirus, and porcine reproductive and respiratory syndrome virus.

Glycyrrhizin has been found to inhibit cellular infection by 11 different flaviviruses, including some of the most damaging: dengue, Japanese encephalitis, tick-borne encephalitis, and yellow fever.

The herb does have a good range of other antimicrobial actions as well, against:

Arthrinium sacchari
Bacillus coagulans
Bacillus megaterium
Bacillus stearothermophilus
Bacillus subtilis
Candida albicans
Chaetomium funicola
Clostridium sporogenes
Enterococcus faecalis
Enterococcus faecium
Enterotoxigenic *E. coli*

Haemophilus influenzae
Helicobacter pylori
Klebsiella pneumoniae
Mycobacterium tuberculosis
Plasmodium spp.
Salmonella paratyphi
Salmonella typhi
Salmonella typhimurium
Sarcina lutea
Shigella boydii

Shigella dysenteriae
Staphylococcus aureus
Streptococcus lactis
Streptococcus mutans
Streptococcus sobrinus
Toxocara canis
Trichophyton mentagrophytes
Trichophyton rubrum
Vibrio cholerae
Vibrio mimicus
Vibrio parahaemolyticus

Use to Treat

Influenza (all types), respiratory viral infections, pneumonia (viral or otherwise), meningoencephalitis, SARS, any viral encephalitis, and as an adjunct in all antiviral herbal combinations. It is a synergist with other herbal medicines, increasing their potency, adds immune-boosting activity, and has numerous other supportive actions specific for many different types of viral infections.

Use licorice also to treat oral bacterial problems, for gums and mucous membranes, as an adjunct for bacterial infections, especially of the GI tract and respiratory tract, especially if there is cramping or ulceration.

Note: Licorice should be used in combination rather than alone. (See the discussion of contraindications and side effects.) I would not recommend this plant be used as a single medicinal.

Other Uses

As a sweetener. *Glycyrrhiza glabra* is also a potent plant remediator for reclaiming saline-heavy soils.

Plant Chemistry

There are hundreds of compounds in licorice, many of which have been intensively studied. These include triterpenoids, polyphenols, polysaccharides, essential oils, flavonoids, saponins, and so on. The primary constituent that everyone talks about is glycyrrhizin, which, supposedly — if you believe stuff on the Internet — can make up to 24 percent of the root by weight. I have not been able to verify this, even after looking at several hundred studies. The WHO (World Health Organization) monograph on the plant indicates that the root ranges only from 2 to 9 percent glycyrrhizin and I tend to believe it. (One of my Chinese materia medica references puts the high number at 14 percent.) The largest concentration I can find in any journal papers from China or Japan on direct study of plants in the field is 6 percent. That was in Uzbekistan, where it ran from 4 to 6 percent by weight in the root. Plants in Spain have run from 0.4 percent to 4.4 percent; in Italy 1.6 to 3 percent. In one paper, for their research, the authors bought licorice root that contained 7.64 percent glycyrrhizin from a supplier in Italy. That is the highest value I have seen that could be verified (so far).

In Japan, the root must have at least 2.5 percent, in China 4 percent, to be considered strong enough for medicine. If 24 percent were at all common, if that figure were even real, it seems that those cultures would be looking at higher figures for their traditional practice, considering that they both consider glycyrrhizin to be the active ingredient in the plant and both use the purified extract medicinally. So, no, not 24 percent. I think the WHO monograph is more accurate.

The glycyrrhizin content can vary considerably depending on species used, where it grows, whether domesticated or wild, and when it was harvested. In general, wild *G. glabra* plants are considered to have the highest glycyrrhizin content.

While there are some minor distinctions in the terms, glycyrrhizin is considered to be a synonym for the terms glycyrrhizinic acid and glycyrrhizic acid.

Some other constituents that people find exciting are glabrin A and B, glycyrrhetinic acid, glycyrrhetol, glabrolide, glabridin, glycidipine, isoglabrolide.

Traditional Uses

Licorice has been used as a food plant and medicinal for between four and five millennia. The genus name, *Glycyrrhiza*, is Greek in origin, *glykys* meaning "sweet" and *rhiza* "root." The root's main constituent, glycyrrhizin, is 50 times sweeter than sugar, as seemingly every article on licorice repeats, ad nauseum. All licorice species have been used as medicine wherever they have grown and by every culture that has had access to them.

AYURVEDA

Variously known as mulathi, yasti-madhu, jasti-madhu, madhuka, mithiladki, and so on. The plant is considered cooling, tonic, demulcent, expectorant, diuretic, and a gentle laxative. It's used for treating poisoning, ulcers, diseases of the liver, bladder, and lungs. It is specific for any inflammation in the mucous membranes anywhere in the body. It is used for cough, sore throat, hoarseness, fevers, and as a general tonic in debility from long-term disease conditions, especially those that are pulmonary or of the GI tract. It is considered a synergist, a specific additive to other herbal formulations.

TRADITIONAL CHINESE MEDICINE

Known as gan cao in Chinese medicine, licorice has been used in China for 3,000 years or so. The herb is considered sweet and mild, to regulate the function of the stomach, to be qi tonifying, lung demulcent, expectorant, latent-heat cleansing, antipyretic, detoxicant, anti-inflammatory, spleen invigorative, and it is a synergist in many herbal formulations. The herb is used in pharyngolaryngitis, cough, palpitations, stomachache due to asthenia, peptic ulcer, pyogenic infection, ulceration of the skin, hepatitis, encephalitis B, measles, and all types of respiratory infections.

WESTERN BOTANIC PRACTICE

The ancient Egyptians used the plant as a major medicinal; the plant has often been found in their tombs. The Greek Theophrastus in the third century BCE noted the plant's use for asthma, dry coughs, and respiratory problems. The Romans called the plant *liquiritia*, which was eventually corrupted to the word *licorice*. It was a primary medicine in ancient Rome for coughs. It was used throughout Europe as a primary medicinal and although harvested in the wild originally, it has been a main agricultural crop for over a thousand years.

The American Eclectics used it intensively, as did most medicinal practitioners in the Americas. The Eclectics used it for coughs, catarrhs, irritation of the urinary passages, diarrhea, and bronchial diseases. It was an early agricultural medicinal, grown by most people in their medicinal gardens. The indigenous tribes of the Americas used the indigenous species similarly, that is, for sore throat, chest pains, swellings, coughs, stomachache, fevers, toothache, skin sores, spitting blood, and as an antidiarrheal and a general tonic.

Scientific Research

The medicinal species have been intensely studied for years; there are over 1,900 citations on PubMed alone. This look will be brief, as a full monograph would run hundreds of pages. And first, given the nature of *this* book . . .

ANTIVIRAL DYNAMICS, MEMBRANE FLUIDITY

Licorice has strong impacts on viruses across a broad range. Licorice and its (strongest?) constituent glycyrrhizin act against a wide range of viruses, specifically by modulating membrane fluidity in both host and viral cells — the herb lowers membrane fluidity significantly.

Enveloped viruses (herpesviruses, poxviruses, hepadnaviruses, flaviviruses, togaviruses, coronaviruses, hepatitis D, orthomyxoviruses, paramyxoviruses, rhabdoviruses, bunyaviruses, filoviruses, and retroviruses) have a viral envelope surrounding them, covering their protein capsids (i.e., their viral shell). The viral envelopes are generally composed of glycoproteins that identify and bind to receptor cells on the surface of host cells the viruses want to enter. Once the proper receptors are identified, the viruses bind to them, fuse with the host cell, create a pore in the cell, and enter the host cell. Voilà! Infection. The viruses take over the cell they have entered, reproduce, burst it open, then spread to other cells.

Licorice and its constituents act by inhibiting the ability of enveloped viruses to fuse with host cells, create pores in the host cell membrane, and enter them. It does this by significantly reducing the membrane fluidity of both the host cell and the virus. As little as a 5 percent reduction in host cell membrane fluidity will reduce HIV infection by 56 percent for instance. An increase of 5 percent will enhance infectivity 2.4-*fold*, more than doubling it.

Interesting speculation: Excess cholesterol in the bloodstream serves to reduce host cell fluidity; the most interesting studies on the effects of licorice and glycyrrhizin on viral infection occurred because glycyrrhizin is similar in shape to cholesterol. The researchers postulated that it might act in a number of instances *because* it was reducing membrane fluidity. This stimulates speculation: Are cholesterol-lowering drugs affecting membrane fluidity across the board in those using them, thus increasing viral infections in that group? (Cholesterol-lowering drugs do affect sterol levels in the body and do reduce, in some circumstances, the levels of steroid hormones that the body produces, especially if combined with a low-cholesterol diet.)

Glycyrrhizin is uptaken fairly quickly into the cell (due most likely to its cholesterol-like shape). It diffuses rapidly across the membrane and concentrates on the inner membrane surface (and possibly within the membrane itself), where it causes the cell membrane to become more rigid, significantly reducing the movement of compounds through the membrane. Due to its nature glycyrrhizin is also

uptaken by the viruses and incorporated into their viral envelope, which also becomes more rigid. At human body temperature the effects on cell fluidity are significant. Once this occurs, a virus's ability to fuse with a host cell and create a pore in the membrane through which to enter the cell is inhibited.

The degree of inhibition is dose dependent. The more licorice or glycyrrhizin, the more inhibition that occurs. Glycyrrhizin also stops the ballooning degeneration that occurs in virus-infected/fused cells. Tests on influenza viruses, vaccinia virus, herpes simplex virus 1, Newcastle disease virus, measles, HIV-1, and SARS have found that it acts in exactly this way with all those enveloped viruses. (It uses different mechanisms with polio, another enveloped virus type.) Of note: Interferon, whose production is stimulated in the body by licorice, also alters membrane fluidity, as well as being directly antiviral. So, licorice acts through multiple mechanisms on membrane fluidity.

Unfortunately, because of improper use and understanding, much of the licorice root in the United States is deglycyrrhized, that is, the glycyrrhizin is removed. Glycyrrhizin is felt to be the constituent that causes most of the side effects of licorice (see the discussion of side effects above). Please note: Deglycyrrhized licorice is worthless as an antiviral (though it does still work for GI tract problems). If you pay attention to the proper use of the herb and its side effects (really! see the side effects section) and use the plant with awareness you really should not have any trouble with the herb. Oddly enough, the Japanese insist that their use of purified glycyrrhizin has produced very few side effects in clinical practice (yes, there have been some). As one researcher noted: "An advantage of GL [glycyrrhizin] is that it is a broad anti-viral agent with few side effects. Although data about the safety of long-term usage and high doses of GL still need to be collected, the best example of safety is a long history of safe use in clinical settings in Japan."[9] Only in the West would they *remove* what is considered by many to be the primary active constituent of the herb.

Note: In general, licorice is rarely used *by itself* for treatment of disease in the countries that do use herbs as part of their health care system, so there are not many studies on its use *by itself*. Glycyrrhizin is, however, used a lot as a potent antiviral (with other actions as well) and there have been a number of studies on it. In Japan, for instance, glycyrrhizin is widely used in clinical practice, has far fewer side effects than pharmaceuticals, and is extensively studied.

PHARMACOKINETICS

Usually, researchers study isolated glycyrrhizin versus licorice root extract pharmacokinetics, with sometimes a variation here and there. Glycyrrhizin is hydrolized (i.e., *changed*) by human intestinal flora by the bacterial enzyme glucuronidase to glycyrrhetinic acid (GA), which is the primary form of glycyrrhizin that is active in the body. Glycyrrhizin is not normally detected in plasma at any time but GA is and is one of the main compounds tested for when looking at plasma concentrations and the pharmacokinetics of licorice.

Rats and rabbits biologically process the herb and its constituents a bit differently. In rats the amount of GA in plasma is a bit less if they are given the herb extract rather than the purified compound. In rabbits that is reversed. Nevertheless, the use of the root extracts themselves do allow most of the glycyrrhizin to enter the bloodstream.

People's bodies work a bit more like rats in this instance. Licorice extract produces a slightly lower glycyrrhizin (glycyrrhetinic acid) profile than the pure extract itself. Peak plasma concentration with the purified extract takes about 6 hours; with the root extract it is 8 hours. Both then decline slowly over the next 24 hours. The level of other licorice constituents such as glabridin are a bit different. They can be detected in plasma within an hour and reach peak within 4 hours. Then they, too, decline slowly over the next 24 hours.

The constituents in licorice do cross the blood-brain barrier. In rats, glycyrrhetinic acid, the metabolite of glycyrrhizin, can be found in plasma, the brain, and the cerebral spinal fluid after oral administration. The amount of glycyrrhizin (glycyrrhetinic acid) in human plasma increases if licorice extracts are taken with Chinese skullcap (which they should be for treating viral infections).

The constituents in licorice root are altered into potent metabolites by gut bacteria and again by the liver, which sends them back into the GI tract in the bile, where the gut bacteria again alter them. Around and around. This is part of the reason that the clearance time of licorice constituents is so long. It is also why licorice is so good for treating viral liver disease; the constituents concentrate in the liver.

In treating viral diseases that are acute, if the amount of the herb and its constituents is increased to a relatively high level and you keep taking them every day, every 3 to 4 hours, then the amounts in the body stay high, essentially bathing the body in those specific compounds. Many of these are uptaken by cells in the body, decreasing their fluidity, which inhibits viral infection. At the very least, the herb needs to be taken until all the virus particles are eliminated, several weeks at minimum. The continual presence of the constituents in the body, especially in the brain, also reduces inflammation and protects neurons from damage, especially during encephalitis infections.

COMPOUND SYNERGY

Studies with licorice have shown, as they invariably do with every plant studied in this fashion, that the constituents of licorice are highly synergistic. For example, licorice extract is strongly reductive of nitric oxide (NO) and inducible nitric oxide synthase (iNOS) in the body. That is, it lowers inflammation by reducing oxidation, one of the reasons it is good for encephalitis, for instance. *However,* *glycyrrhizin, by itself, has no effect on NO or iNOS.* Further, a licorice extract with the glycyrrhizin removed has, as the researchers put it, "significantly attenuated" impacts on NO and iNOS; that is, it barely reduces inflammation. But if they add the glycyrrhizin, which has no effect on NO or iNOS itself, back into the extract, the impacts on NO and iNOS return to their previous levels.

ANTIVIRAL ACTIONS

Licorice prevents viral replication across a wide range of viruses, inhibits viral growth, and inactivates virus particles. In vitro studies have found that licorice inhibits influenza A uptake into cells and inhibits RANTES secretion by bronchial cells infected with influenza A. In vitro, glycyrrhizin is more active against SARS-associated coronavirus than ribavirin, 6-azauridine, pyrazofurin, and mycophenolic acid.

Protection from influenza death in vivo: Glycyrrhizin significantly reduced morbidity and mortality in mice infected with lethal doses of influenza virus (H2N2). There were no survivors in the control group; all the licorice-treated mice survived. Pulmonary consolidations and virus titers in the lung tissues of the licorice group were significantly lower than in the tissues of the control group. When splenic T cells from the licorice mice were transferred to nonlicorice mice, survival rate increased to 100 percent.

Another in vivo study found that glycyrrhizic acid inhibited influenza virus and Newcastle virus growth in embryonated eggs.

Glycyrrhizin is strongly protective of mice with induced herpes simplex encephalitis. Mortality was significantly reduced (from 60 to 25 percent), and glycyrrhizin directly inhibited the virus replication in vivo and markedly reduced the expression of iNOS, significantly alleviating autoimmune reactions to the disease.

Glycyrrhizin has been found to be 10 times more potent in reducing the infectivity of hepatitis A viruses than ribavirin. Both licorice and glycyrrhizin have been found to irreversibly inactivate herpes simplex viruses.

Glycyrrhizic acid cream, applied six times daily in people with acute oral herpetic infections (HSV1), resolved pain and dysphagia within 24 to 48 hours.

Three HIV patients were given IV glycyrrhizin six times over 1 month. HIV p24 antigen was present in all at the beginning of the trial; by the end it had either decreased or become negative.

In infants infected with cytomegalovirus who were given IV glycyrrhizin, liver enzymes normalized and the virus disappeared sooner than in controls. Oral glycyrrhizin worked similarly.

NEUROPROTECTIVE/CNS ACTIONS

Stronger Neo-Minophagen C, a glycyrrhizin-containing preparation used in Japan for treating hepatitis, showed potent neuroprotective effects after induced middle cerebral artery occlusion in the postischemic rat brain. Motor movement, neurological deficits, and infarct volume all improved. (Whole licorice preparations are more effective along this line than purified glycyrrhizin.)

Glycyrrhizic acid is strongly neuroprotective in postischemic rat brains via anti-inflammatory activity through the inhibition of HMGB1 phosphorylation and secretion.

Albendazole and diammonium glycyrrhizinate (DG) were used to treat eosinophilic meningitis in mice infected with *Angiostrongylus cantonensis*, a parasitic roundworm that normally causes this condition in people and animals. Albendazole is a pharmaceutical used to kill the worms, DG is a form of glycyrrhizin. When DG was added to the treatment, survival time increased, mortality was reduced, neurological dysfunction was significantly reduced, weight loss decreased, levels of IgE, IL-5, and eotaxin all decreased.

Glycyrrhizin was found to reduce secondary inflammatory processes in mice after spinal cord compression injury. NF-κB, NO, iNOS, and Bax were reduced. Bcl-2 was increased.

An aqueous extract of licorice given to mice (150 mg/kg) significantly improved learning and memory. It also reversed the amnesia induced by diazepam and scopolamine.

IMMUNE IMPACTS

Licorice and glycyrrhizin enhance interleukin-10 (IL-10) production in the body. IL-10 is also known as cytokine synthesis inhibitory factor; it is an anti-inflammatory cytokine. It essentially downregulates other cytokines and blocks NF-κB activity. In other words, if an infectious organism begins a cytokine cascade by initiating NF-κB activity (common), increasing

IL-10 will begin to normalize cytokine levels in spite of what the bacteria or viruses are doing. Another component of licorice root, isoliquiritigenin, also has potent effects on cytokines, especially NF-κB. Specifically it blocks the induction of VCAM-1 (vascular adhesion molecule-1), E-selectin, and PECAM-1 (platelet endothelial cell adhesion molecule-1). It interferes with THP-1 monocyte adhesion to TNF-α-activated endothelial cells, and abolishes many of the cytokine effects of TNF-α. It does this by blocking the nuclear translocation of NF-κB, essentially acting as an upstream cytokine cascade blocker in bacteria- or virus-initiated inflammatory processes.

A double-blind, repeated-within-subject, randomized trial with *Echinacea purpurea, Astragalus membranaceus,* and *Glycyrrhiza glabra* found that licorice increased CD25 expression on T cells. It also increased CD69, CD4, and CD8 expression on T cells.

SORE THROAT TREATMENT

Forty adults about to undergo elective lumbar laminectomy were split into two groups. One received water as a preoperative gargle, the other water with licorice. The use of licorice gargle performed 5 minutes before anesthesia was effective in reducing or eliminating the incidence and severity of postoperative sore throat in patients.

SYNERGY IN TUBERCULOSIS TREATMENT

Licorice enhances outcomes in the treatment of tuberculosis: A randomized, double-blind, placebo-controlled study with 60 people with sputum positive pulmonary tuberculosis was conducted. They were split into two groups, one taking placebo, the other licorice — in addition to their regular therapy. Sputum conversion was seen in 80 percent of the licorice group, 70 percent of the placebo group. Fever was relieved in all of the licorice group, 80 percent in the placebo group. Cough was relieved in 96 percent of the licorice group, 81 percent of the placebo group. GI side effects were seen in 20 percent of the placebo group, none of the licorice group. ALT and AST levels were raised in 6 percent of the licorice group, 30 percent of the placebo group. Elevated uric acid in serum was observed in 3 percent of the licorice group, 16 percent of the placebo group.

HEPATITIS

A single compound, an interferon stimulator, from licorice was used to treat patients with subacute hepatic failure. The survival rate was 72 percent compared to 31 percent in those who received traditional therapies.

In 13 cases of infectious hepatitis treated with licorice, the icterus index normalized in 13 days, urinary bile pigments were negative in 10 days, marked reduction of hepatomegaly took 9 days, pain over the liver disappeared in 8 days.

Glycyrrhizin has been used in Japan for more than 60 years in the treatment of hepatitis C. In several clinical trials it has been found to significantly lower AST, ALT, and GGT concentrations while reversing histologic evidence of necrosis and inflammatory lesions in the liver. And glycyrrhizin improves clinical picture, improves liver function, and reverses viral infection during chronic hepatitis B infection.

OTHER STUDIES

Atopic dermatitis. A licorice gel was used to successfully treat atopic dermatitis in a double-blind clinical trial, with 30 people in each group. The gel significantly reduced erythema, oedema, and itching over the 2-week trial.

Aphthous stomatitis. Bioadhesive patches containing licorice were used to control the pain and reduce healing time in recurrent aphthous ulcer. Licorice patches caused a significant reduction in the diameter of the inflammatory halo and necrotic center compared with placebo. (There have been three of these trials, all successful.)

Pharmaceutical side effects. In a comparative trial, licorice, when used along with spironolactone in the treatment of polycystic ovary syndrome, significantly reduced the side effects compared to spironolactone when used alone.

Peptic ulcer. Licorice was found in a trial with 100 people with peptic ulcer (86 of whom were unresponsive to conventional treatment) to be effective: 90 percent experienced good effects, 22 were cured, 28 were significantly improved.

Lichens planus. In a clinical trial of lichens planus, 66 percent of people who took glycyrrhizin were cured.

Miscellaneous. There have been a number of trials using licorice in combination with other herbs. It reduced risperidone-induced hyperprolactinemia in patients with schizophrenia. Reduced hyperuricemia in vegetarians. Was effective in the treatment of advanced pancreatic and other gastrointestinal malignancies. Was successful in the treatment of 138 cases of intestinal metaplasia and 104 of atypical hyperplasia of the gastric mucosa.

In vivo studies have found licorice to be potently antioxidant, to stimulate immune activity, to be anticonvulsant, to be potently anti-inflammatory on skin eruptions, to be liver protective, to be cerebroprotective, to heal aspirin-induced ulcers, to be antispasmodic to the lower intestine, to be strongly antitussive, and to protect the mitochondria from damage.

Lomatium

Family: Apiaceae, the carrot family.

Species used: There are 70 or maybe 80 species in this genus — trying to pin a taxonomist down is like gluing feathers on a donkey so it can fly. They are indigenous to the United States (lomatiums, not taxonomists) and grow from the Mississippi River region throughout the West, Southwest, and Northwest. A number of them can be used medicinally but information on the genus and its medicinal uses is very sparse. *Many of the species are exceptionally rare and are endangered so be highly conscious if you are wildcrafting. Only harvest if the species is very common in your area or is not endangered.* The most commonly used lomatium is *Lomatium dissectum* but several others can be used identically and grow in enough abundance, here and there, to be harvested and are (usually) not considered endangered: *L. ambiguum, L. bicolor, L. cous, L. foeniculaceum, L. grayi, L. macrocarpum, L. nudicaule, L. orientale, L. simplex, L. triternatum.*

L. dissectum, L. cous, L. bicolor, L. foeniculaceum, L. macrocarpum, and *L. orientale* have the widest range, some of them extending into Iowa, Minnesota, and Missouri. *L. nudicaule,* though confined to the Northwest, has a particularly long history of medicinal use and is considered by some to be stronger than *L. dissectum.*

There are, just to make things harder, two varieties of *L. dissectum, L. dissectum* var. *dissectum* and *L. dissectum* var. *multifidum.* The former is more prevalent east of the Cascade mountain range, the latter west. The former likes more rain and lower altitudes, the latter likes it semiarid and grows as high as 7,000 feet (2,200 m). I have generally used *multifidum;* it appears to be somewhat stronger in its medicinal effects. Almost no source you order from will be able to tell you which variety of *dissectum* they are selling you.

Synonyms: The *Lomatium* genus used to be the genus *Leptotaenia.* It was reclassified during World War II — shortly before it was inducted. *Lomatium dissectum,* for example, used to be *Leptotaenia dissecta.*

For some reason *Lomatium dissectum* was also once called *Ferula dissoluta*, *ferula* meaning "rod" and *dissoluta* meaning "debauched, unrestrained by convention or morality," ergo, debauched rod (there's a really good joke here but . . .). In any event, it appears that botanists and taxonomists are closely related, perhaps from an ancient debauchery.

Common names: Lomatium, biscuit root, cough root, Indian consumption plant, desert parsley, Indian parsnip. *Lomatium dissectum* is sometimes known as fernleaf biscuitroot.

Biscuit root, desert parsley, and lomatium are the general common identifiers and will usually be combined with a descriptive to create a particular species' common name in a geographical area, e.g., northern Idaho biscuit root, Bradshaw's desert parsley, California lomatium.

Parts Used

The root is normally what is used, but the seeds are highly active. They often contain considerably more constituents than the root and may be used instead (though hardly anyone does).

Preparation and Dosage

Lomatium is generally used as a tincture (at least these days).

TINCTURE

Fresh root: 1:2 herb:liquid ratio. Chop the wilted root as finely as possible with a very sharp knife, place in a jar, add the tincturing medium (70 percent grain alcohol, 30 percent water), cover, and let macerate 2 weeks. Dosage: 10–30 drops up to 5x daily. In acute conditions, take 10–30 drops each hour.

Dry root: Same as for the fresh root, except powder the root and use an herb:liquid ratio of 1:5.

Fresh seeds: Same as for the fresh root.

Dry seeds: 1:3, 50 percent alcohol. Dosage: 1 dropperful 3–5x daily or once per hour in acute conditions.

Common influenza tincture blend: Combine equal parts of lomatium, red root, licorice, and pleurisy root (*Asclepias tuberosa*) tinctures. In acute conditions with debility (bedridden, lingering loss of energy, failure to thrive, pneumonia) take up to 1 teaspoon 6x daily. You should make up 16 or so ounces to keep on hand. When the flu hits you won't want to make it. (I do, however, prefer the more extensive formulation described in chapter 2; see page 46.)

INFUSION OR DECOCTION

You can try it, it worked for the indigenous peoples. I have tasted and used the tea myself and its impact on the tongue is nearly as strong as that of the tincture. Somehow, in spite of not being water soluble, the aromatics are indeed getting into the tea. (It is prepared by pouring hot water over the root and leaving it covered for an hour or so. This does help keep the aromatics in there.)

Add 1 teaspoon of the powdered root to 6 ounces hot water, cover, and let steep.

Influenza decoction blend: Robin Seydel's influenza blend (via Northwest herbalist Ryan Drum): Combine 1 ounce each of lomatium seeds, lobaria lichen, licorice root, Oregon grape root, echinacea blossoms, red clover blossoms, and rowan berries. Grind all the herbs into a powder (or as close as you can get). Add to 1 quart hot water, and boil for 2–4 minutes. Remove from the heat, cover, and let steep for an hour. Then strain, add lemon juice and honey to taste, and drink hot, 1 quart per day.

STEAM INHALANT

Pour boiling water over some of the freshly chopped root or seeds (which should be in a hot-liquid-tolerant container). Drape a towel over your head and the container, and breathe in. This works a treat for influenzal infections. Take the tincture, too.

Side Effects and Contraindications

Pregnancy and a nasty rash. (Actually, that should be "Nasty rash and pregnancy" — you won't get pregnant from taking the tincture.)

From what is known, the plants are exceptionally nontoxic. Injections of isolates of the plants at 2.5 percent of the weight of mice were not toxic in any way — no observable differences at all. *However*, the plant is contraindicated in pregnancy *and* about 1 percent of people using the herb get a rather nasty rash. The rash appears to be associated only with *Lomatium dissectum*; the use of other species has apparently not produced it.

As far as anyone knows, this *is* an allergic reaction to the plant but it is a rather unusual one — there is no itching, no discomfort other than the visual. Herbalist Michael Moore reports that he found it occurring *only* with the fresh root tincture and only then if the tincture was taken as a single, i.e., not blended with anything else.

The rash usually begins within 8 hours of taking the tincture. It can cover the whole body — warm baths often make it worse. The rash is a deep to dark red, even purplish. It can cover the entire body (most people stay home to avoid encountering the human subspecies *Homo staris*). There is rarely, if ever, any itching or discomfort. It's just there. *Nothing* will make it better, not steroids, not Benadryl, not calamine lotion, not Pepcid, not herbs, not herbal washes, not doctors or hospitals. So save your money and skip the emergency room visit — besides physicians don't know squat about plant medicines, or their side effects. (Though they are often highly prejudiced against them.) It's grin-and-bear-it time. The rash will disappear within a week or so after its initial occurrence.

To avoid the rash use lomatium as part of a mixture, not singly, and use the dried root, not the fresh root, for tinctures. Oh, and don't spend a lot of time looking in the mirror.

Herb/Drug Interactions

None known.

Habitat and Appearance

The lomatiums are called desert parsleys for a reason; their leaves and stems often look very similar to those rarely purchased parsley bunches you see in the grocery store and sometimes buy and use a tiny bit of for an experimental recipe before the rest decays into a dessicated phytomemory (often found months later) in the bottom of the vegetable drawer in the refrigerator. Some of the species are small, like that parsley bunch, while others are much larger; *L. dissectum* is one of the giants.

Like most of this family, *L. dissectum* begins as a fernlike bunch of basal leaves that, as the plant matures, sends up a rather substantial flowering stalk. The fernlike leaves of this species may be up to a foot long, with a dozen or so leaves spreading out from the root core. The flowering stalks can be from 2 to 5 feet in height. They are usually leafless. The plant flowers in early spring, the seeds mature in late summer or early fall.

The roots are 3 or so inches in diameter and up to 2 feet long (*L. nudicaule*: 6 inches in diameter, up to 3 feet long); they're big. Herbalist Michael Moore describes the root in his typical fashion:

> The root is fleshy, thick at the top, lumpy, and irregular, like a mutant cross between a carrot and rutabaga, with odd parts left over. The skin is pearly grey, with many oil glands spread throughout the variously cream- and yellow-colored flesh.[10]

Most lomatiums grow in well-drained, sandy or rocky soil — basically a certain kind of deserty-sandy-dryish-hard-to-get-to, hard-to-dig-in, old volcanicy or decomposed granity terrain and soil. There are a few exceptions — such as *L. nudicaule*. But herbalist Ryan Drum comments that *that* particular plant was most likely brought to the island on which he lives in Puget Sound by the Salish who settled there. The plant only grows near old Salish settlements on extensive beach sand flats with few other plant competitors, a terrain similar to the desert homeland it was transplanted from.

The lomatiums are semiarid plants of the Great Plains, deserts, high mountains, and northwest United States. That's where you will find them.

Properties of Lomatium

Actions

Analgesic	Antimicrobial	Antiviral
Antibacterial	Antiseptic	Expectorant
Antifungal	Antispasmodic	Mucous membrane tonic

Active Against

There have been few studies on the activity of the lomatiums against microorganisms and virtually none on their activities against viruses. The two most comprehensive studies occurred in 1948 and 1949 in the United States. Both focused on the antibacterial activities of extracted aromatics of the root, one isolated through steam distillation, the other through ethyl acetate extraction and filtration. The range of activity was fairly broad. Fractions of the steam distillate were found active against the following:

Achromobacter lacticum
Agrobacterium spp.
Aspergillus spp.
Bacillus spp.
Candida albicans
Clostridium spp. (mildly)
Coccidioides immitis
Corynebacterium diphtheriae
Diplococcus pneumoniae
Eberthella typhosa

Escherichia coli (mildly)
Fusarium spp.
Haemophilus influenzae
Histoplasmosis capsulatum
Micrococcus tetragenus
Microspermum trichoderma
Mucocus capsulatus
Mucor culmorum
Mycobacterium spp.
Mycoderma spp.

Neisseria spp. (mildly)
Pestallotia funera
Proteus spp.
Pseudomonas spp.
Pythium debaryanum
Rhizoctonia spp.
Serratia marcescens
Shigella spp.
Staphylococcus spp.
Streptomyces griseus
Trichophyton spp.
Zooleal spp.

In the ethyl acetate extracts study, several different forms were used at varying degrees of strength. They were found active against the following:

Bacillus subtilis
Corynebacterium diphtheriae
Diplococcus pneumoniae
Escherichia coli (mildly)

Micrococcus aureus
Neisseria catarrhalis
Proteus vulgaris (mildly)
Pseudomonas aeruginosa (mildly)

Serratia marcescens (mildly)
Streptococcus pyogenes
Vibrio comma (a.k.a. *V. cholerae*)

The ethyl acetate extracts were not active against *Klebsiella pneumoniae*, *Salmonella schottmuelleri*, *Aerobacter aerogenes*.

Both studies found the steam and ethyl acetate isolates much more active against Gram-positive organisms than Gram-negative (as usual). Even at concentrations of 10^{-3} the Gram-positive organisms were completely inhibited. Some of the Gram-negative organisms were, however, highly susceptible to the isolates, e.g., *Vibrio comma*, *Neisseria catarrhalis*.

There have been no in-depth studies on the antiviral properties of lomatium, however a few researchers looking a bit more broadly report the plant roots to be active against rotavirus and HIV as well as *Bacillus subtilis*, *Staphylococcus aureus*, *Colletotrichum fragariae*, *Mycobacterium tuberculosis*, *Pseudomonas aeruginosa*, *Trypanosoma cruzi*, and *Propionbacterium acnes*.

In spite of the lack of viral studies, I, and many others, have found the plant highly active against most viral and bacterial respiratory infections, including pneumonia. I haven't found anything better for serious, debilitating influenza, avian flu, swine flu, West Nile, or incapacitating pneumonia. In some instances the people were bedridden, very weak and debilitated; in others, ER physicians had diagnosed them with severe pneumonia. In all cases focused treatment (i.e., high, frequent doses) worked well, though in the more debilitated instances, it took weeks to turn it around. Normally, people begin to show improvement within a day or two.

Use to Treat

Upper respiratory viral infections, all influenza strains, SARS, viral encephalitis, pneumonia. Lomatium is most effective, in my opinion, if combined with other herbs such as red root, licorice, pleurisy root. Nevertheless, it is very potent by itself and can be used as a single (however, see the section "Contraindications and Side Effects"). The taste is intense though you can get used to it.

Clinicians have reported good success in using the plant for other viral infections, for instance, Epstein-Barr and cytomegalovirus (in chronic-fatigue-like situations), hepatitis C (lowering viral load), and HIV. Some (Michael Moore) have used it in the treatment of shigella and other bacterial infections with good success.

There is a tendency to look at the plant as a systemic antibacterial due to the early studies. I think the plant is better thought of as a systemic

Continued on next page

Continued from previous page

antiviral, especially for respiratory infections, most especially the emerging influenza strains. See "Western Botanic Practice" (page 242).

Other Uses

The roots of many lomatiums, before they attain maturity, are highly edible (though the taste may take some getting used to). The roots have traditionally been eaten fresh, steamed, roasted, boiled, in soups and stews, canned, or dried to crispy, and very tasty, sticks (if the roots are small enough). Larger immature roots or the sweeter varieties were peeled, pounded into cakes, and dried in the sun, hence the "biscuit" part of the common name. Lewis and Clark compared the taste of the dried cakes to bread. Most lomatium species were apparently used similarly.

Finding It

You can order the sliced and dried roots rather easily online. I prefer Pacific Botanicals for most herbs that I have to order in bulk; their quality is supreme.

Cultivation and Collection

The lomatiums don't cultivate easily though a few agricultural groups are insisting they are indeed growing the plant and at least one commercial company describes its tincture as being from organically grown roots. Still, germination of the seeds is reportedly difficult. The plant *could* grow in similar terrain any place on Earth but it would take work to get it to take in a new location. Transplanting may be a better option.

If you are wild-harvesting, you need to be aware of a couple of things. The first is the terrain: Lomatium likes it tough. *Lomatium dissectum*, and its variants, likes to grow around impossibly difficult rocky outcrops and the roots are tenacious. Find some in soil and skip the rocky ones. The second is the *nature* of the root itself: It appears in different forms depending on its age, the time of year, and which species it is from. Michael Moore comments:

> In the spring the roots ooze milky aromatic sap; by fall the sap is more resinous and balsamic; but in any case, the sticky bitter aromatic sap and the soft, fibrous flesh (not at all woody) differentiate this big Lomatium from the others of the genus. The Lomatium clan is huge, with eighty closely related species in the western states. For many years the large size of a few of these plants (most Lomatiums are quite small) caused botanists to classify them apart in the genus Leptotaenia. The larger Lomatiums, by whatever name, are an amorphous group, and I have found several strikingly varied stands whose roots are typical of *L. dissectum* in their morphology and constituents, which act like *L. dissectum* when tinctured, have identical constituents as measured by TLC (think-layer chromatography), but don't particularly look like *L. dissectum*. I have found these plants in such varied locations as Modoc County, California, northwestern Wyoming, and the front range of Colorado.... Most of the other large Lomatiums that grow in the range of *L. dissectum* have sweet, starchy parsniplike roots and could not be confused with this bitter, aromatic, oily- and waxy-rooted giant.[11]

Moore lists the species that he has found to be usable as *L. dissectum, L. multifidum, L. eatonii,* and *L. occidentalis.* Ryan Drum comments that *L. nudicaule* is just as good if not better. *Lomatium grayi* and *L. dissectum* overlap in their range and the two are often confused.

In any event, the root you are harvesting must be strongly aromatic, bitter, and oily if it is to be antiviral. Normally this is seen *only* in mature plants. If it is not, then it probably won't work as a medicinal though it will work as a rather good food source.

You can harvest the roots at any time of the year. They are easier to identify in the spring, a bit easier to dig after spring rains.

Dry the roots for a few days, then cut them up (they are a bit too resinous if you don't let them dry a little first). *Make sure you cut them up.* Generally they are sliced into wheels as you would slice a carrot. If you dry them whole, you will need a chainsaw to reduce their size later. (Just an FYI on that one.) Once the root circles are well dried store them in well-sealed plastic bags inside a well-sealed plastic tub out of direct sunlight in a coolish location. They will last several years. At least.

Moore likes the spring roots for making a fresh root tincture, and the fall roots for dried root tincture. I tend to prefer spring roots in this family; they are much bigger in my experience and, I feel, more potent. That is because the roots of all perennials grow throughout the winter, albeit very slowly. By spring they are full of stored nutrients and tend to be juicy and fat. By fall they have used those stores to send up stalks and set seed. Fall roots are stringier, a bit dryish and beef-jerkyish.

The big lomatiums are perennials; it takes them years to mature — often as much as a decade before they can be harvested. *Many sources put the minimum period of growth before the plants can be harvested for medicine at 20 years.* Some of the lomatiums in the wild are very old indeed — several hundred years; old-growth plants are not just trees.

Ryan Drum notes that the young *L. nudicaule* roots are sweet and starchy, very tender and highly edible, much like a plant candy. Only the older plants, when matured, will present with the typical oily, resinous, aromatic medicinal constituents needed in this species. Numerous other sources indicate that the same is true of *L. dissectum* and its variants — the plants need somewhere near a decade at minimum before they begin generating their volatile, and potently antiviral, oils and become useful for medicine.

If you harvest a root and it is sweet and starchy, then eat it but don't use it for medicine. However, all indications are that the seeds can be used no matter how old the plant is; they possess a similar chemistry to the root. This is borne out in part by the traditional uses of the seeds of *L. nudicaule* by the Salish in northwestern Washington State. They used *only* the seeds for medicine (the root was a food staple) and their traditional uses of the seeds are for the same range of problems that the roots are now used for in conventional practice.

Plant Chemistry

One of the main problems with scientific studies on the lomatiums (there haven't been many) is that researchers rarely make any distinctions between older plant roots that are highly aromatic and younger plant roots that are not. (It took highly schooled plant specialists *decades* to realize that some plants they had listed as perennials — or biennials — were in fact unique monocarpic plants, *Frasera speciosa* being an example. That plant may take anywhere from 20 to 100 years before it sends up a stalk and flowers and once it does, it dies. These specialist guys, they are a bit slow. And no, they didn't think to look at any of the Native American data on that plant.)

Comparison studies on the lomatiums should only occur with plants of similar ages; the differences in the percentage of compounds found in various subspecies of *Lomatium dissectum* could easily be from differences in the age of the roots tested. The current chemistry studies, which are nice to have, are nevertheless suspect in some of their conclusions about the species studied due to the failure of the researchers to indicate the age of the plants or to be certain the plants were of a similar age before comparisons.

Nevertheless, many members of the *Lomatium* genus (and the carrot family of which it is a member) have a number of similar chemistries, e.g., apiol, a calcium antagonist widely present in the carrot family and strongly present in the seeds and roots of *Lomatium californicum* and *Ligusticum hultenii*. The antiasthmatic and antispasmodic compound Z-ligustilide is common in many of the lomatiums as well.

Most of the chemical studies on the lomatiums have been conducted by butterfly researchers since butterflies are strongly attracted to this genus (the researchers are looking for the exact chemical attractants so they go deep). The nearest to a comprehensive look at the chemistry of the main medicinal species has occurred with the essential oils of two variants of *Lomatium dissectum*. The roots, seeds, and stems all were found to contain a number of terpenoid hydrocarbons, among other things.

The seeds of *Lomatium dissectum* var. *dissectum*) were found to contain 113 compounds; the seeds of *Lomatium dissectum* var. *multifidum* contained 138. The leaves and upper stems of variety *dissectum* contained 137 compounds; those of variety *multifidum* contained 173.

The root of variety *dissectum* had 68 compounds; oddly, the study doesn't reveal the number of root compounds of variety *multifidum*. Variety *dissectum* is particularly rich in esters, specifically the 2-methylbutyrates; the primary compounds found are: phellandrene, limonene, beta-caryophyllene, palmitic acid, E-beta-ocimene, linolenic acid, octanol, octyl acetate, myrcene, 4-methylpentyl 2-methylbutyrate, alpha-bisabolol, cuparene, Z-S-hexenol, decyl acetate, longifolene, palmitoleic acid, Z-ligustilide, and E-2-methyl-3-octen-5-yne. The roots of the two closely related forms of *Lomatium dissectum* have very similar chemistries but they do differ, e.g., *Lomatium dissectum* var. *multifidum* has about 20 percent longifolene (a major constituent of many pines) in its complex of essential oils, while *Lomatium dissectum* var. *dissectum* has only about 3 percent.

Studies with other lomatiums have found similar compounds. The best in-depth look at species other than *dissectum* comes from Philip S. Beauchamp, et al. ("Essential Oil Composition of Six *Lomatium* Species Attractive to Indra Swallowtail Butterfly [*Papilio indra*]: Principal Component Analysis Against Essential Oil Composition of *Lomatium dissectum* var. *multifidum*," *Journal of Essential Oil Research* 21 [2009]: 535–42). They identified over 200 constituents in the plants. While all of the plants did not have the same constituents, they were similar in their compounds. The principal components of the six species (*brandegei, eastwoodiae, graveolens, howelii, junceum,* and *parryi*) are (in order or prominence): alpha-pinene, beta-pinene, camphene, alpha-phellandrene, alpha-terpinene, beta-phellandrene + limonene, Z-beta-ocimene, gamma-terpinene, p-mentha-2,4(8)-diene, linalool, dehydrosabina ketone, terpinen-4-ol, cryptone, alpha-terpineol, methyl chavicol, citronellol, methyl thymol, linalyl acetate, lavandulyl acetate, citronellyl acetate, beta-bourbonene, benzyl-2-methylbutyrate, beta-elemene, italicene, dodecanal, beta-caryophyllene, gamma-elemene, alpha-humulene, 7-epi-e,2-dehydrosesquicineole, gamma-muurolene, germacrene D, beta-selinene, bicyclogermacene, germacrene A, alpha-cadinene, germacrene B, epi-alpha-cadinol, alpha-muurolol. There are a number of highly antimicrobial tetronic acids in the root.[12]

Other species (*californicum, dasycarpum, grayi, lucidum, macrocarpum, nuttallii, rigidum, suksdorfii, utriculatum*) contain large amounts of similar constituents: falcarindiol, coniferyl ferulate, ferulic acid, Z-ligustilide, senkyunolide, trans-neocnidilide, apiol, suksdorfin, osthol, chromones, sibiricin, macrocarpin, beta-phellandrene/limonene, decanal, dodecanal, bornyl acetate, germacrene D, alphahumulene, bicyclogermacrene, alpha-pinene, beta-pinene, peucenin 7-methyl ester, beta-caryophyllene, Z-3-hexenol, palmitic acid, linoleic acid, E-2-hexenal, sabinene, terpinen-4-ol, myrcene, various coumarins, glycosides, and flavonoids. Z-falcarinol levels are particularly high in most lomatium species' roots.

The chemistry of the lomatiums, as with most plants, is complex and poorly understood. The seeds and aerial parts do have a great many more compounds than the roots, the seeds appearing nearly as active as antimicrobials as the roots. However, the roots do possess a number of compounds unique to them and are generally, in traditional practice and conventional herbal circles (though not in indigenous), considered to be the most potent antiviral parts of the plants.

Again: Only as the plant roots age do the major aromatics become highly concentrated in the roots; the seeds possess them from the beginning.

Traditional Uses

I have spread what would normally be in this section throughout this monograph. Read on.

AYURVEDA

Unknown.

TRADITIONAL CHINESE MEDICINE

Unknown.

WESTERN BOTANIC MEDICINE

All the lomatiums were known to the indigenous cultures that lived among them. All of them used the plants similarly: roots for food, seeds and roots for medicine (among other things). Lewis and Clark knew of the plants' uses for food, as they used them on their trek across the country once they were introduced to them. They almost certainly would have known of the plants' uses as medicine. Many of the trappers who lived in the region would have known as well. They didn't seem to have written about them, however. Lomatium only came to the awareness of the medical community during the influenza epidemic of 1918–1919.

The Washoe tribe in Nevada used the plant to treat members of the tribe who had fallen sick with the disease. A report on their use of the plant was printed in the *Bulletin of the Nevada State Board of Health*, in January 1920, by a physician, Ernst Krebs. If you have read, in depth, the description of just what the 1918 influenza virus did in the bodies of those it infected and then compare the outcomes in practice from lomatium during the pandemic, the effects of the herb are considerable.

The Indians gather this root in the late fall, November being considered the proper month for gathering. The root is used in the fresh or dry state. It is cut up and a decoction is made by boiling the root in water, skimming off the top and giving large doses of the broth. A pound of root is considered about the proper dose to treat a case of fever for 3 days, which is the longest time needed to break up a fever due to influenza or pulmonary disease, although the Washoes used it as a panacea. Whether a coincidence or not, there was not a single death in the Washoe tribe from influenza or its complications, although Indians living in other parts of the State where the root did not grow died in numbers. It was such a remarkable coincidence that the root was investigated by a practicing physician who saw apparently hopeless cases recover completely without any other medication or care of any kind.

A preparation was prepared and employed in a great many cases among the whites, from the mildest to the most virulent types of influenza, and it proved itself to be a reliable agent in preventing pulmonary complications. Other physicians were induced to give it a trial with the same results. It is beyond the experimental stage, as its therapeutic action in this direction is established and beyond any doubt. The cases in which it has been used run into the hundreds. There is probably no therapeutic agent so valuable in the treatment of influenzal pneumonia and, as far as being tried, in ordinary lobar pneumonia if started early. Its action on coughs is more certain than opiate expectorants and its benefit is lasting. It acts as a powerful tonic to the respiratory mucus membranes. It is a bronchial, intestinal and urinary antiseptic and is excreted by these organs.[13]

Interestingly, the aromatic constituents in the root are only mildly soluble in water, are better soluble in alcohol, and are lost when boiled (making a decoction). Given the traditional indigenous preparation methods, there are obviously a number of other compounds in the root, water soluble and heat resistant, that are, inescapably, strongly antiviral.

For a while, the reports of the efficacy of the plant stimulated study of its actions but the emergence of pharmaceutical antibiotics stopped research on the plant until Michael Moore began speaking about it in the early 1970s. It is now considered (among many herbalists) to be *the* primary antiviral medicine in the U.S. herbal community.

Scientific Research

Most of this section has been spread throughout the rest of this monograph, so, just a couple of notes here:

The lomatiums contain a large number of chemically unique coumarins (pyranocoumarins, furanocoumarins, prenyloxycoumarins, prenyloxyfuranocoumarins, and so on) that have been found in a number of studies to be powerfully antiviral against both RNA and DNA viruses ("remarkable" is how one research team put it). The compounds penetrate the viral coat and inhibit ribonucleo-protein-complex-associated activity among other things. They have been found exceptionally potent against influenza viruses (H1N1, etc). *Ferula assa-foetida*, once considered a close relative of *Lomatium dissectum* (formerly *Ferula dissoluta*), is especially rich in the same compounds; they are more potent against influenza viruses than amantadine. (Specifically, they inhibit the M2 ion channel.) The compounds in lomatium are in fact some of the most potent M2 ion channel inhibitors known.

Lomatiums also have high levels of longifolene, which is an exceptionally active antimicrobial. It is as active as the pharmaceutical nifurtimox against *Trypanosoma cruzi*, which causes Chagas' disease. It is primarily active against Gram-positive bacteria.

Honorable Mentions

There are a few other herbs that are showing potent antiviral actions that I think warrant closer examination over time. They are *Ampelopsis brevipedunculata, Forsythia suspensa, Sophora flavescens, Strobilanthes cusia,* and boneset (*Eupatorium perfoliatum*). The only one I will offer any depth on here is boneset. (And, yes, there are *lots* of other plants with antiviral actions; this is just a beginning. And yes, I do know about *Ocimum sanctum*.)

AMPELOPSIS BREVIPEDUNCULATA

Ampelopsis brevipedunculata, a.k.a porcelain berry, is an invasive, especially in the eastern United States, and is native to Asia. It's a woody vine that grows to 25 feet in length with an extensive root system. It mimics kudzu root in a lesser, porcelain berry sort of way, covering whatever it can as it spreads. It is on the lists of most phytoaryans; it is considered armed and dangerous, to be exterminated with extreme prejudice.

The herb is active against a number of viruses, including enterovirus 71, hepatitis, and varicella zoster. The stem, roots, and leaves are all used, though the stem and roots are the most commonly used for treating viral diseases. A water/ethanol extract of the roots and stems was found to be the strongest medicinal plant compound, of any tested, for treating four strains of enterovirus 71. The plant is traditionally used in Japan and parts of Asia as a major anti-inflammatory, hepatoprotective, and analgesic.

It has a number of immune modulation effects and has proved effective in treating liver fibrosis. It protects the liver from various toxic substances, is active against breast cancer cells, is a fairly potent antioxidant, is decidedly anti-inflammatory, and is analgesic. Because the plant is an invasive, its use really should be further explored.

FORSYTHIA SUSPENSA

Forsythia suspensa is one of the 50 fundamental herbs in Chinese medicine. It is a weeping forsythia, a large shrub, and quite pretty. It has escaped cultivation and is moderately invasive throughout the United States.

It is called either qing qiao or huang qiao in Chinese medicine, depending on whether the green or fully ripe yellow fruit is used as medicine. The unripe fruit is considered to be the strongest. (Rarely, the stem bark and leaves are used.) The dried fruit, whatever its ripeness, is used for fever, headache, restlessness, delirium, lymph gland enlargement, erysipelas, boils, and inflammations.

The herb is highly active against influenza A viruses, avian infectious bronchitis virus, cytomegalovirus, and respiratory syncytial virus. A number of the compounds in the plant have a fairly wide range of antiviral action (ursolic acid, oleanolic acid, quercetin, rutin, pinoresinol) and the plant really should be tested further. Studies on the leaves have found them to be stronger in their impacts than the flowers.

It is anti-inflammatory, antioxidant, vasorelaxive, antibacterial (against staph, *Helicobacter pylori*, *E. coli*), antiemetic, cytoprotective, and diuretic (antiedema).

SOPHORA FLAVESCENS

Sophora flavescens is also an herb used in traditional Chinese medicine, in which it is called ku shen. It is used for the treatment of viral hepatitis, viral myocarditis, gastritis, enteritis, cancer, and various skin diseases. The root is usually used. The plant is considered specific for jaundice, dysentery, leukorrhea, itching, scabies, eczema, and dysuria when used in combination with other plants.

The herb has been found active against a range of viruses: hepatitis B, respiratory syncytial virus, Coxsackie B3, HHV-6, coronavirus, influenza A (H1N1), rotavirus, herpes simplex virus 1 and 2, HIV, and various cancers. It is a potent neuraminidase inhibitor and also has some antibacterial (staph, enterococci, resistant and nonresistant) and antifungal (*Aspergillus niger*) actions.

STROBILANTHES CUSIA

Strobilanthes cusia is a plant that deserves more attention as an antiviral in that it contains many of the same compounds (e.g., tryptanthrin, indigo, indirubin) as isatis. (One of the plant's common names is actually Assam indigo and it was once used, as isatis was, as a source of indigo dye.) And, not surprisingly, it is a pretty good antiviral, too. In Chinese medicine it is called da-chang-yeh. The roots and leaves are used.

The plant is active against a number of viruses including influenza A (H1N1) strains, hepatitis B, herpes simplex virus 1, Sindbis virus, eastern equine encephalitis virus, Getah virus, and tobacco mosaic virus. Studies *in planta* found it increased innate resistance in plants to virus infections.

The plant contains some fairly potent compounds that target the subgenomic RNA of alphaviruses and alphavirus-like RNA viruses. This viral group, when it infects people, causes rashes and arthritis and encephalitis.

The plant has also shown antiplasmodial and antifungal activity.

In Chinese medicine, the plant is used for influenza, epidemic cerebrospinal meningitis, encephalitis B (Japanese viral encephalitis), viral pneumonia, and mumps. It is used for sore throats, aphthae, inflammatory diseases of the skin, and to reduce fever. The plant is considered antinociceptive, anti-inflammatory, and antipyretic.

Because the plant has so many of the same potent antiviral compounds as isatis and because it is widely grown throughout the world as an ornamental, its antiviral actions should be studied in more depth. One hope: Because the plant is in a different family, maybe it won't taste like isatis, i.e., spoiled cabbage.

Boneset

There have been extremely few studies on boneset; most of them are very old and what newish ones there are mostly quote nineteenth-century texts. Recently Mareike Maas, in Germany, has been doing some very good in-depth research on the plant, much of which is very hard to get in English. Her work is showing that the plant has a much wider range of antiviral actions than was formerly understood. I suspect the plant is going to be a more useful antiviral than previously suspected.

Family: Compositae.

Species used: There are 36, or 60, or pi? species in the *Eupatorium* genus, taxonomists being troublesome again. Nearly all are native to the Americas, *Eupatorium cannabinum* being an exception. Many of the species in the genus are medicinal, and some do have a very similar range of action. However, this is the one I know best, so *Eupatorium perfoliatum* it is.

Common names: Boneset, common boneset, throughwort, agueweed, feverwort, sweating plant — but no one has used those last three names since 1885. (And it's pronounced A-gyew-weed, not aaagh-weed, big fella.)

Parts Used

Aerial parts, in flower or just before flowering, depending.

Preparation and Dosage

The herb is bitter and about as much fun to drink as a tea made from earwax. Honey helps considerably . . . and if you have the kind of flu where you can't taste anything. Generally, the herb is taken as tea or tincture but few take the tincture directly on the tongue. Too bitter.

TEA

Cold tea: Combine 1 ounce of herb with 1 quart boiling water, and let steep overnight. Strain and drink throughout the day. The cold infusion is better for the mucous membrane system and as a liver tonic. If you want to help fevers, you need to take the tea hot.

Hot tea: Combine 1 teaspoon herb with 8 ounces hot water, and let steep 15 minutes. Take 4–6 ounces up to 4x daily. Boneset is only diaphoretic when hot and should be consumed hot for active infections or for recurring chills and fevers.

TINCTURE

Fresh herb in flower: Use a 1:2 herb:liquid ratio, with 95 percent alcohol. Dosage: 20–40 drops in hot water up to 3x daily.

Dry herb: Use a 1:5 herb:liquid ratio, with 60 percent alcohol. Dosage: 30–50 drops in hot water up to 3x daily.

For acute viral or bacterial upper respiratory infections: Take 10 drops of tincture in hot water every half hour up to 6x daily.

For chronic conditions: When the acute stage has passed but there is continued chronic fatigue and relapse, take 10 drops of tincture in hot water 4x daily.

Side Effects and Contraindications

For some reason the phytohysteria surrounding elder is not present with this herb. Boneset is an emetic when taken in large doses, so an early sign that you may be taking too much is *nausea*. Generally, the cooler the tea the less nausea. However, the tea really must be taken hot to help fevers. The herb *may* be contraindicated in pregnancy but no one really seems to know why. *Sometimes* some people have an allergic reaction to plants in this family (chamomile, feverfew, ragwort, tansy), so if you are allergic to those, careful with this one.

Herb/Drug Interactions

None noted.

Habitat and Appearance

The plant is pervasive in the eastern half of the United States and Canada, from Texas, Oklahoma, North Dakota, and so on eastward. However, every place I've seen it grow has been wettish, humid, with good soil.

Boneset grows up to 3 feet tall, they say. I've never seen it get that big, but most of my experience of the plant has been in the tiny state of Vermont. Two feet seems about average, just as with hominids. The plant grows in a straight stalk, the leaves going north-south, then east-west, then north-south again. The leaves continue on through the stalk, hence throughwort; it basically looks like the opposing leaves were glued together at the wide end and the stalk just punched through them. Once seen, never forgotten.

Cultivation and Collection

The plant is a perennial and likes full or partial sun in moist to wet conditions, on the edges of swamps, along streams, in wet meadows, in marshlands, basically anyplace mosquitos like to breed except maybe old tires. It spreads by seed; there are a lot of sources on the Internet.

If collected at flowering and allowed to dry the plant will usually go to seed as it dries. It should only be collected in flower (August or September) if being tinctured fresh and *right now*. If you are going to use it as a tea, it should be picked just prior to flowering, hung upside down in a shaded place, and allowed to thoroughly air-dry. If you pick it in flower and try to dry it then, it will go to seed as it is hanging there, like a bat, upside down, waiting to come suck your blood late in the night, and there will be a mess.

Finding It

Fields and streams in the eastern United States, the Internet, herb stores here and there. Horizon Herbs sells the seeds.

Properties of Boneset

Actions

Analgesic	Emetic (mild)	Mucous membrane tonic
Antibacterial (mild)	Febrifuge	
Anti-inflammatory	Gastric bitter	Peripheral circulatory stimulant
Antiviral	Immunostimulant	
Cytotoxic	(increases	Smooth muscle relaxant
Diaphoretic	phagocytosis)	

Active Against

There hasn't been a lot of testing of this plant as an antimicrobial. It is mildly active against some Gram-positive bacteria such as *Staphylococcus aureus* and *Bacillus megaterium*. It is stronger in its actions against malarial parasites (*Plasmodium* spp.), making it essentially a midlevel anti-plasmodial herb. It has pretty good activity as an antiviral against influenza A (H1N1). Although not tested for it, I do believe this species is active against some, if not all, serotypes of dengue.

The eupatoriums do have a range of action against viruses but there has been much too little work on them. *Eupatorium patens* is active against dengue-2, HSV-1, and HSV-2; *Eupatorium articulatum* against HSV-1 and vesicular stomatitis virus (VSV); *Eupatorium glutinosum* against

Plant Chemistry

Methylglucuronoxylan, astragalin, eufoliatin, eufoliatorin, eupatorin, euperfolin, euperfolitin, euperfolide, euccannabinolide, eupatoriopicrin, hyperoside, rutin, polysaccharides, a number of guaianolides, and a bunch of other stuff. Many of those are sesquiterpene lactones, common in the eupatoriums. There are a number of caffeic acid derivatives in the plant, at least five flavonoid glycosides, and a number of dicaffeoylglucaric acid derivatives that are considered unusual. (And if David

VSV; *Eupatorium bunifolium* against herpes simplex viruses. Most of these eupatoriums have been used similarly to boneset.

Note: Because of the common name *boneset* some people think this eupatorium good for setting bones. Others, however, insist that the name came from a common, ancient name for dengue, breakbone fever, and that the herb has never been used for setting bones and, more, indigenous peoples never used it for that either. (Feelings run high.) I have taken various sides in this over the years but did think it highly amusing a number of years ago when a well-respected indigenous herbalist (from the United States) who had used the herb for over 50 years (and who had learned its use from *her* teacher when she was very small) informed a rather self-satisfied group of herbalists that she used the herb primarily for setting broken bones (as a compress/poultice) and had done so all of her life. (So, now, I read fiction novels and don't think about why it is called what it is called.)

Use to Treat

Influenza, dengue fever, malaria, all viral infections with intermittent fever (hot, then cold, then hot, then . . .), and aches and pains. Comment: I consider the plant a useful adjunct botanical for intermittent viral infections (flu, malaria, dengue), not a primary treatment botanical. It will really help lower fevers. It will help with the aches and pains of viral infections. It *will* make you sweat (if taken hot as a tea, as it should be).

Hoffmann is reading this that means: depsides of hydroxycinnamic acids with hexaric acids.) These unusual compounds are particularly high in the flowers.

Traditional Uses

AYURVEDA
Nope, but there are other eupatoriums used in this system.

TRADITIONAL CHINESE MEDICINE

No, but there are other eupatoriums used in this system.

WESTERN BOTANIC PRACTICE

The plant, indigenous to North America, has been used by native peoples for millennia, specifically for intermittent fevers and chills, with pain in the bones, weakness, and debility. The American Eclectics used it for intermittent (i.e., malarial), typhoid, and remittent fevers, for general debility, pneumonia, cough, epidemic influenza, colds, catarrh, and pains accompanying those conditions. It was one of their primary remedies.

Scientific Research

The sesquiterpene lactones in boneset have a large range of actions. They are highly immunostimulatory and very active against cancers. One study found the herb itself to be potently cytotoxic, in essence comparable to the strength of the pharmaceutical chlorambucil.

The specific lactone active against the malarial parasite is considered to be a dimeric guaianolide. It has a range of antiplasmodial actions but is strongest against *Plasmodium falciparum*. The action is mild (compared to herbs such as cryptolepis) but if the plant is added to a traditional antimalarial that is strong, such as cryptolepis, the effects are mutually supportive. A homeopathic formulation of boneset was found to significantly inhibit plasmodial replication (60 percent inhibition). And an in vivo study with mice found that the homeopathic preparation of the herb did inhibit plasmodial parasites but not completely.

South and Central American healers have been using homeopathic preparations of boneset to try and minimize the impacts of dengue fever outbreaks. In Rio in 2008, a homeopathic preparation containing phosphorus (30c), *Crotalus horridus* (30c), and *Eupatorium perfoliatum* (30c) was given to nearly 160,000 people. The incidence of the disease, compared to the same time period the year before, fell by 93 percent. In comparison, in areas not using the homeopathic preparation the disease incidence increased 128 percent. (Note: A few other, much smaller studies with the homeopathic of eupatorium itself for the common cold and dengue fever — though the people who were ill were not actually tested for dengue [the researchers guessed based on symptoms] — did not find any usefulness from the preparation.)

Clinical trials have shown that boneset stimulates phagocytosis better than echinacea, is analgesic (at least as effective as aspirin), and reduces cold and flu symptoms. In mice it has shown strong immunostimulant activity and cytotoxic action against cancer cells.

The herb is a decent anti-inflammatory. It is anti-inflammatory for lipopolysaccharide-stimulated macrophages, primarily by inhibiting NO and iNOS expression. CSF-3, IL-1α and ß, and the chemokines CCL2, CCL22, and CXCL10 are all inhibited. TNF-α is moderately inhibited. Indications are that it inhibits NF-κB.

Again, despite boneset's long use and potent reputation little research has occurred with the plant.

ANTIVIRAL SUPPLEMENTS

While there are a number of supplements that do help during viral infections (vitamin C, vitamin B complex) zinc seems the most crucial, while monolaurin has shown some good antiviral activity in vitro and users report help from its addition to viral protocols.

ZINC

Zinc has been found active against a number of viruses (alphaviruses) and supportive in treatment for others (influenza, HIV). Studies have found that zinc supplements can triple the survival rate for children with pneumonia, for example, and that it significantly reduces the duration of the common cold.

Dosage: 10–25 mg daily depending on age and weight; 25–40 mg daily during acute episodes.

MONOLAURIN

Monolaurin is one of the major constituents of coconut oil and one of the factors in "the coconut oil miracle." It has been found, in vitro, to be active against measles, HIV, HSV-1 and HSV-2, hepatitis, Epstein-Barr, infectious bronchitis virus, rubella virus, Newcastle virus, dengue (four serotypes), lymphocytic choriomeningitis, vesicular stomatitis virus, visna virus, cytomegalovirus, influenza viruses, pneumonovirus, and respiratory syncytial virus. Caveat: Most of these in vitro studies are hard to find; many of the assertions come from people connected with products, or are merely repetitions of other sources. There are very few in vivo studies, and even fewer with people. However, the constituent is considered safe (it's on the FDA's "Generally Recognized as Safe" list) and it has shown some very good effects against HIV in in vivo studies. I have seen some people experience good healing with it.

Dosage: 2–4 grams per day.

SUPPORTING LYMPH FUNCTION

During many viral infections, especially those that affect the lungs, the lymph system can become overloaded, the nodes severely inflamed, the spleen enlarged. Herbs that stimulate lymph action are very important to use. My favorite one is red root.

Red Root

Family: Rhamnaceae.

Species used: *Homo dissertationus* has determined that there are
50 or 60 or 4³ species of *Ceanothus* in the Americas, from Canada to
Guatemala. The genus doesn't grow anyplace else, at least not *natively*,
though it is an ornamental throughout most of the world in one species
shape or another.

Most species can be used medicinally; the most common are *C.
velutinus*, *C. cuneatus*, *C. integerrimus*, *C. greggii*, and *C. americanus*.
All species are apparently identical in their medicinal actions. My personal favorite is *Ceanothus fendleri*, a.k.a Fendler's ceanothus, which
grows in my region and which I have been using for over 25 years.
The important part is the color of the bark — see "Cultivation and
Collection" on page 256.

Common name: Red root mostly, but in the old days it was supposedly called New Jersey tea (so they say; I never heard anyone say that
phrase, at least when referring to something that does not inebriate).

Part Used

The root or inner bark of the root.

Preparation and Dosage

Red root can also be used as a tincture tea, strong decoction, gargle, or
capsules (but really, I think the tincture is best).

TINCTURE

Dry root, in a 1:5 herb:liquid ratio, with 50 percent alcohol. Dosage:
30–90 drops up to 4x daily.

TEA

1 teaspoon powdered root in 8 ounces water, simmer 15 minutes,
strain. Dosage: Drink up to 6 cups daiy.

STRONG DECOCTION

1 ounce herb in 16 ounces water, simmer slowly for 30 minutes, covered. Dosage: 1 tablespoon 3x or 4x per day.

GARGLE

In cases of tonsillitis or throat inflammation gargle with strong tea 4–6x per day.

CAPSULES

Take 10–30 "00" capsules per day if you must.

Side Effects and Contraindications

No side effects have been noted; however red root is contraindicated in pregnancy.

Herb/Drug Interactions

Should not be used with pharmaceutical coagulants or anticoagulants.

Habitat and Appearance

The various species in this genus seemingly grow everywhere in North and Central America, from Canada to Guatemala, from sea-level coastal scrublands to pine forests at 9,000 feet (2,750 m) or higher. They can grow in hot, humid locations and semiarid desert areas. They are widely divergent in appearance, too, from tiny deciduous ground covers (up to 12 inches tall) to large evergreen bushes (to 9 feet tall) to "small" trees to 25 feet in height. Their foliage ranges from tiny leathery leaves to large broad softies. Some species' branches have "spines," some don't. They do all have leaves though, so identification should not be a problem.

The flowers grows in tufted clusters and are intensely fragrant. (Yummy to my nose — at least with *C. fendleri.*) The seed capsules are identical on all species I have seen, three-lobed triangular things that, again in all species I have seen, turn a reddish color, the exact color of the root bark (and tincture), when mature. That and the flowers, once you have seen them, are the easiest ways to identify the genus.

Cultivation and Collection

This genus has been intensively cultivated and there are scores if not hundreds of cultivars and hybrids. Adding to the confusion, the plants mix with abandon in the wild and . . . well, basically they just have sex whenever and with whomever they wish and the result is a very variable genus. In any event, you can get a large number of types if you wish to grow the species yourself. The genus should grow in just about any geographical location and it has made a home in other places than the Americas by masquerading as an ornamental; it is common in the UK and the EU. It will soon (I hope) escape into the wild, where it will be found to be invasive, for in ceanothus habitat, there are some two million seeds produced per acre once the plants establish themselves. They are propelled under great force out of the capsules (to extend their range) and can remain viable for centuries. I really love these guys.

The plants are propagated by seed or cuttings. The seeds need to be scarified first (show them horror films?) and then stratified. They are usually soaked in water for 12 hours followed by chilling for 3 months — mimicking winter.

The roots/inner root bark should be harvested in the fall or early spring — whenever the root has already had a good frost. The inner bark of the root should be a bright red and this color should extend through the white woody root as a pink tinge after a freeze. The root must look like this to be actively medicinal. If you get the roots in the late spring, summer, or early fall, they will be white throughout with just a hint of pink in the inner bark. They just will not work like that. It takes that cold snap to stimulate the production of the chemical constituents that you need the plant for.

Caution: The root is extremely tough when it dries. It should be cut into small 1- or 2-inch pieces with plant snips while still fresh or you will regret it. Really. Trust me on this one thing.

Store the cut and dried roots in plastic bags in large plastic bins in a cool place and they will last you for years.

Properties of Red Root

Actions

First and foremost red root is a lymph system stimulant and tonic. It is anti-inflammatory for both the liver and spleen. It is also an astringent, mucous membrane tonic, alterative, antiseptic, expectorant, antispasmodic, and exceptionally strong blood coagulant.

Finding It

North and Central America, the Internet, herb stores. In gardens nearly everywhere. It is commonly planted throughout the UK and the EU — though the herbalists in those regions, for the most part, have not yet cottoned on to that fact. It will grow well in those regions, or . . . you can sneak into a garden some night and dig some. Just be really, really quiet.

Alternatives: Poke root (*Phytolacca*) is an excellent alternative. Dosage however should be one-third that of red root. As well, poke itself contains some fairly potent antiviral compounds in the fruit, root, and so on. The pokeweed antiviral protein has been shown to cure mice of HIV infection and is apparently active against a wide range of viruses. I have a feeling about poke . . . it may turn out to be a much more important medicinal than we have thought it to be.

Cleavers will have some of the same effects but the dosage should be four times that of red root. The fresh juice of the plant is best. Cleavers, additionally, strongly inhibits elastase (by about 60 percent) and is useful for bacteria that use elastase as part of their infection strategy.

Plant Chemistry

Betulin, betulinic acid, bacteriohopanetetrol, ceanothic acid, ceanothenic acid, ceanothine, ceanothamine, ceanothane, americine, integerressine, integerrenine, integerrine, methyl salicylate, a lot of tannins, flavonoids, flavonol glycosides, flavonones, dihydroflavonols. The leaves have a somewhat different profile, but I won't include it here as the root is what we are dealing with. The plant is fairly high in protein, iron, copper, zinc, magnesium and very high in calcium. The roots are nitrogen fixers and possess nitrogen-filled nodules.

Traditional Uses

Red root is an important herb in many disease conditions in that it helps facilitate clearing of dead cellular tissue from the lymph system. When the immune system is responding to acute conditions or the onset of disease, as white blood cells kill bacterial and viral pathogens they are taken to the lymph system for disposal. If the lymph system clears out dead cellular material rapidly the healing process is enhanced, sometimes dramatically. The herb shows especially strong action whenever any portion of the lymph system is swollen, infected, or inflamed. This includes the lymph nodes, tonsils (entire back of throat), spleen, appendix, and liver.

AYURVEDA

Nope.

TRADITIONAL CHINESE MEDICINE

Not remotely.

WESTERN BOTANIC PRACTICE

Red root has a very long history in the Americas. The indigenous cultures used the plant for a wide range of complaints from arthritis to influenza, primarily as an astringent. The early American herbalists picked it up and the Eclectics then developed the use of the plant considerably, using it as an astringent, expectorant, sedative, antispasmodic, and antisyphilitic. It was used specifically for gonorrhea, dysentery, asthma, chronic bronchitis, whooping cough, general pulmonary problems, and oral ulcerations due to fever and infection.

Its primary use, however, was for enlarged spleen and, to some extent, enlarged liver.

Scientific Research

There hasn't been much study on the plant, however, and really nothing looking in depth at its actions on the lymph system, including the spleen, though there are some nice hints here and there.

In recent years there has been a minor amount of exploration on the antimicrobial actions of red root. Several of the root compounds have been found active against various oral pathogens including *Streptococcus mutans, Actinomyces viscosus, Porphyromonas gingivalis*, and *Prevotella intermedia*. The flowers are active against *Staphylococcus aureus* and a couple of candida species; the roots probably are, too.

Betulin and betulinic acid, which are fairly prominent in the root, have a broad range of actions, both in vivo and in vitro: antiplasmodial, antiviral, anti-inflammatory, anthelmintic, antioxidant, antitumor, immunomodulatory. Ceanothane is a fairly strongly antistaphylococcal, antiplasmodial, and antimycobacterial. These various actions are going to have some effect on bacterial and viral diseases but exactly what and how much is not clear.

There is some evidence that red root's activity in the lymph nodes also enhances the lymph nodes' production of lymphocytes, specifically the formation of T cells. Clinicians working with AIDS patients, who have historically low levels of T cells, have noted increases after the use of red root.

It is especially effective in reducing inflammation in the spleen and liver from such things as excessive bacterial garbage, white blood cell detritus in the lymph, and red blood cell fragments in the blood in diseases like babesiosis. There is evidence, clinical, that it has broad action throughout the lymph system and helps reduce not only the spleen but also the appendix when inflamed and that it stimulates lymph drainage as well in the intestinal walls.

A number of human trials have occurred using the herb as a tincture extract (usually 10–15 ml per person). The trials focused on heavy bleeding including excessive menstruation, and the plant was found to be a powerful coagulant and hemostatic in all studies. A marked reduction of clotting time was noted.

In one study, a single oral administration of 3.5–7.0 ml of a hydro-alcoholic (tincture) extract of ceanothus (species *americanus*) resulted in an interesting effect: At low doses accelerated blood clotting occurred within 10–20 minutes after administration. However, at higher doses coagulation *decreased* 1 hour after administration. This raises interesting speculations about the herb's range of actions.

In vivo studies have shown marked hemostatic activity and hypotensive action. In vitro studies have also found a strong reverse transcriptase inhibition and a broad antifungal activity.

6

STRENGTHENING THE IMMUNE SYSTEM

It is the body which ultimately controls infections, not chemicals.
Without underlying immunity, drugs are meaningless.

— Marc Lappé

One of the great lessons from the AIDS epidemic is the realization, among the medical establishment, of the necessity for a healthy immune system. Among those with infections such as tick-borne encephalitis, influenza, Lyme, mycoplasma, and bartonella (as examples) researchers have constantly noted that the healthier the immune system, the less likely one is to be infected and, if infected, the less severe the course of the disease.

The immune system is an "organ" just as our lungs and livers are and there are things you can do to keep the immune system healthy. Regular touching is one of them, such as receiving Swedish massage on a weekly or monthly basis. Certain foods do help immune health as well. Some of the best foods that support immune health are:

- **Yogurt.** Regular intake does result in fewer sick days. The body's white blood cell count increases substantially and the GI tract bacterial community remains very healthy, which also helps. Kefir can also be used.

- **Oats and barley.** Farm animals given a mix of the two have many fewer infections, including those from influenza. (And yes, in spite of rumors to the contrary, we actually are animals, too.)

- **Garlic.** Although not as strong an antibiotic as I had formerly thought, regular garlic intake does boost immune function — in one study, those taking garlic were much less likely to catch colds and flu.

- **Selenium-rich foods** have been found to help clear influenza infections from the body. Selenium is found highest (in descending order) in Brazil nuts, fish (tuna, cod, halibut, sardines, flounder, salmon), poultry (chicken and turkey), sunflower seeds, shellfish (oysters, mussels, shrimp, clams, scallops), meat (liver, beef, lamb, pork), eggs, mushrooms, whole grains, wheat germ, onions, garlic, asparagus, broccoli, tomatoes. One ounce of Brazil nuts (usually just called "nuts" in Brazil) will supply 544 mcg of selenium — you don't need many; one Brazil nut can supply a whole day's supply of selenium. To give a comparison, tuna fish contains 68 mcg per ounce, cod 32 mcg per ounce, turkey 27 mcg, sunflower seeds 23, oysters 22, and so on.

- **Chicken soup.** Yes, it does work.

- **Black tea.** It significantly increases the immune system's interferon levels. Green tea will also be of benefit.

- **Zinc-containing foods.** Zinc is an essential mineral, especially in immune function. It enhances the actions of many of the immune system's actors, including T cells. Zinc is highest in oysters, wheat germ, liver, seeds (highest in sesame, tahini, pumpkin, squash, and watermelon seeds), roast beef, dark chocolate and cocoa, lamb, peanuts, garlic, chickpeas. To give you an idea of levels: Oysters concentrate zinc (and copper as well). One medium oyster contains about 13 mg of zinc, 3 ounces of wheat germ contains 17 mg, calf liver has about 12 mg per 3 ounces, sesame seeds contain about 8 mg per 3 ounces, and so on.

- **Mushrooms.** But not the usual store-bought variety. Shiitake and maitake can both be used in cooking, and they are both very good for raising immune function, primarily due to their high levels of polysaccharides. Their polysaccharides raise immune function considerably when taken as a regular part of the diet.

- **And of course:** ginger in the diet, broccoli and other members of that family (all have some of the same properties as isatis), red bell peppers (which are, gram for gram, higher in vitamin C than anything else on the planet), and oregano.

And then there are the herbs.

Immune Herbs

These are my favorite three herbs for optimizing immune function. All three are tonic herbs, can be taken in large quantities, and help the immune system respond to any adverse events that may occur. They tend to act as adaptogens, that is, substances that alter the body's responses to stressors (either internal — think "illness" — or external — think "my job") in such a way as to maximize healthy functioning. If you have low energy, or a low-functioning element of the immune system, these will raise them. If you have an overabundance of energy (stressed out) or an overactive immune system, these will lower or calm function.

Of special note: These herbs also have some activity against viruses, including influenza and encephalitis viruses, making them nicely synergistic with the herbal antivirals in this book. They also very specifically reduce the cytokine cascades many of these viruses initiate *and* raise just the right immune markers necessary to reduce the viral invasion of the body. They are very good herbs. They are: astragalus, cordyceps, and rhodiola.

Astragalus

Family: Leguminosae.

Species used: This is a huge genus of some 3,000 species, prevalent throughout the world. The primary species used is *Astragalus membranaceus*, a.k.a. *A. membranaceus* var. *mongholicus*, a.k.a. *A. mongholicus*. Sigh . . . now that the number of species in this genus has been, almost, settled, the number of variants is in question. (*Yes*, this one is *Astragalus membranaceus* but it looks funny. I found it in Mongolia, therefore …)

There is not much information on whether any of the other species in the genus can be used similarly. Most sources say not. However the Chinese are doing some good work with different species and finding a range of antibacterial, antiviral, anti-inflammatory, analgesic, and some immunomodulatory actions in them that are similar to those of the main medicinal species. The species they are looking at are *A. adsurgens*, *A. aksuensis*, *A. brachystachys*, *A. siculus*, *A. strictus*, *A. verrucosu*, and *A. verus*, so there are quite a few out there that are possibly good medicinals.

Synonyms: *Astragalus propinquus* is, in some circles, a synonym for *A. membranaceus*. However, a number of sources now insist (cue shocked expression) that *this* is the correct name for the plant. And of course, *Astragalus mongholicus* is just the aromatic reproductive expression of a woody perennial of the genus *Rosa* by any other name.

Common names: Astragalus (English), huang-qi (Chinese).

Part Used

The plant is a perennial with a long fibrous rootstock. The root, which is the part used for medicine, is often found thinly sliced and dried (a traditional preparation in Chinese medicine) and most closely resembles a yellow (medical) tongue depressor. Bulk quantities of the powdered or coarsely ground organic root are commonly available through herbal suppliers to Western botanic practitioners.

Preparation and Dosage

Many astragalus formulations are standardized, though I'm not sure that the literature really supports standardization with this herb.

The root is sometimes standardized for 7,4′-hydroxy-3′-methoxyisoflavone-7 (or just hydroxy-3′-isoflavone-7) but the reasons are not entirely clear for doing so. No literature exists that I can find that lays out why in fact this particular constituent was singled out and not the astragalosides. (Astragaloside IV, for instance, is one of the primary active ingredients of the plant in heart disease. It increases exercise tolerance, reduces chest distress and dyspnea, and optimizes left ventricular function.) The methoxyisoflavone constituent for which the plant is often standardized is an anabolic-type compound that enhances strength and muscle formation and may have some protective actions in upper respiratory infections and on digestive function. Data on its functions are somewhat unclear and hard to come by; I have been unable to locate any clinical or laboratory studies on the constituent — though they must exist somewhere. Their rarity stimulates speculation. A number of manufacturers, however, seem to have cottoned on to this and are now standardizing for astragalosides.

The whole root contains constituents that are essential for treating carditis and enhancing immune function. And, indeed, the majority of the Chinese studies — clinical and laboratory — were with the whole herb.

The herb may be taken as tea, powder, capsules, tincture, or in food.

TINCTURE

Tincture preparations vary considerably in their herb:liquid ratio, from 1:2 and 1:3 up to 1:5, and with alcohol concentrations ranging from 25 to 60 percent. There doesn't seem to be a lot of data on why nor what is the best tincture preparation procedures. However, there is some good data suggesting it be done this way . . .

In general, many of the most potent actions of the plant come from its polysaccharides, and polysaccharides are most efficiently released from the root cells by hot water. This is, in part, why many traditional uses of astragalus involve cooking it or using it as a tea. So, if you are making an extract of, let's say, 5 ounces of astragalus powder, you would then use anywhere from two to five times that amount of water. Many of the manufacturers whose products I think are good use from 40 to 50 percent alcohol for their astragalus tinctures in either a 1:3 or 1:5 tincture ratio. For this example, let's do it this way . . .

Start with 5 ounces of astragalus root powder and 25 ounces of liquid (this makes it a 1:5 ratio). The liquid should be half water and half pure grain alcohol, which will give you a 50 percent alcohol extraction medium. You would be using 12.5 ounces of water. Combine the root with the water *only* in a pot, and bring it to a boil (starting with cold water). As soon as it comes to a boil, turn off the heat and cover. Let it steep overnight. In the morning, put the whole mess in a jar, add the alcohol (12.5 ounces), and tighten the lid. Leave for 2 weeks, shaking when you remember to do so. Then decant.

As for dosages:

As a tonic: 30–60 drops up to 4x daily.

In chronic illness conditions: 1 teaspoon 4x daily.

As a preventive (from viral infection): 1 teaspoon 4–6x daily.

In acute conditions: 1 teaspoon 4–6x daily, generally every 3 hours.

TEA

Put 2–3 ounces of herb in 1 quart of hot water, let steep for 2–3 hours, strain, then drink throughout the day.

POWDER

In chronic conditions: 1 tablespoon 3x per day.

In acute conditions: 2 tablespoons 3x per day.

Your body's own bile and stomach acids will extract the constituents. You can go higher on these doses if you wish. The Chinese use very large doses of the powdered root, from 15 to 60 grams per day, essentially ½ to 2 ounces per day.

FOOD

Astragalus has been used for centuries as an additive to meal preparation. The sliced root is placed in soups and removed before eating or a strong infusion of the root is made and used to cook rice or as a stock for soups.

IMMUNE-ENHANCING BROTH

Robyn Landis and K. P. S. Khalsa share a tasty recipe (below) for an immune-enhancing astragalus broth in their book *Herbal Defense* (Warner Books, 1997).

Immune-Enhancing Broth

INGREDIENTS

3 cups water or vegetable broth

1 ounce astragalus (five "tongue depressor" lengths of the sliced root)

1 bulb (5–10 cloves) fresh garlic, sliced or whole

Salt and pepper to taste

Combine the water, astragalus, and garlic and simmer for several hours, until the garlic is soft. Season with salt and pepper to taste. Consume all the broth if you feel an infection coming on, or take a cup or two several times during the week to prevent infection. Consume the cooked garlic separately, leave in the broth, or use as a spread on toast.

Immune-Enhancing Rice

INGREDIENTS

4 cups water, plus more as needed

1 1/2 ounces sliced astragalus root

2 cups brown rice

Directions

Combine the water and astragalus, bring to boil, and simmer for 2 hours, covered. Remove from the heat and let stand overnight. Remove the astragalus, and add enough water to bring the broth volume back up to 4 cups. Add the rice, bring to a boil, then reduce the heat and simmer, covered, until done, approximately 1 hour. Use this rice as you would any rice, as a base for meals throughout the week.

Side Effects and Contraindications

No toxicity has ever been shown from the regular, daily use of the herb nor from the use of large doses. The Chinese report consistent use for millennia in the treatment of colds and flu and suppressed immune function without side effects.

Astragalus is contraindicated, however, *for some people*, in certain kinds of late-stage Lyme disease because it can exacerbate autoimmune responses in that particular disease. For others it can alter the Th1/Th2 balance and reduce the autoimmune dynamics. Whether or not it acts as a modulator seems to depend on individual reactions to the herb; I haven't been able to find a reason why, for some people, it exacerbates their condition and for others it does not.

Herb/Drug Interactions

Synergistic actions: Use of the herb with interferon and acyclovir may increase their effects. The herb has been used in clinical trials with interferon in the treatment of hepatitis B; outcomes were better than with interferon alone. It has also shown synergistic effects when used with interferon in the treatment of cervical erosion; antiviral activity is enhanced.

Drug inhibition: Use of the herb with cyclophosphamide may decrease the effectiveness of the drug. Not for use in people with transplanted organs.

Herb/Herb Interactions

Synergistic with echinacea and licorice in the stimulation of immune function.

Habitat and Appearance

There are over 3,000 species of astragalus in the world, 16 of which grow in the United States. The leaf structure looks like that of a typical member of the pea family. It is a short-lived, sprawling perennial and grows up to 4 feet in size.

The medicinal astragalus is native to northeast China though it has been planted a great many other places, including the United States. Wild populations are still rare in the West though astragalus is under wide cultivation as a medicinal in the United States and escape to the wild will occur sooner or later.

Cultivation and Collection

Astragalus is started from seeds in the early spring indoors. The seed coat needs to be scored with something like sandpaper prior to planting. Growers (e.g., Elixir Farm in Missouri) have found that it prefers a sunny location with, as the Elixir Farm website notes, "deep, sandy, well-drained, somewhat alkaline soil. It does not like mulch or deep

Properties of Astragalus

Actions

Adaptogen	Diuretic	Immune modulator
Antibacterial	Enhances function in	Immune restorative
Antihepatotoxic	lungs, spleen, and	Immune stimulant
Antiviral	GI tract	Tonic
Cardioprotective	Hypotensive	
	Immune enhancer	

Astragalus is an immune potentiator and modulator. It strongly regulates interferon-gamma and interleukin-2 levels. If interferon-gamma levels are high, it is strongly active in lowering them. Enhances CD4+ counts and balances the CD4:CD8 ratio. Astragalus is specific for immune atrophy and enhances function in the spleen and thymus.

Active Against

While not specifically an antimicrobial herb, astragalus does possess some antimicrobial actions. Most important for this book, it does have antiviral activity. It is active against influenza A (H1N1, FM1), human adenovirus type 3, herpes simplex 1, Coxsackie virus B3, infectious bursal cultivation. The crowns of the emerging plants are very sensitive to compost and respond well after they have gained some momentum in the spring." Not surprisingly, given the plant's medicinal actions, it is highly resistant to insect damage, crown rot, mildew, and drought.

The plant grows larger and more woody each year, with the roots harvested beginning in the fall of the third year or spring of the fourth. Spring and fall harvests occur in China. The root is generally considered too weak a medicinal if harvested prior to that time.

disease virus, cytomegalovirus, Punta Toro virus, Japanese encephalitis virus, porcine parvovirus, hepatitis B and significantly reduces the effects of canine distemper virus in vivo. The herb is strongly protective against infection with Japanese encephalitis virus and bunyavirus if taken prophylactically. Most of its actions come from antivirus stimulation of the immune system.

The herb does have some other antimicrobial effects. It is active against *E. coli*, *Arbiter aerogenes*, *Proteus vulgaris*, *Staphylococcus aureus*, *Salmonella enteritidis*, *Shigella dysenteriae*, *Campylobacter*, *Streptococcus hemolyticus*, *Diplococcus pneumoniae* (a.k.a. *Streptococcus pneumoniae*), *Aeromonas hydrophila*, and *Candida albicans*.

Use to Treat

All viral infections as an immune adjuvant. Many people are beginning to view the herb as a primary immunomodulator to prevent viral infection and illness. It is specific for that purpose.

It is also specific for treating myocarditis from Coxsackie B3 infection. It is specific for reducing the impacts of Japanese encephalitis virus. It is specific as a preventive for reducing the likelihood of infection from Lyme bacteria and reducing the severity of the disease.

Finding It
Herb stores everywhere and the Internet.

Plant Chemistry

Astragalosides 1 through 7, astraisoflavin, astramembranagenin, astrapterocarpan, beta-sitosterol, betaine, formononetin, GABA, isoastragaloside (1, 2, and 4), isoliquiritigenin, linoleic acid, linolenic acid, soyasaponin I, kumatakenin, choline, glucuronic acid, 4'-hydroxy-3'-methoxyisoflavone-7, a couple of dihydroxydimethylisoflavones, 3'-hydroxyformonentin, calcium, folic acid, copper, iron, magnesium, manganese, potassium, sodium, zinc.

Traditional Uses

Astragalus, first mentioned in the 2,000-year-old Chinese text *Shen Nong Cao Jing*, is considered to be one of the superior tonic herbs in Chinese medicine. The plant has become one of the primary immune herbs used worldwide over the past four decades.

AYURVEDA

Five species of astragalus are used in the materia medica of India, none of them this species. They are minor herbs, used primarily as emollients.

TRADITIONAL CHINESE MEDICINE

Astragalus has been a major herb in Chinese medicine for between 2,000 and 4,000 years. It is one of the 50 fundamental herbs in Chinese medicine. Its traditional uses are for spleen deficiency with lack of appetite, fatigue, and diarrhea. It is specific for disease conditions accompanied by weakness and sweating, stabilizes and protects the vital energy (qi), and is used for wasting diseases, numbness of the limbs, and paralysis. Other uses are: for tonifying the lungs, for shortness of breath, for frequent colds and flu infections; as a diuretic and for reduction of edema; for tonifying the blood and for blood loss, especially postpartum; for diabetes; for promoting the discharge of pus, for chronic ulcerations, including of the stomach, and for sores that have not drained or healed well.

WESTERN BOTANIC PRACTICE

The herb was not used to any extent in Western botanic practice until the tremendous East/West herbal blending that began during the 1960s. It is now one of the primary immune tonic herbs in the Western pharmacopoeia.

Scientific Research

A considerable amount of scientific testing has occurred with astragalus, including clinical trials and both in vivo and in vitro studies. PubMed now lists over 5,700 citations for studies with astragalus and this does not include the many Chinese studies that have never been indexed for it. The Chinese database CNKI now has over 16,000 entries on the herb. What follows is merely a sampling.

IMMUNE FUNCTION

Most of the clinical studies and trials regarding immunostimulation have been focused on the use of astragalus in the treatment of cancer and/or as an adjunct to chemotherapy to help stimulate chemo-depressed immune function. A number of other studies have examined its immune effects with a range of different conditions.

The herb has been used with children suffering tetralogy of Fallot after radical operation to correct the condition. Tetralogy of Fallot is a complex of four heart abnormalities that occur together, generally at birth. Surgery is used to correct it. Astragalus was found to decrease abnormal levels of IgG, Igm, C3, C4, CD8+, and CD19+ while increasing levels of CD4+ and CD56+. The ratios of CD4:CD8, CD3:HLA-DR, and CD3:CD16 normalized between the second and third weeks of use. IL-6 and TNF-α both began decreasing in the first week and by the fourth week were in the normal range.

When astragalus was used in the treatment of herpes simplex keratitis levels of Th1, including IL-2 and IFN-γ, increased and Th2 levels, including IL-4 and IL-10, decreased, showing that the herb modulated Th1 and Th2 levels. This same kind of effect has been found in the treatment of numerous cancers. For example in a study of 37 lung cancer patients astragalus was found to reverse the Th2 status normally present in that condition. Th1 cytokines (IFN-γ and IL-2) and its transcript factor (T-bet) were enhanced and Th2 cytokines were decreased.

A clinical study with 63 people suffering serious abdominal traumatic injury found that the addition of astragalus to the treatment regimen significantly increased cellular immunity.

In clinical trials with a number of different cancers and congestive heart conditions, astragalus has been found to increase CD4+ levels, reduce CD8+ levels, and significantly increase the CD4:CD8 ratio. The plant has been found to have a broad immunostimulatory effect. Use of the herb with cancer patients undergoing chemotherapy found that white blood cell counts improved significantly (normalizing). The herb has been found to be specifically useful in preventing or reversing immunosuppression from any source: age, bacterial, viral, or chemical. It enhances phagocytosis and increases superoxide dismutase production from macrophages.

RESPIRATORY INFECTIONS

Eighty-eight children with recurrent respiratory infections were split into two groups. One received astragalus, the other did not. The children were followed for 1 year. Those in the astragalus group had significantly fewer occurrences.

HEART DISEASE

There have been numerous clinical trials with the herb for treating heart disease. The herb has been found specific for inhibiting Coxsackie B infections, both as an antiviral and as a heart protector. It will reverse damage to the heart in a number of conditions. With respect to Lyme carditis probably the most important of its impacts are those on left ventricular function, angina, and shortness of breath. While it is not completely protective for atrioventricular (AV) block it does improve electrophysiological parameters and ameliorates AV block to some extent.

In a trial of astragalus for 2 weeks with 19 people with congestive heart failure, 15 people experienced alleviation of symptoms of chest distress and dyspnea, and their exercise tolerance increased substantially. Radionuclide ventriculography showed that left ventricular modeling and ejection function improved, and heart rate slowed from 88.21 to 54.66 beats/minute.

In another trial, 43 people suffering from myocardial infarction were tested with astragalus. Left ventricular function strengthened. Superoxide dismutase activity or red blood cell levels increased, and lipid peroxidation of plasma was reduced.

In a study with 366 cardiac patients astragalus was found to be effective when compared to lidocaine and mexiletine (which were not found effective). With astragalus the duration of ventricular late potentials shortened significantly.

In the treatment of 92 patients suffering ischemic heart disease, astragalus was more successful than nifedipine. Patients were "markedly relived" from angina pectoris. EKG test results improved 82.6 percent.

ANTI-INFLAMMATORY ACTIVITY

Astragalus has been found to possess anti-inflammatory activity by inhibiting the NF-κB pathway and blocking the effect of IL-1ß in leukotriene C production in human amnions. The constituent astragaloside IV inhibits increases in microvascular permeability induced by histamine. The whole herb decoction has been found to reduce capillary hyperpermeability. It is strongly inhibitive of TGF-ß as well.

NEUROLOGICAL ACTIONS

Astragalus was found to improve anisodine-induced impairment of memory acquisition and alcohol-elicited deficit of memory retrieval. After use of the herb the number of errors were reduced. The plant has been found to exert potent antioxidant effects on the brain, helping to prevent senility.

In one study, 106 newborns with neonatal hypoxic ischemic encephalopathy were separated into two groups. One received oral astragalus granule for 7 months, the other nimodipine for 3 months, then pyritinol for an additional 4 months. There was better recovery in the astragalus group with less long-term negative effects from the initial condition. The incidence of cerebral palsy was markedly reduced. (Another study used injection, with similar outcomes.) Studies on the use of astragalus injection in the treatment of cerebral palsy in children found that it significantly reduced symptoms.

FATIGUE

Astragalus has been found effective in alleviating fatigue in heart patients and in athletes. In one trial, 12 athletes were randomly separated into two groups, and six were given astragalus. Astragalus was found to positively influence anaerobic threshold, enhance recovery from fatigue, and increase fatigue threshold.

A double-blind, randomized, controlled trial with 36 adults with chronic fatigue found that a mixture of astragalus and Salviae Radix significantly decreased fatigue scores.

RENAL EFFECTS

In one study, injection of astragalus was found helpful in reducing negative parameters in patients with chronic glomerulonephritis. In another study astragalus injection was used in the treatment of renal syndrome of hemorrhagic fever. One hundred forty-six people were separated into two groups. One group received ribavirin, the other astragalus. Both groups received IV glucose. The course of the disease was shorter in the astragalus group; renal function was restored more quickly.

HEPATITIS

A number of trials have found the herb effective in the clinical treatment of hepatitis B and liver disease. Liver function is improved, the liver is protected from damage, and regeneration is stimulated.

Cordyceps

Family: Ummm, errrr, uhhhh, well, let's see . . . (Counts on fingers — can I use the thumb? Is it a finger? Or not?). Ophiocordyceps? (Taxonomists really are the most irritating of people.)

Rant

As usual taxonomists are creating trouble for everyone who accepted their formerly completely-accurate-and-no-doubt-about-it descriptions of the natural world. Remember all those lectures we tried not to sleep through, the notes we took that concretely identified parts of the world as this and not that, the tests that we passed (or didn't), and the degrees we got (or didn't) that proved how much we knew? Well, none of it, it turns out, had much to do with the real world. (Cue shocked expression.)

In previous years — well, centuries actually — plants, and ultimately most living organisms, were classified by the system that that irritating man Carl Linnaeus developed. He spent a lot of time looking up plant skirts and describing their sexual organs and physical appearance and then putting them into groups — as did his legions of obedient automatons, I mean, followers. The classification system used in most plant field guides is still oriented around the basic framework he laid down centuries ago.

But . . . with the advent of DNA analysis everything in the natural world is being relabeled, creating a huge shift in the human lens through which the natural world is segmented into its various boxes. In the old model, hippos and whales were very different animals. In the new one, they are each other's closest living relatives. The closest living relatives of birds are now crocodiles and alligators (you can tell by the feathers). The closest living relative of the hyrax, a guinea-pig-like animal (weighing 8 pounds) is now the elephant (which is the only animal that can't jump — my mind's a junkyard). And the closest living relative of the taxonomist is the measuring tape. (Who knew?)

Close examination shows that this new lens is likely to be, ultimately, as unworkable as the old one. There really isn't a basic underlying reality upon which all other things rest that will allow us to conquer our fear of the wild (allowing us to feel in control of all the lesser-evolved organisms on the planet). And as some of the new generations of naturalists are beginning to say (and as Darwin himself said long ago) evolution is not

Species used: *Cordyceps sinensis* almost always though *C. militaris* is considered interchangeable (and by some, stronger), and many of the others in the genus are usable as well.

In total, there are 140 or 480 or 670 members of the *Cordyceps* genus or the *Ophiocordyceps* genus or the *Metacordyceps* genus, or the

an escalator going from there to there (with us riding triumphantly on the top step) but in reality a tremendously tangled bush all woven about itself, every branch equidistant from the center (and all equally important). As those involved in deep, perceptual observations of the real world will find, this new DNA system of ours will itself be found to be flawed (because under every cause is another cause, ad infinitum), which will lead in time to a new classification system that will, again, make all our previous maps unworkable once more.

These classification systems, again, are only *maps*. And maps are not, and never have been, the real world. (Hmmm, the GPS says that this road *does* go through, where the hell did this swamp come from? Hey! Is that an alligator? I mean a bird?) Nevertheless . . .

Once upon a time, there was a large grouping of mushrooms called the cordyceps. (And no, they really aren't mushrooms but are in fact *ascomycetes* and yeah, tomato is a fruit — but no one cares.) And for hundreds of years there were scores, nay, hundreds of mushrooms in the genus. Then came a plague of DNA scientists upon the land and one of them, after much thought, putteth down his tools and he looketh upon the multitude and sayeth, "This is so wrong." And he taketh up his measuring tape and toucheth his chalk to the board and then he writeth for those among us who haveth ears . . .

"The Species *Cordyceps sinensis* of the Genus that we have known as *Cordyceps* of the Family called *Clavicipitaceous* is no more. It is casteth out and we place it now in the Family *Ophiocordycipitaceae* and we rename the Genus *Ophiocordyceps*. And the one that was formerly called *Cordyceps sinensis* shall henceforth be known as *Ophiocordyceps sinsensis*."

And drawing the sacred dagger along the ground he declared, "So mote it be." Then a great cry went up throughout the land in-the-year-of-our-DNA-scientist 2007 and thus was this thing done. Woe be to he that heedeth it not.

Still . . .

Elaphocordyceps genus, or all of them together ... or something. (I read the whole 55-page peer-reviewed journal article — three times — but despite having opposable thumbs and a degree in advanced basket weaving, I still can't follow it. Let's see, the seraphim are the ones that hang from the top of the cave ...?).

All of these (prefix)cordyceps mushrooms are endoparasitoids (as distinct from elastoparanoids, i.e., taxonomists). This 10-dollar word simply means that they are parasitic on other living organisms, mostly insects, though a few parasitize other fungi (*turning* on their own kind). The fungus invades and takes over the host's body, replacing its tissues with its own. The main medicinal species that most people use, *Prefix-or-not-cordyceps sinensis*, is a parasite on caterpillars, specifically the larvae of the ghost moth (which is why it is sometimes called the caterpillar fungus). The fungal spores invade the caterpillar (which lives underground), and they sprout into active mycelia (which spread throughout the caterpillar body via the circulatory system), eventually killing the caterpillar (which then mummifies). The mycelia ultimately fill the corpse, leaving the exoskeleton intact, and the mushroom sprouts from the body (via the head) the next summer, and, hey, we got medicine. (Yum!)

Cordyceps species of one sort or another are common throughout the world. Each species is a parasite of either a different arthropod or the one particular mushroom species it likes to parasitize. The range of insect hosts is large: beetles, moth and butterfly pupae and larvae, ants, spiders, grasshoppers, locusts, cicadas, centipedes, bees, and cockroaches, and probably more that no one has found out about yet. Each species of cordyceps has somewhat different medicinal actions, no doubt coming, in part, from what kind of host species it infects (and no, no one has studied this as yet either).

This particular species of *I-guess-it's-a-cordyceps* that we are talking about, the primary one used in medicine, is specific to the Tibetan plateau and the Himalayas in India, Nepal, and Bhutan. It is generally hand-harvested by the local people and is, at this point in time, tremendously expensive (a recent estimate I was given — in 2012 — was

US$1,600 to $2,000 per pound; prices are increasing about 20 percent per year). Cordyceps mushrooms provide a major source of income for people in those regions. Several hundred tons are harvested each year, making up about half the yearly income of the local peoples and about 10 percent of Tibet's GDP.

To lower the cost and to make the herb more available, the mycelia, in China, are now grown (fermented) in vats much like penicillin and other pharmaceuticals. Those manufactured in the West are usually grown on grains (*vegan* cordyceps?). All the commercial varieties of cordyceps you are likely to find are grown, not wild.

Synonyms: *Sphaeria sinensis, Cordyceps sinensis, Ophiocordyceps sinensis.*

Common names: Cordyceps, caterpillar fungus, yartsa (or yatsa) gunbu (Tibetan), keera jhar (India), dong chong xia cao (Chinese, and it translates as "worm in winter, herb in summer"), chong cao (Chinese again, but this term usually refers to species other than *C. sinensis*), tochukaso (Japanese), aweto (Maori, New Zealand), club mushroom (United States — we are a poetic people but we walk really softly).

Part Used

Grown varieties: the mycelium. Wild-harvested: the whole damn thing — caterpillar body, fruiting mushroom, and all.

Preparation and Dosage

Cordyceps needs to be viewed as a medicinal *food*, not a raw drug to be taken in minute doses. The Chinese tonic dosages are normally rather large, 3 to 9 grams per day, and during acute disease conditions they can go as high as 50 grams, nearly 2 ounces, per day.

If you think of the herb as a food, then eating 2 ounces, say, as you do of asparagus or potatoes, doesn't seem like all that much. In China, cordyceps is often added to soups and stews (just as astragalus is) as a food ingredient for chronic illness. Sometimes the Chinese decoct it in water and drink it as a tea; however traditional healers for millennia in

Tibet and India (and in parts of China) used the herb only after soaking it in an alcohol/water combination, usually the local alcoholic drink. And in fact a number of the constituents are only extractable in alcohol.

The best way to use the herb is either as a powder preparation, taken directly by mouth (allowing the stomach acids and bile, etc., to extract for you), or as a tincture.

For acute viral infections, especially in the brain and CNS, and systemic mycoplasma, especially with brain/CNS involvement, I would recommend you buy the powder in bulk from someone such as 1stChineseHerbs.com and then take 3–4 tablespoons of the powder blended in water or juice three times daily.

The tepid U.S. dosages, 500–1,000 mg daily, are useless for any active disease condition.

CAPSULES

The Chinese brands, if you buy capsules, run around 900–1,000 mg per capsule and the suggested dose is 6,000 mg (6 grams) per day — just for a tonic dose. If you want to use the capsules for active viral infections in the brain and CNS I would double that.

TINCTURES

As a tonic: $^{1}/_{4}$–$^{1}/_{2}$ teaspoon 3x daily.

For active infections: $^{1}/_{2}$–1 teaspoon 3–6x daily.

Note: If you are going to make your own tincture from cordyceps powder, then use a 50 percent alcohol solution in a 1:5 herb:liquid ratio. Add the cordyceps powder to the water *only*. Starting with cold water, bring the mixture to a boil, then cover and let steep overnight. *Then* add the alcohol and let it steep for a few weeks. This will more efficiently extract the polysaccharides from the root.

Some sources recommend taking cordyceps with vitamin C to help assimilation. There isn't anything in the scientific literature on this and the Asians used the herb (and noted its beneficial effects) for thousands of years before vitamin C was discovered, so . . . not sure where that urban legend came from.

Side Effects and Contraindications

There are no side effects noted in the literature. Up to 5 grams per kilogram of body weight per day have been used in rats long term with no side effects. That would be 350 grams — i.e., about 12 ounces or $3/4$ pound — in a person weighing 150 pounds. Double that dose was used with rabbits for 3 months with no side effects.

The only reported side effects I can find are occasional reports of dry mouth, nausea, diarrhea. One case of an allergic reaction that subsided when the herb was discontinued.

Herb/Drug and Herb/Herb Interactions

Cordyceps sinensis is synergistic with cyclosporine A and the amount of the drug needed is lessened if cordyceps is taken. The hypoglycemic actions of the herb also reduce the dosage needs for those on antidiabetic medications. There is some concern as well that cordyceps might be synergistic or additive with antiretroviral drugs, thus affecting dosage requirements, but nothing has yet been reported in the literature.

Habitat and Appearance

The most common cordyceps medicinal species are what are called club mushrooms by all the mushroom hunters I know, though some mycofanatics are given to Latinizing, often rolling the consonants trippingly across their tongues. They are generally brownish-to-orangish in color (the mushrooms, not the tongues, though if the tongues *were* brownish-to-orangish this medicine would help clear them up). They look somewhat like a tiny club, narrowing at the bottom, widening at the top, up to 5 inches or so tall (the mushrooms, not the mycologists, though there was this one guy . . .). Basically a very tiny version of something Fred Flintstone might use. Normally they are a bit wrinkled along the sides. There are some other species that have a cap, like other mushrooms, but I have never seen one in person; they tend to be a bit rare in my part of the woods. *Cordyceps militaris* is the one most often found in the United States; it's the only one I have met, and collected, personally, in the Rocky Mountains at 8,000 to 10,000 feet. (*C. sinensis* develops at high altitudes between 10,000 and 16,000 feet, on and in prairies rather than in forests, and tends to be more brownish; *C. militaris* tends more toward orange.)

Most of the cordyceps species specialize in their preferred hosts but *Cordyceps militaris* (go figure) parasitizes the pupae and larvae of numerous moth species and, I have heard, beetles as well. All of the cordyceps tend to sprout from the head of whatever insect they infect. (What *is* this about anyway? Doctrine of signatures? Good for treating mental disorders?) *Cordyceps*, by the way, means "club head," *cord* being club, *ceps* head, while *y* is a query referent, e.g., why.

Most of the species that have been found exist in Asia (about 100 in China alone) but there are somewhere between 5 and 20 in the United States depending on how many digits the taxonomists are using to count them. The U.S. species commonly parasitize cicadas, beetles, and moth larvae and pupae. *Cordyceps cardinalis* for example is moderately common in the southern Appalachian mountains of the eastern United States (and also in southeastern Japan). It is closely related to *C. militaris* (or *C. pseudomilitaris*, which only pretends to be violent), the species that has the largest geographical distribution, having been found on all continents except Antarctica. (Antarctica means "no bears," another useless fact I can't get out of my brain.)

C. militaris grows throughout the United States and is especially common in the Rocky Mountains, the Carolinas, and along the East Coast, often in mountainous regions. It is the primary medicinal species that is easy to find wild in this country. It is used similarly to *C. sinensis* and there have been some decent studies on its effects (150 or so on PubMed, versus 300 on *C. sinensis*).

Properties of Cordyceps

Actions

Adrenogenic	Antitumor	Immunomodulator
Antiasthmatic	Antitussive	Insecticidal
Antibacterial	Bronchial regulator	Mitochondrial
Anticonvulsant	Cardiotonic	adaptogen
Anti-inflammatory	Expectorant	Nerve sedative
Antimetastic	Hepatoprotective	Neuroprotective
Antimicrobial	Hypoglycemic	Renoprotective
Antioxidant	Hypolipidemic	Sleep regulator
Antipyretic	Immunoadaptogen	Steroidogenic

Cordyceps is a rather potent immunoadaptogen. If immune activity is high, it reduces it; if low, it enhances it. When taken regularly, if the immune system is stressed by, say, a bacterial organism, the herb will stimulate the immune system in just the right way to respond to the stressor while lowering the levels of or inhibiting entirely the bacterial-induced cytokines that are generated.

As a mitochondrial adaptogen, it increases oxygen utilization in the mitochondria, stimulates ATP production by the mitochondria, and protects mitochondria from adverse events. As a hepatoprotective, it offers autoimmune protection, reduces fibrosis, reduces and inhibits cirrhosis, and protects against hepatitis B. As a renoprotective, it protects from toxicity, inhibits renal failure, and reverses glomerulonephritis. And as a cardiotonic, it is hypotensive, strengthens heartbeat, is antiarrhythmic, and improves myocardial ischemia.

Active Against

Cordyceps is not primarily an antibacterial but is rather a systemic tonic and adaptogen. Still it does have some antimicrobial actions. It is active against some viruses, a few strongly so — influenza virus (H1N1, H9N2), herpes simplex virus 1, HIV-1 protease, hepatitis B, Newcastle virus — and a number of other microbes such as *Mycobacterium tuberculosis*, *Plasmodium* spp., *Clostridium* spp., *Staphylococcus aureus* (resistant and nonresistant), *Enterococcus faecalis*, *Bacillus subtilis*, *Candida albicans*, and various cancers (breast, thyroid, kidney, bladder, prostate, lung, Leydig cell tumor, melanoma). Its antiviral actions make

Continued on next page

Continued from previous page

it a perfect immune adjunct for use in treating most major viral infections.

The herb, while not generally active against bacteria, is, however, highly protective of the human body when bacterial infections occur. For example, in one study, mice were fed either phosphate buffered saline (PBS) or *Cordyceps sinensis* mycelium for 3 days and then infected with *Streptococcus pyogenes.* The PBS group showed bacterial dissemination throughout their bodies, while those in the cordyceps group did not. Only 40 percent of the PBS group survived until day 8, while at day 10 70 percent of the cordyceps group were still alive. In addition the PBS group showed extensive skin necrosis, none in the cordyceps group did.

Survival was significantly increased if the cordyceps group received more cordyceps every other day. In fact, *all* of the cordyceps-treated group then survived while ALT and AST levels remained normal. Use of the extract, in vitro, against the same bacterial strain showed *no* direct anti-bacterial activity at all.

Use to Treat

Any respiratory viral infection, any inflammation in the brain or CNS — especially encephalitis and meningitis, fatigue and weakness, especially after long illness or in chronic infections, poor mitochondrial function, chronic wasting, unproductive cough from no known cause, joint inflammation, mental fog and confusion, low libido, lung infections, kidney infections, thick mucus in the lungs that will not move, immune dysregulation, dizziness, tinnitus, nocturia, cancer. It is especially effective for mycoplasma infections.

Finding It

You can get bulk powder and capsules from 1stChineseHerbs.com (www.1stchineseherbs.com) as well as many other places on the Internet. If you want to spend enormous amounts of money, you can also buy the wild-crafted mushroom itself. Or . . . you can join the local mycological society (find a fun one, usually it *won't* include guys with mathematically shaven beards) and learn to find it in the wild.

Cultivation and Collection

I have seen photos of *Cordyceps militaris* being intentionally grown on grain. In fact, the main method to develop fruiting bodies of cordyceps, rather than just the mycelium, is to use grains as a substrate — the first used, and still most common, is rice. There is also a company in Texas, called Unicorn Bags, that sells *C. militaris* spores with detailed inoculation information on how to use live pupae (that is the stage between caterpillar and butterfly). Not my thing really but if you are excited about it look them up (www.unicornbags.com). (First, grasp the pupa firmly, then take your hypodermic needle and . . .)

There is some speculation, but there is little research on it as yet, that the fruiting mushrooms grown on grain have different medicinal actions and chemistry than those found wild and this is true of the vat-grown mycelium as well.

Studies of the gross constituents show a high similarity between the grown and wild species and, when tested, the grown varieties do have very similar impacts in the body. The one in-depth study I have seen does show a variation in chemistry — the same compounds are in both but in differing quantities, the grown having much more of some, less of a few others. One other analysis found that there were some particular compounds in the insect-host-grown cordyceps that were not in the vat-grown. Those compounds tend to be named after the insect host itself, e.g., cicadapeptins. And those compounds do have medicinal actions themselves. Nevertheless, most studies have been with the grown varieties, not the wild, and they have been shown to have range of action very close to that of the wild species.

If you wish to harvest wild cordyceps, especially in the United States, you will most likely find *C. militaris*. I, personally, don't know any of the others in their wild state though some mycofanatics do know of them, find them, and utilize them with supposedly good results. *C. militaris* does have the best research outside of *C. sinensis*; I don't think there is any doubt that the two can be considered interchangeable in action. The Chinese, in practice, apparently agree, and some even think *C. militaris* is better. So, if you want to hunt the wild

cordyceps, look for *C. militaris*. (Easiest way? Join the local mycological society and go hunting with them.)

The best time to harvest the mushroom is in the summer after a
good wet winter or spring — depending on the local climate they can be
found from April to August. I have found them only in the mountains,
in pine forests, usually in July/August. Once you've located one, carefully dig the entire mushroom, including the host insect, which will be
belowground or embedded in rotted wood (or something). Bag it separately from all the other mushroom species you have collected, take
it home, and dry it on an open-air tray in the dark. Watch it carefully
to make sure it does not decay as mushrooms are wont to do (though
these generally are not as wet as most of the other types and so are less
prone to decay once picked). When dry, store in whole form in plastic
bags in plastic tubs, out of the sun.

Plant Chemistry

Three constituents are, at present, considered to be the major active
chemicals in cordyceps: cordycepin (a.k.a. 3′-deoxyadenosine, a
purine alkaloid and a derivative of adenosine), cordycepic acid (a.k.a.
D-mannitol), and cordyceps polysaccharide. Some commercial formulations are standardized for cordycepic acid (usually 10 percent),
others for 7 percent cordycepin or 0.1 percent adenosine (sort of the
same thing). Most are made from cordyceps mycelium and will state
as much on the label.

Vat-fermented cordyceps mycelium contains a lot more cordycepin than the wild mushrooms, 40 mcg per gram versus 5 mcg/g.
Cordycepic acid varies in wild populations, comprising anywhere
from 7 to 29 percent by weight depending on time of year, location,
and so on. The fruiting bodies contain from 30 to 85 mg per gram of
cordycepic acid; the mycelial content is much higher (which is part of
the reason the whole caterpillar is harvested for medicine, not just the
club mushroom itself).

Cordyceps, like most mushrooms, has a very high polysaccharide
content. The main one is considered to be cordyceps polysaccharide

and is primarily composed of D-mannose and D-galactose in a ratio of 3:5. It runs from 3 to 8 percent by weight of the harvested fungus. Most of the rest of the polysaccharides in the herb are simply labeled by identifiers such as P70-1, CPS-1, and so on. As with many mushrooms, there are a lot of them, 36 so far.

The fungus is very high in nucleotides, the molecular components of the nucleic acids RNA and DNA. The main ones are guanosine, adenosine, and uridine in that order. The nucleotides tend to be higher, often much more so, in vat-grown cordyceps mycelium than in the wild fungus.

There are various sterols. Ergosterol is a primary one, a precursor of vitamin D_2. It is much higher in the fruiting body itself (10 mg/g) than in the grown mycelium (1.5 mg/g). Others are sitosterol, daucosterol, and campesterol.

Cordyceps has very high levels of 18 different amino acids. The mycelial powders have the highest content. Glutamate, arginine, and aspartic acid are the highest.

The mushroom also has very high levels of fatty acids, in this order: linoleic acid, oleic acid, palmitic acid.

It also contains substantial quantities of 13 different minerals (and traces of 7 more), in this order: potassium, phosphorus, magnesium, calcium, sodium, iron, aluminum, zinc, manganese, silicon, boron, copper, selenium.

And, of course, vitamins: E, K, B_1, B_2, B_{12}.

There are a few other compounds in the fungus including cordymin, various aminophenols, some unusual cyclic dipeptides, various dihydroisocoumarins, cordypyridones A and B, various diphenyl ethers, myriocin, various polyamines (cadaverine, spermidine, spermine, putrescine and so on).

The constituents of *C. militaris* are very similar.

Note: Research is showing that some of the active compounds in the various cordyceps species are specific to the insect host upon which they form, e.g., cicadapeptins 1 and 2 that *Cordyceps heteropoda* creates from the chemicals in the cicadas upon which it develops. Again, this type of research is very new and very uncommon.

Traditional Uses

Cordyceps was first recorded in Tibet in the fifteenth century in the medical text *Mennag chewa rinsel* by Zurkhar Namnyi Dorje. Oddly enough, in spite of the fact that cordyceps first appeared in Tibetan healing texts, and continued to do so through the nineteenth century, it is rarely used as a medicine there. Those who do use it do so primarily as a liquid tonic that they take throughout the day for increasing vigor and strength and as an aphrodisiac. Generally, the liquid is prepared by placing four or five cordyceps mushrooms in arak (a rice or barley liquor) and leaving it to steep in a cool, dark place for 2 to 3 months (sometimes up to a year).

While rarely mentioned in Tibetan texts, and not considered all that important an herb in that tradition, its range of actions in that system are increasing the energy of the body, increasing and restoring semen, increasing kidney strength. It is considered specific for altitude sickness.

Though the Tibetans didn't find cordyceps to be a major medicine, the Chinese did. It has, since its discovery, been a major trade item with China, sometimes worth more than gold.

The herb came to Western prominence in 1994 when a Chinese track coach insisted that his team won so handily in the 1994 Asian Games in Hiroshima, Japan, beating the world records in the 1,500-, 3,000-, and 10,000-meter events, because he had them use the herb regularly as part of their training regimen.

AYURVEDA

In spite of cordyceps being indigenous in India, there is little, if any, mention of the herb in traditional Ayurvedic texts. There is some speculation that the herb "sanjivani" mentioned in the older texts is cordyceps, but it's a guess.

In India, the use of cordyceps primarily occurs in community herbal practice, not in formal Ayurvedic healing. It is commonly used among traditional healers in Sikkim, a landlocked Indian state in the Himalayan mountains that borders both Nepal and Tibet. It is recommended as a tonic for all illnesses, improving energy, appetite, stamina, libido, endurance and normalizing sleep. It is considered to be a longevity herb and specific for colds and flu, coughs, asthma, cancer, tuberculosis, diabetes, erectile dysfunction, BHP, jaundice, and hepatitis. Although occasionally prepared as a water extraction it is generally infused in an alcoholic liquor, as in Tibet.

TRADITIONAL CHINESE MEDICINE

Cordyceps is described variously as having a neutral property and sweet taste or as being sweet/acrid with a warm property. It acts on the lung and kidney channels, is lung nourishing, kidney vital essence and vital energy tonifying, hemostatic, and phlegm resolvent, that is, a mucolytic. It is generally prescribed for overall debility after sickness and for the aged. It is considered to be one of the three primary invigorating medicinals in Chinese medicine along with Asian ginseng and deer antler.

It is specific for tonifying the lungs, arresting bronchial bleeding, dispelling phlegm, chronic cough, asthma, wasting, and tonifying the kidneys. It is also used for impotence, low libido, poor seminal emissions, aching of loins and knees, and as a tonic for spontaneous sweating, aversion to cold, tinnitus, chronic nephritis, general weakness, and sexual hypofunction.

WESTERN BOTANIC USE

Until 1994, none. Now, lots of interest, primarily based on the Chinese and Japanese research and cordyceps's reputation as a longevity herb and aphrodisiac. (We seek our youth and we will not be denied.)

Scientific Research

Most of the scientific studies have occurred since 1995, after the Asian Games, and the numbers of published articles are increasing every year. There were four studies published in 1995, by 2011 there were 80. And those are just the ones accessible through PubMed; there are scores more in the Chinese, Japanese, and Korean databases, most not translated into English.

Of those 80, only 13 were not Korean, Japanese, or Chinese and about half of those 13 were not studying the medicinal actions of the plant. The Western world is still betting that those buggy whip orders will pick up again ... any day now.

The majority of the studies I am citing were with *C. sinensis* or *C. militaris* herbs or their isolated compounds.

IN VITRO STUDIES

Cordyceps downregulates a number of inflammatory cytokines and upregulates others such as IL-10, TGF-ß, and IL-1ra that are specific for controlling overactive inflammation responses in the body. In underactive immune systems, it will upregulate cytokines to help the body deal with disease. In overactive immune circumstances it will downregulate them.

It downregulates or inhibits NF-κB, TNF-α, IL-1ß, IL-12, NO, iNOS, SOD, elastase, luceriferase, ERK, JAK-2 (Janus kinase-2), JNK, p38, PGE2, spleen tyrosine kinase (Syk), STAT-1, AP-1, MMP-3, MMP-9, and H_2O_2 hemolysis, and it scavenges hydroxyl radicals.

When cells are challenged by lipoproteins from the bacterial cytoplasmic membrane cordyceps strongly downregulates TNF-α, IL-12, and NO. In lipopolysaccharide-activated macrophages it inhibits NF-κB, NO, TNF-α, IL-1ß, IL-6, IL-12, IFN-γ, AP-1, COX-2, the phosphorylation of p38 MAPK and Akt, as well as inhibiting PGE2 levels and suppressing Syk/NF-κB, IKKε/IRF-3, and p38/AP-1 pathways.

Treatment with cordyceps or the cordyceps constituent cordycepin, or adenosine, causes lipopolysaccharide-stimulated macrophages to return to their original inactivated shape. This dynamic is dose dependent and needs relatively high levels of the herb.

Cordycepin suppresses TNF-α and MMP-9 expression in human bladder cancer cells, inactivates the phosphoinositide 3-kinase (PI3K) pathway in LNCaP cells, and increases levels of TIMP (tissue inhibitor of metalloproteinase) 1 and 2, and thus downregulates MMP-3 and MMP-9 in prostate cancer cells.

Cordyceps possesses a potent sphingomyelinase inhibitor that inhibits the breakdown of sphingomyelin in the body, especially in the brain, making it specific for mycoplasma. It strongly inhibits hydrogen peroxide oxidation and activity against cells and actively protects the mitochrondria (reducing oxidative stress and mitochondrial depolarization). It acts as an intracellular antioxidant and is a strong hydroxyl radical scavenger. All these actions are dose dependent.

Cordycepin strongly inhibits lipopolysaccharide-activated inflammation in microglia cells. It significantly inhibits the production of NO, PGE2, and proinflammatory cytokines in the microglia. It suppresses NF-κB translocation by blocking IkappaBalpha degradation and inhibits phosphorylation of Akt, ERK-1 and ERK-2, JNK, and p38 kinase. A compound of cordyceps, coptidis rhizoma, and Chinese skullcap was shown to have powerful neuroprotective effects on lipopolysaccharide-activated microglial cells. It inhibited NO, iNOS, COX-2,

PGE2, gp91 phox, iROS (intracellular reactive oxygen species), TNF-α, IL-1ß, and IkappaBalpha degradation. It upregulated heme oxygenase-1 and increased cell viability and mitochondrial membrane potential. The three-herb compound was found to strongly protect neural cells from toxicity.

Cordyceps is strongly modulatory on immune cells. In vitro it acts as an activator and maturation stimulant to monocytes and immature dendritic cells by stimulating the expression of costimulatory molecules and pro-inflammatory cytokines, enhancing dendritic-cell-induced allogeneic T cell proliferation and reducing the endocytic ability of dendritic cells. *However*, during lipopolysaccharide stimulation cordyceps suppresses the proinflammatory cytokines involved. It suppresses the lipopolysaccharide-induced, dendritic-cell-elicited allogeneic T cell proliferation and shifts the immune response from a potent Th1 to a Th2 dynamic. In the absence of infection, it potentiates Th1 immune activity. During active infection, it actively modulates the extreme upregulation of lipopolysaccharide cytokines and balances the overreactivity of the Th1 response.

Cordyceps has a lot of effects on airway epithelial cells. It acts to normalize cellular function in airway epithelia by normalizing ion transport. It blocks airway inflammation by blocking NF-κB production in airway epithelial cells. It significantly reduces epidermal-growth-factor-stimulated mucous hypersecretion in lung mucoepidermoid cells by downregulating COX-2, MMP-9, and MUC5AC gene expression through blocking NF-κB and the p38/ERK MAPK pathways. It strongly regulates the inflammation that occurs in the bronchii and regulates bronchoalveolar lavage fluids by doing do. It downregulates IL-1ß, IL-6, IL-8, and TNF-α. It is highly protective of epithelia and normalizes the function of the surface epithelium.

In rheumatoid arthritis synovial fibroblasts it inhibits IL-1ß-induced MMP-1 and MMP-3 expression. MMP-1 degrades fibrillar collagens, MMP-3 the extracellular matrix. It also inhibits MAPK activation, specifically p38 and JNK. It is a fairly potent inhibitor of p38 phosphorylation.

Cordyceps is highly protective of renal tubular epithelial cells in vitro. It is antiadipogenic. It is antiatherogenic by blocking MAPK, specifically ERK, JNK, and p38. It suppresses the expression of diabetes-regulating genes. It reduces platelet aggregation.

Cordyceps stimulates ATP generation by mitochondria and also antioxidant activity, and it modulates immune responses intracellularly. It protects mitochondria from ROS and enhances the mitochondrial antioxidant defenses. The effects are dose dependent.

IN VIVO STUDIES

Cordyceps militaris, grown on soybeans, was used to prepare a hot water extract that was then given to mice infected with influenza A virus. Significantly reduced virus titers in lung tissue were observed after 3 days when compared with mice not given cordyceps. A polysaccharide, presumed to be the most active antiviral agent, was extracted and given intranasally to mice infected with lethal strains of influenza A. Mortality dropped from 70 to 18 percent. The polysaccharide was determined to be a type of arabinogalactan, similar to those extracted from larch and juniper.

In rats, cordycepin attenuated neointima formation (a thickened layer of arterial tissue) in vascular smooth-tissue muscle cells by inhibiting ROS. Cordymin, a constituent of cordyceps, was found to be strongly anti-inflammatory in induced gastric inflammation in mice by inhibiting IL-1ß, TNF-α, and total oxidant levels. It was also found to be strongly analgesic. Cordyceps (*militaris*) extract suppressed induced acute colitis in mice and significantly reduced the production of inflammatory cytokines from macrophages and mast cells. NO, iNOS, and TNF-α were all strongly inhibited. Cordyceps extract inhibited airway inflammation in rats by blocking NF-κB. It significantly inhibited ovalbumin-induced airway inflammation in sensitized guinea pigs and rats that mimics the human condition of asthma. Likewise, *Cordyceps militaris* reduced airway inflammation in a mouse asthma model.

Lipopolysaccharide-injected mice, experiencing induced inflammation, showed a remarkable reduction of IL-1ß, TNF-α, iNOS, COX-2, and PGE2 when given an extract of *Cordyceps pruinosa*.

Cordyceps extract increased CD4+ and CD8+, IL-4, and IL-10 in mice, especially in mesenteric lymph node lymphocytes. Regular daily doses of cordyceps extract prevented disuse-induced osteoporosis in rats. And

an extract increased glutathione levels, reduced oxidants, and lowered blood glucose levels in rats with streptozotocin-induced diabetes.

Cordyceps extract significantly improved learning and reduced memory impairment in mice. *Cordyceps militaris* extract (and cordycepin) protected hippocampal neurons in gerbils from ischemic injury. Cordycepin was found to be strongly protective of neurons against cerebral ischemia/reperfusion. It considerably lowered levels of MMP-3 in the brain, increased SOD, and decreased malondialdehyde, significantly reducing oxidation. In one study *Cordyceps sinensis* mycelium strongly protected rat neurons from ischemic injury by inhibiting NF-κB, PMNs (polymorphonuclear neutrophils), IL-1ß, iNOS, TNF-α, ICAM-1, and COX-2. A cordymin extract pretty much did the same thing in another study. In still another study cordyceps extract protected the brain from injury after middle cerebral artery occlusion-induced cerebral ischemia in rats. And in yet another study cordycepin prevented postischemic neuronal degeneration in mice.

Cordyceps sinensis extract significantly reduced renal ischemia/reperfusion injury in rats. Various forms of renal injury in rats were ameliorated by the use of several types of *Cordyceps cicadae* extracts.

Mice exposed to ionizing radiation experienced restored immune function from a polysaccharide of *C. sinensis* through modulation of the secretion of IL-4, IL-5, and IL-17. A butanol extract of *Cordyceps bassiana* was shown to inhibit induced atopic dermatitis in mice. And in hamsters, cordycepin was shown to prevent hyperlipidemia.

Other studies have shown cordycepin to be strongly steroidogenic. It stimulated testosterone production in mouse Leydig cells. And serum testosterone and sperm count and motility were strongly increased in rats after supplementation with *Cordyceps militaris*.

HUMAN CLINICAL STUDIES AND TRIALS

Cordyceps extract inhibits the proliferation and differentiation of Th2 cells and reduces the expression of related cytokines by downregulating GST-3 mRNA and upregulating FOXP3 mRNA and relieves chronic allergic inflammation by increasing IL-10 in the blood of children with chronic asthma.

In one study, 60 asthmatic patients were split into two groups. Thirty used an inhaler, the rest used *Cordyceps sinensis* (CS) capsules. IgE, solubal ICAM-1, IL-4, and MMP-9 were all lowered in the cordyceps group (though not as much as in those using an inhaler). Another study at the Beijing Medical University with 50 asthma patients found that the symptoms in the group treated with CS were reduced by 81 percent in 5 days versus 61 percent over 9 days in the pharmaceutical group.

There have been a number of other trials of the herb in the treatment of chronic obstructive pulmonary disease (COPD), asthma, and bronchitis that have not been translated into English. The herb was effective for all these conditions; it is especially indicated for COPD.

One trial split 65 renal dialysis patients into two groups. The 33 in the second group took cordyceps (330 mg) and ginkgo (230 mg) three times daily for 3 months. At the end of that period microinflammation, a problem in renal hemodialysis, was significantly lowered in the herb group. Levels of hs-CRP (high-sensitivity C-reactive protein), IL-6, and TNF-α were all much lower.

In one study with 51 patients suffering chronic renal failure, the use of 3–5 grams/day of CS significantly improved renal function and increased immune function. Another study with 57 people suffering gentamicin-induced renal damage split the subjects into two groups; one received CS, the other conventional pharmaceuticals. After 6 days those in the CS group had recovered 89 percent of their kidney function versus 45 percent in the other group.

Sixty-one people with lupus nephritis were split into two groups. One received 2–4 grams of cordyceps (before meals) and 600 mg of artemisinin (after meals) three times daily for 3 years. They were observed for an additional 5 years after treatment. Twenty-six had no recurrence, four had mild, and for one the herbs did not work.

A randomized trial of cordyceps in the treatment of 21 aged patients (divided into two groups) found that cordyceps ameliorated aminoglycoside nephrotoxicity.

Cordyceps sinensis (CS) was used in the long-term treatment of renal transplant patients. Long-term survival was no different in the treated and untreated groups, however the incidence of complication was significantly lower in the CS group. The CS group needed much lower doses of cyclosporine A and serum levels of IL-10 in the CS group were much higher. Another renal transplant study with 200 transplant patients showed the same outcomes.

Three separate studies with a combined patient population of 756 men and women who were experiencing reduced sex drive found that after 40 days 65 percent of those taking cordyceps reported improved libido and performance versus 24 percent of those taking placebo. In another study with elderly patients complaining of decreased libido, impotence, and other sexual malfunctions 3 grams/day of cordyceps was administered for 40 days. Increased sperm survival time, increased sperm count, and decreased numbers of malformed sperm were all found in the majority of males. Improvements in hypoleukorrhagia, menoxenia, and sex drive were reported in a majority of the women.

There have been a number of clinical studies of the herb in cancer treatment, along with chemo and radiation. In one study of 50 patients taking cordyceps, tumors reduced in 23. In another, after 2 months, most patients taking cordyceps reported improved subjective symptoms. White blood counts stayed at $3000/mm^3$ or higher. The use of cordyceps during radiation and chemo has been found to counteract the negative immune effects of those procedures.

There have been a number of Chinese studies on using the herb for treating heart conditions, liver problems, hypercholesterolemia, and male/female sexual dysfunction but few of them have been translated into English. There have also been a few studying exercise tolerance and improvement, e.g., 20 adults aged 50 to 75, in a double-blind, placebo-controlled trial showed improved exercise performance while taking cordyceps. However, the main studies in the United States have been on exercise tolerance with young athletes, and they all showed no improvement. The dosages were extremely low.

. . . .

The best overall look at the herb, its history, and its medical uses is probably John Holliday and Matt Cleaver, *On the Trail of the Yak: Ancient Cordyceps in the Modern World* (June 2004). I have only found it online and downloaded it from the website of Earthpulse Press (www.earthpulse.com).

Note: To be effective for anything, cordyceps *must* be dosed appropriately.

That means a minimum dose of 3 grams daily but the best results occur with 6 grams daily as the baseline, especially in acute conditions. The renal studies usually used from 3 to 4.5 grams. This dose range can also work for lung problems, except in truly acute conditions when it should be 6 to 9 grams (in mycoplasma treatment as well).

Rhodiola

Family: Crassulaceae.

Species used: There is, as usual, confusion among those with advanced degrees in plant science as to just how many species of rhodiola there are: 36, or maybe 60, probably 90. It's like stamp collectors ("No, look at that tiny ink spot on the edge, that's what makes it rare."); I just want to scream.

The primary medicinal that most people use is *Rhodiola rosea*, but many of the related species are used medicinally in the regions in which they grow. Because of the interest in *R. rosea*, the genus is being intensively studied for activity: I have found medicinal studies of one sort or another on *R. crenulata*, *R. quadrifida*, *R. heterodonta*,, *R. semenovii*, *R. sachalinensis*, *R. sacra*, *R. fastigiata*, *R. kirilowii*, *R. bupleuroides*, *R. imbricata*, *R. rhodantha*, and *R. integrifolia*.

There have been some extravagant claims (easily found on the Internet) that *only* Russian *Rhodiola rosea*, harvested near the Arctic Circle (presumably by fasting virgins as the northern lights first emerge over the rim of the Earth), contains the necessary active constituents for the herb to be useful. However, *all* the *Rhodiola rosea* plants, irrespective of where they grow or in what country, have nearly identical chemistry. They are all perfectly usable as medicine.

But please note: The exact chemical profile of the *R. rosea* plants themselves differs depending on time of year, time of day, and geographical location (this valley in Russia or *that* one) irrespective of whether they are harvested at the Arctic Circle in Russia by fasting virgins or not. In other words, you can pick *R. rosea* from this location in May and again in September and the chemical profile of the plant *won't* be the same. The same is true of every species in the genus — and of every medicinal plant on Earth. Part of the art of herbalism is being able to determine medicinal potency of the plants you are harvesting by using the most sophisticated scientific instrument ever discovered — the focused power of human consciousness. Machines just aren't a reliable substitute for the capacity to reason *and* feel simultaneously. Furthermore ... oops! Sorry. Got carried away again.

Studies on 14 other species in the genus have found the same constituents in them as in *R. rosea*. They can all be used medicinally, they all do pretty much the same things, they all work identically to the usual commercial variety *R. rosea* — see "Scientific Research" (page 300) for more. *Rhodiola integrifolia,* by the way, is considered to be a natural hybrid between *Rhodiola rhodantha* and *R. rosea*; you can consider it pretty much identical to *R. rosea.*

Synonyms: The rhodiolas look much like sedums and were once included in that genus, so you will see *rosea* sometimes listed as *Sedum rosea* and so on.

Common names: Rhodiola, golden root, roseroot, stonecrop, arctic root. The fresh roots smell a bit like roses, hence the origin of that name. They are golden in color, thus golden root.

Part Used

The root.

Preparation and Dosage

Generally used as capsules or tincture.

TINCTURE

Use the dried root, in an herb:liquid ratio of 1:5, with the liquid being 50 percent alcohol. Some people use a 1:3 formulation. I am not sure it is necessary.

Tonic dose: 30–40 drops 3x of 4x daily, usually in water.

In acute conditions: $^1/_2$–1 teaspoon 3x daily for 20–30 days, then back to the tonic dose. There really isn't an upper dosage limit that I can find.

CAPSULES

The root is most often used in capsule form, 100 mg each. Usual dose is 1 or 2 capsules per day. In acute conditions up to 1,000 mg a day can be taken. The capsules are often standardized to contain 2–3 percent rosavins and 0.8–1 percent salidroside. They are usually taken just before meals.

Side Effects and Contraindications
Some people experience jitteriness from the herb; you should not take it at night until you know if you are one of them.

Herb/Drug Interactions
None noted.

Habitat and Appearance
Rhodiolas are plants that like high altitude and cold; either will do. They are a circumpolar genus of the subarctic and cool, mountainous regions of the northern hemisphere and are common in eastern Russia, parts of China, Tibet (which has many species), the mountains and northern climes of Europe, Canada, the mountainous and colder regions of the United States. The United States, Europe, and Tibet appear to have the largest populations, with Tibet having the most species.

The rhodiolas are typical succulents with fleshy, moisture-filled, grayish-green leaves. The plants grow to about 12 inches and they will have, depending on the species, a cluster of yellow, pink, red, or orange flowers at the top of the stalk. *R. rosea*'s flowers are yellow.

The root system is fairly large if the plants grow in a nutrient-rich environment. The farther north they grow, and the poorer the soils, the smaller the root.

There are three species of rhodiola in North America: *Rhodiola rosea*, which grows in the mountains of North Carolina, and in Pennsylvania through New England into Canada and all the way to the Arctic Circle; *R. rhodantha*, which grows in the Rocky Mountain states from New Mexico and Arizona up to the Canadian border; and *R. integrifolia*, which has the widest distribution in North America. It ranges from the Rocky Mountain spine (New Mexico, etc., westward) up into Canada and into the Arctic. There are populations as well in Minnesota and New York State. Most of the eastern rhodiolas are considered endangered.

If you are in the western United States and wanting to wild-harvest your own roots, look for *R. integrifolia*; it is just as useful as *R. rosea* medicinally *and* it is not endangered as many of the eastern U.S. *R. rosea* populations are.

Cultivation and Collection

Due to the popularizing of the plant as an antiaging and chronic fatigue medicinal, wild populations of rosea are becoming endangered; the Russians have put them on their red list of threatened plants. The largest populations of the plant were formerly in the Altai region of southern Siberia. However, over 45 companies have been harvesting the plant for export ("*Real* Russian rhodiola") and those plant populations have been severely reduced.

If you live in a region in which rhodiola grows, you can harvest your own roots; you won't need to harvest much for yourself and your family. Commercial harvesting, except for very limited amounts in abundant areas, is highly discouraged.

If you find the plant in your area, harvest the roots in the fall after seeding or in the spring just as it is coming up. The roots will be bigger and, in my opinion, more potent in the spring. Slice the bigger roots; the interior of the root will change from white to a brown or reddish color as it begins to dry.

Due to the heavy worldwide demand for the plant, there are increasing efforts to make the plant an agricultural staple in regions where it will grow; Bulgaria, Canada, and Finland are early innovators in growing the crop. The yields are low, only about 3 tons per hectare, and they are labor intensive. Since the roots are taken, and only after 5 years, agricultural production of the plant demands a minimum of five fields, planted in rotation so they can be harvested in successive years in order to keep up continual production.

The seeds are tiny; 1,000 of them weigh only 0.2 gram. The germination rates are low, 2 to 36 percent; they are happier with a little stratification. Thirty days at –5°C (23° F) will increase germination rates to 50 to 75 percent. Soak the seeds in water overnight, mix into moist soil, store for 1 month at a temperature of 2° to 4°C (36–39° F). You will then get about a 75 percent germination rate.

In Finland they get 95 to 100 percent germination if they sow the seeds on the surface of a sand/peat mix and keep the trays outside all winter under the snow. In April/May the boxes are brought into a greenhouse at a temperature of 18° to 22°C (64–72° F). Germination begins in 3 days to 1 week.

If you keep the seedlings inside for a year before transplanting, yields are significantly higher. They like sandy, loamy soil, neutral or slightly acidic. NPK: 50/50/70. They don't need additional fertilizer after the first year. The easiest method, however, is to divide the roots of an established plant and plant the root cuttings, much like potatoes.

The plant takes a minimum of 3 years to mature but the roots should not be harvested for 5 years. Dig in the fall, slice, let dry out of the sun. Store in plastic bags, inside plastic containers, in the dark.

Plant Chemistry

Most people think that salidroside (a.k.a. rhodioloside) is the most important compound in the root, while others insist it is the rosavin. Others say, yeah those and . . . rosin, rosarin, and tyrosol. Studies have found, as usual, that salidroside is much more effective when combined with rosavin, rosin, and rosarin. So, I'm guessing, just a wild shot here, that it's the whole root that is most active.

There are, of course, a great many other compounds in the root, at least 85 essential oils and another 50 water-soluble nonvolatiles. Many of the usual plant compounds are present.

Traditional Uses

Rhodiola, as far as I can tell, and in spite of assertions that it is a long-standing medicinal in traditional Chinese medicine, was a contribution to the medicinal plant world by the Russians due to their interest in adaptogens. This is pretty much a Russian-introduced category of medicinal herb — a plant that enhances general overall functioning, somewhat like a tonic but one that increases the ability of the organism to respond to outside stressors of whatever sort, diseases included. It enhances an organism's general resistance to multiple adverse influences or conditions.

The Russians have done a lot of great work on the medicinal actions of plants and deeply developed some unique categories of herbs, such as the adaptogenics. I see a lot of comments here and there picking on them, insisting that they are a dour people. But the Russians themselves say they smile and laugh only when there is truly something to smile or laugh about (which is almost never). Contrariwise they comment, "Have you ever wondered why the first thing Americans do when they meet you is show you their teeth?" And, of course, they did not laugh when they said that (but I did, it's really funny).

Rhodiola, like the stronger preparations of eleutherococcus (another Russian-developed herb), is considered to be not just adaptogenic but an adaptogenic stimulant — part of the reason it can cause jitteriness and wakefulness in some. I like it and it tastes yummy (yes, that is a technical Russian term).

A few of my obscure herb reference sources reveal that rhodiola was used in traditional Russian folk medicine to increase physical endurance, work productivity, longevity, resistance to altitude sickness, fatigue, depression, anemia, impotence, GI tract ailments, infections, and nervous afflictions. But they seem to be the only people who used it regularly.

Finding It

You can buy it pretty much everywhere. If you live in the right climate you can probably find it wild or grow it yourself.

Properties of Rhodiola

Actions

Adaptogen	Ergogenic	Muscular stimulant
Adrenal protectant	Hippocampal	Nervous system tonic
Anticancer	protectant and tonic	Neural protectant
Antidepressant	Hypoxia antagonist	Rhodiola is also
Antifatigue	(potent)	possibly a synergist;
Antioxidant (strong)	Immune tonic	the plant is strong
Antistressor	Mental stimulant	inhibitor of CYP3A4
Cardiotonic (potent)	Mitochondrial tonic	and P-glycoprotein.
Endocrine tonic	and protectant	

Active Against

Again, this herb is not primarily an antimicrobial but it does have some antiviral actions. It is active against influenza viruses due to its neuraminidase inhibitory activity. It has been found active against H1N1 and H9N2 viral strains. It is also active against the hepatitis C and Coxsackie B3 viruses. One of its constituents, kaempferol, is specific against Japanese encephalitis virus and enterovirus 71. It has some antibacterial activity as well, against *Staphylococcus aureus* (strong), *Bacillus subtilis* and *Mycobacterium tuberculosis* (moderate), *E. coli* (weak).

Use to Treat

Chronic long-term fatigue, recurrent infections, recovery from long-term illness and infections, nervous exhaustion, chronic fatigue syndrome, chronic disease conditions with depression, low immune function, brain fog, and to accelerate recovery from debilitating conditions.

Note: The plant is specific for the kinds of damage that occur during encephalitis infections. It is highly neuroprotective and strongly anti-inflammatory in the brain and CNS. It should be used in all encephalitis infections.

Other Uses

The leaves of most species can be eaten, chopped finely and added to salads, or cooked as a pot herb. The plants are very high in vitamin C, with 33 mg per gram of fresh plant.

AYURVEDA AND TRADITIONAL CHINESE MEDICINE

I just can't find much mention of the herb.

Rhodiolas *have* (supposedly) been used in Chinese medicine, Tibetan medicine, and Ayurveda for a very long time — according to many reports. But my library, extensive, doesn't list the genus in any of my source books for those systems of healing. I did find some indigenous uses in Tibet, however. The plant is a part of traditional Tibetan medicine for promoting blood circulation and relieving cough. In central Asia the tea has been used for a long time as the most effective local treatment for colds and flu. Mongolian physicians use it for tuberculosis and cancer.

WESTERN BOTANIC PRACTICE

The plant never was a huge medicinal in the West even though there are traces of its use as far back as the seventeenth century in the Scandinavian countries. *Rhodiola rosea* and *R. integrifolia* were used by the indigenous tribes of Alaska as food, and the root was eaten for sores in the mouth, tuberculosis, stomachache, and GI tract troubles. The Eclectics recognized a couple of the sedums but none of the rhodiolas before their name change.

Scientific Research

There is a lot of research on this plant right now, and more studies are occurring daily. There have been, unlike the case for many other newish medicinal plants, a lot of human clinical trials with this herb. I am primarily going to look at the neuroprotective/neuroregenerative, immune, and antistress/antifatigue actions of the plant — they are strongly interrelated. The potent antioxidant actions of the plant are deeply interrelated with those as well.

NEUROPROTECTIVE/NEUROREGENERATIVE

In vitro: Compounds in both *Rhodiola sacra* and *R. sachalinensis* protect neurons against beta-amyloid-induced, stauroporine-induced, and H_2O_2-induced death. Salidroside, a common compound in many rhodiolas, protects cultured neurons from injury from hypoxia and hypoglycemia; protects neuronal PC12 cells and SH-SY5Y neuroblastoma cells against cytotoxicity from beta-amyloid and against hypoglycemia and serum limitation; and protects neurons. It does so by inducing the antioxidant enzymes thioredoxin, heme oxygenase-1, and peroxiredoxin-1, downregulating the pro-apoptotic gene Bax, and upregulating the anti-apoptotic genes Bcl-2 and Bcl-X(L). It also restores H_2O_2-induced loss of mitochondrial membrane potential and restores intracellular calcium levels.

In vivo: *Rhodiola rosea* enhances the level of 5-hydroxytryptamine in the hippocampus, promotes the proliferation and differentiation of neural stem cells in the hippocampus, and protects hippocampal neurons from injury. *R. rosea* protects against cognitive deficits, neuronal injury, and oxidative stress induced by intracerebroventricular injection of streptozotocin. Salidroside protects rat hippocampal neurons against H_2O_2-induced apoptosis. A combination of rhodiola and astragalus protects rats against simulated plateau hypoxia (8,000 m/24,000 feet). It inhibits the accumulation of lactic acid in brain tissue and serum.

Human clinical trial: A double-blind, placebo-controlled, randomized study with 40 women, ages 20 to 68, who were highly stressed, found that a *Rhodiola rosea* extract increased attention, speed, and accuracy during stressful cognitive tasks. Similarly, *Rhodiola rosea* was used with 120 adults with both physical and cognitive deficiencies (exhaustion, decreased motivation, daytime sleepiness, decreased libido, sleep disturbances, concentration deficiencies, forgetfulness, decreased memory, susceptibility to stress, irritability); after 12 weeks, 80 percent of patients showed improvements. In another study, a combination formula (Xinnaoxin capsule) of *Rhodiola rosea*, *Lycium chinense* berry, and fresh *Hippophae rhamnoides* fruit juice was given to 30 patients with chronic cerebral circulatory insufficiency; after 4 weeks the condition was significantly improved. A double-blind, crossover 3-week study on stress-induced fatigue on the mental performance of healthy physicians during night duty found that *Rhodiola rosea* extract decreased mental fatigue and increased cognitive functions such as associative thinking, short-term memory, calculation and concentration, and speed of audiovisual perception.

ANTIFATIGUE/ANTISTRESS

In vitro: Salidroside stimulated glucose uptake by rat muscle cells. *Rhodiola rosea* extract stimulated the synthesis or resynthesis of ATP and stimulated reparative processes in mitochondria.

In vivo: *Rhodiola rosea* extracts increased the life span of *Drosophila melanogaster*, lowered mitochondrial superoxide levels, and increased protection against the superoxide generator paraquat. Four weeks' supplementation with *R. rosea* extract significantly increased swimming time in exhausted mice — it significantly increased liver glycogen levels, SREBP-1 (sterol regulatory element binding protein 1), FAS (fatty acid synthase), heat shock protein 70 expression, the Bcl-2:Bax ratio, and oxygen content in the blood. Salidroside protected the hypothalamic/pituitary/gonad axis of male rats under intense stress — testosterone levels remained normal rather than dropping, secretory granules of the pituitary gland increased, and mitochondrial cells were strongly protected. *R. rosea* extract completely reversed the effects of chronic mild stress in female rats — that is, decreased sucrose intake, decreased movement, weight loss, and dysregulation of menstrual cycle. Rhodiola suppressed increased enzyme activity in rats subjected to noise stress — glutamic pyruvic transaminase, alkaline phosphatase, and creatine kinase levels all returned to normal, and glycogen, lactic acid, and cholesterol levels in the liver also returned to normal. *R. rosea* reduced stress and CRF-induced anorexia in rats. And so on.

Human clinical trial: Twenty-four men who had lived at high altitude for a year were tested to see the effects of rhodiola on blood oxygen saturation and sleep disorders; rhodiola was found to increase blood oxygen saturation significantly and increase both sleeping time and quality. In a double-blind, placebo-controlled study of the effects of *R. rosea* on fatigue in students caused by stress, physical fitness, mental fatigue, and neuro-motoric indices all increased (other studies found similar outcomes). *R. rosea* intake in a group of healthy volunteers reduced inflammatory C-reactive protein and creatine kinase in blood and protected muscle tissue during exercise. *Rhodiola rosea* in a placebo-controlled, double-blind, randomized study was found to increase physical capacity, muscle strength, speed of limb movement, reaction time and attention — in other words it improved exercise endurance performance. A similarly structured study found that 1 week of rhodiola supplementation decreased fatigue and stress levels but more interestingly decreased photon emissions on the dorsal side of the hand. In another study *Rhodiola rosea* increased the efficiency of the cardiovascular and respiratory systems and prevented fatigue during an hour of continuous physical exercise. A phase three clinical trial found that rhodiola exerts an antifatigue effect that increases mental performance and concentration and decreases cortisol response in burnout patients with fatigue syndrome; other studies have found similar outcomes including the amelioration of depression and anxiety.

IMMUNE ACTIONS

In vitro: *Rhodiola imbricata* protects macrophages against tert-butyl hydroperoxide injury and upregulates the immune response. Additionally it potently stimulates the innate immune pathway and initiates strong immunostimulatory actions, increasing Toll-like receptor 4, granzyme B, and Th1 cytokines. *R. sachalinensis* extract enhances the expression of iNOS in macrophages. *R. quadrifida* stimulates granulocyte activity and increases lymphocyte response to mitogens. *R. algida* stimulates human peripheral blood lymphocytes and upregulates IL-2 in Th1 cells and IL-4, IL-6, and IL-10 in Th2 cells.

In vivo: *Rhodiola kirilowii* enhances cellular immunity, stimulating the activity of lymphocytes and increasing phagocytosis in response to microbial organisms. *R. imbricata* enhances specific immunoglobulin levels in response to tetanus toxoid and ovalbumin in rats — the plant has adjuvant/immunopotentiating activity in both humoral and cell-mediated immune response.

Human clinical trial: *Rhodiola rosea* (in combination with schisandra, eleuthero, and leuzea) significantly increased both cell-mediated and humoral immune response in ovarian cancer patients. Rhodiola significantly reduced problems and infection after the treatment of acute lung injury caused by massive trauma/infection and thoracic-cardio operations. A combination formula of rhodiola, eleuthero, and schisandra significantly enhanced positive outcomes in the treatment of acute nonspecific pneumonia. *R. rosea* increased the parameters of leukocyte integrins and T-cell immunity in bladder cancer patients.

OTHER ACTIONS

Rhodiola, various species, has been found effective in the treatment of breast cancer. It inhibits the tumorigenic properties of invasive mammary epithelial cells, inhibits superficial bladder cancer, suppresses T241 fibrosarcoma tumor cell proliferation, and reduces angiogenesis in various tumor lines. *R. imbricata* is highly protective in mice against whole-body lethal radiation.

The plant has also been found highly antioxidant in numerous studies, to be liver protective, and to be highly protective of the cardiovascular system.

The plant is adaptogenic; that is, it increases the function of the organism to meet whatever adverse influences are affecting it, whether stress or illness. Most of the attention has been paid to its ability to increase endurance and mental acuity but its effects on the immune system, though less studied than eleuthero's, are similar.

303

WHAT THE FUTURE HOLDS

Once your life is saved by a plant
Things are never the same again.

We live in interesting times. Although most of us, in the West, were trained to see the world around us as stable, unchanging year after year, that is an anomaly in the long history of this planet. The Earth goes through long periods of stability, then, rather abruptly, things change. The ecological parameters of climate alter and I am not just talking about "climate change" here. Wind patterns shift, currents in the ocean change, animal migration patterns, rainfall, snowfall, soil composition, insect density, mouse populations, and so on — all of them shift. They shift for reasons that few reductionist scientists understand — or want to. There are patterns inside the living physical world that few of us look for or notice, invisible patterns, and upon them our survival depends.

We are just one part of that incredibly large, complex, deeply inter-woven ecological scenario, one organism among trillions, interwoven into an ecological matrix that has lasted billions of years. We aren't, and never have been, in charge. So, things change, as they are wont to do, and they are in the process of changing drastically. None of us will escape the consequences of it.

One of those consequences happens to be the emergence of new dis-ease organisms, their unique movements through the ecological fabric of the world, and their infection of new species, most especially us.

The medical paradigm that most of us in the West know emerged out of a certain historical context operating against the background of a stable ecosystem. It has been shaped by that unique situation *and* by the interests, and hubris, of powerful corporations, educational organizations, government bureaucracy, nongovernmental activist groups, and self-interested trade unions (i.e., medical doctors) — all of whom still assume that the planet is a stable background against which they can operate. It has most certainly not been shaped by the needs of those who become ill or a genuine understanding of disease organisms and the ecological matrix in which all life forms on this planet are embedded. For anyone who looks, the fraying fabric of that stability is clear to see, and so also the crumbling of the Western medical paradigm.

The Western medical paradigm is failing. It is failing because it is inherently dysfunctional and most especially because it does not accurately understand the nature of disease, most especially the nature of the organisms it has considered responsible for most of those diseases. In the coming decades, within 10 years if some bacterial and viral researchers are to be believed, we will see not only the emergence of microbial diseases more potent than any our species has heretofore experienced but the failure of most antimicrobial pharmaceuticals that medical science uses — primarily due to resistance problems. This means that the kind of complacency that has been in place for most of us throughout most of our lives will have to change. We will no longer be able to go to a physician to cure microbial disease; we will be forced back on our own resources. This is a scary prospect for the emotionally dependent, which all of us have been, at one time or another, when it comes to illness.

And so, we enter difficult times. But as old systems fail, out of the shards, and out of the human capacity that our species has always possessed, we will, of necessity, create something new, something that really does work better and that does reflect the world in which we live more accurately. Ironically, that will include a return to plant medicines as our primary healing agents for infectious diseases.

Some of my ancestors, powerful political physicians, actively worked to destroy the Western tradition of herbal medicines, feeling that they were the outmoded and tragic remnants of a superstitious past. They felt that science would offer the answers, *all the answers,* that through science we could defeat all disease organisms on this planet. It is fascinating to me that in the midst of the failure of that utopian and very psychological projection the plants are returning once again to help us in our lives and with our diseases. They have been here 700 million years, some of them, others a mere 170 million. And they have learned a thing or two in that time. We, here a few hundred thousand years (or perhaps a million or two if you take into account earlier expressions of *Homo* spp.), have a great many things yet to learn, among them humility. It is no accident, I suspect, that the Cherokee peoples have repeated a legend for generations to their children, a legend that tells of the time plants were asked by the animals and insects (whom the humans had harmed by their lack of awareness) to turn on humans and give them diseases (just as the animals and insects were doing). The plants thought it over and said, "No, we will not, for they are our children. And for every disease you create for them, we will make a cure. And when they come to us in their need, we will heal them."

We face difficult times, but interesting ones as well. A new paradigm of healing is emerging, one partly based in the older healing systems of the human species (including technological medicine) but one that also contains elements never known before. In *your* own genius resides aspects of that new paradigm. I invite you to bring it, in whatever form it manifests, into the world. We are all going to need each other's help, you know, and we might as well start now.

In veriditas veritas
Silver City, New Mexico
July 2012

APPENDIX A

A BRIEF LOOK AT HERBAL MEDICINE MAKING

[Our bodies] are not distinct from the bodies of plants and animals, with which we are involved in the cycles of feeding and the intricate companionships of ecological systems and of the spirit. They are not distinct from the earth, the sun and moon, and the other heavenly bodies. It is therefore absurd to approach the subject of health piecemeal with a departmentalized band of specialists. A medical doctor uninterested in nutrition, in agriculture, in the wholesomeness of mind and spirit is as absurd as a farmer who is uninterested in health. Our fragmentation of this subject cannot be our cure, because it is our disease.

— Wendell Berry, *The Unsettling of America*

Tremendous empowerment comes from learning to recognize the medicinal plants that surround us, even more in learning how to make them into medicines for healing. And though it takes time, as your knowledge increases, as you learn how to tend to your illnesses and those of your family, the sense of helplessness that so many of us have experienced when we become ill, often ingrained since birth, begins to dissipate.

We have been trained to place our health in the hands of outside specialists who, very often, know neither ourselves nor our families, not the fabric of our lives nor the communities in which we live. They have no understanding of, and often no interest in, the complexity in which we live and from which our illnesses emerge. But for most of us, those specialists are the *only* place we know to go when we are ill, uncertain, and afraid, to seek help — for ourselves or our loved ones.

The world, however, is a great deal more complex than that frame allows and there are many more options to healing than that system acknowledges. All of us live, all the time, in the midst of a living pharmacy that covers the surface of this planet. And that living pharmacy is there for you, or anyone, to use — anytime you wish. Once you *know* that, once you have been healed by the plants in that living pharmacy, often of something that physicians said could not be healed, things are never the same again. You begin to break the cycle of dependence on which the health care system depends.

Taking back control over personal health and healing is one of the greatest forms of personal empowerment that I know. It does take time and effort, this kind of learning, but the learning goes quickly. Harder, perhaps, is learning to trust the plants with your life. It is a truly frightening moment, that moment of decision, when trust is extended in that way, for, before it occurs, there is no way to experientially *know* what the outcome will be. Most people on this planet, though, people who do not live in the Western, industrialized nations, make that decision every day of their lives. It is a trust they extend every moment of every day. Trusting the healing capacities of the plants is not a new experience to the human species.

The next step is learning how to turn the plants you are learning about into medicines for yourself and your family. It isn't that hard — people all over the globe have been doing it for a hundred thousand years. At least.

This is a brief look at herbal medicine making. It is condensed from a much larger exploration in the second edition of my book *Herbal Antibiotics*.

The Different Kinds of Herbal Medicines

Herbal medicines, in general, fall into two groups: 1) those for internal use, and 2) those for external use.

The main forms of herbal medicines for internal use are:
- Water extracts (infusions and decoctions)
- Alcohol extracts (tinctures)
- Percolations (water or alcohol)
- Fluid extracts
- Syrups/oxymels/electuaries
- Glycerites
- Fermentations
- Vinegars
- Fresh juice (stabilized or not)
- Powders (plain or encapsulated)
- Food
- Suppositories/boluses
- Douches
- Essential oils
- Steams
- Smokes

The main forms of herbal medicines for external use are:
- Oil infusions
- Salves
- Evaporative concentrates
- Washes
- Liniments
- Lotions
- Compresses/poultices
- Essential oils
- Smudges

Most of these you can make yourself. In this condensed version, I will primarily look at alcohol and water extractions.

A Comment on Solvents

Unless you are using the plant itself in some form — as powder, food, juice, or so on — what you will be doing when you make your medicines is extracting the chemical constituents of the plant in some kind of liquid solvent. (When you take the whole herb internally, the stomach acids, bile salts, and so on *are* the solvent media. They leach out the active constituents of the plants for you.)

Every solvent has its own properties and people use different ones for many different reasons, some of which I will go into here. Generally, a solvent is referred to as a *menstruum.* The term comes from *menstruus*, a Latin word meaning "month." It was felt, in the old days, that the moon and its cycle of 28 days had an influence on liquids, just as it does on the tides. So, herbs were placed in liquids — on particular days by the fanatical — and left in there for one cycle of the moon. Hence *menstruum.* Though derided as superstition by scientists there is some legitimacy to this kind of thinking. Plants really are stronger when harvested on certain days, the moon does affect the underground aquifers of the Earth, just as it does the oceans (causing the ground to breathe out moisture-laden air), leeches really are useful (surgeons use them regularly now), maggots really do clean gangrenous wounds better than anything else, and . . . oops, sorry, got carried away again.

Anyway, the solvent is called the *menstruum*, herbs are placed in the menstruum, and once there they begin to *macerate.* Maceration is the soaking of something — usually a plant of some sort — in a solvent until the cell walls begin to break down so the compounds in the herb will leach into the solvent, where they are held in suspension. When you later separate the liquid (containing the medicinal compounds) from the solids, the solids that are left are called the *marc.* The liquid is called whatever kind of medicine you were making: tincture, infusion, or so on.

Water is considered to be *the* universal solvent; it works for most things to some extent. For most of human history it has been the primary solvent people have used. Alcohol is the next most effective solvent. Combining them will give you the most comprehensive solvent medium that exists.

Just as with the plants you harvest, use the best-quality solvents you can get. Your water, especially, should be well, spring, or rain water — if you can get it. If you use tap water, have a filter on the water line if you are at all able to do so. Or else buy a good-quality water. The better the water, the better the medicine. (Tap water is, as well, filled with minute quantities of pharmaceuticals — you really don't want to ingest them. They are highly bioactive.)

Another thing to understand is that the more finely powdered your herb, the more surface area is exposed to the solvent. This allows more of the chemical constituents to leach into the solvent.

When you are making extracts, part of what you learn, and develop in your practice, is knowledge of just what kinds of solvents are right for which herbs and in what combinations. The goal is to get as many of the medicinal compounds as possible into the extractive medium. Each herb is different and needs different combinations of water and alcohol — that is, a different formula for preparation. Some do better in pure alcohol, some in pure water. Some need oils to extract the active constituents (*Artemisia annua* is an example of this; artemisinin is more easily soluble in fats than in either alcohol or water). Some need boiling, some prefer cold liquids.

Pharmacists, prior to World War II (before pharmaceuticals began to dominate medicine) were extensively trained in very sophisticated forms of herbal medicine making — many of which are beyond the scope of this book (and of most pharmacists these days). This is why pharmacists are still called "chemists" in England and the drugstores there the "chemist's shops." Distressingly, that kind of training no longer occurs; it is now a lost art. I doubt there is a medicinal pharmacist in practice anywhere in the world who can prepare a tincture of *Colchicum officinale* and determine, exactly, the amount of colchicine in it — as all pharmacists could do in 1920.

In becoming an herbal medicine maker, you are learning how to be a practical dispensing pharmacist. Part of what that means is discovering how to best prepare the herbs and with which solvents. A brief description follows; my book *Herbal Antibiotics* includes an herbal formulary that will give you the ratio of alcohol and water for several hundred plant tinctures.

Water Extractions

The two most common forms of water extractions are infusions and decoctions.

Infusions

Teas are, at heart, weak infusions. When making medicine, however, you are usually working with what would formally be called an infusion. Infusions are stronger than teas since the herbs sit, or *infuse*, in the water for a much longer period.

An infusion is made by immersing an herb in either cold or hot (not boiling) water for an extended time. Again, the water you use should be the purest you can find, *not* tap water. Water from rain, a healthy well, or a spring is best.

The weakness of infusions, cold or hot, is that they do not keep well; they tend to spoil very quickly. Refrigeration will only slow the process a little. Infusions, unless you stabilize them with something like alcohol, need to be used shortly after you make them. Their strength is that nearly everyone has access to enough water to make them without resorting to the expense of buying alcohol.

HOT INFUSIONS

The following guidelines are for hot infusions and will work with most herbs. Although these guidelines use short timelines for hot infusions, I often make my infusions at night just before bed and let them infuse overnight. I usually make enough for 1 day, then drink the infusion throughout the next day.

Most *hot* infusions are consumed, confusingly, not hot but warm or at room temperature; the infusion periods are too long for the water to stay hot. *Hot infusion*, in this sense, is a description of the extraction process, not of its temperature when used.

Some herbs, however, are best consumed while still hot, often these are diaphoretics that stimulate sweating. Yarrow, if being used to stimulate sweating to help break a fever, is best consumed hot (steeped 15 minutes, covered). If being used for GI tract distress or to stimulate menstruation it is best prepared as a hot infusion (covered), then consumed hours later at room temperature.

To prepare a hot infusion, bring water to a boil, then pour it over the herb in the following manner:

For leaves: 1 ounce per quart of water, let steep 4 hours, tightly covered. Tougher leaves require longer steeping. The more powdered the leaves (if dried), the stronger the infusion. If you are using fresh leaves, cut them finely with scissors or chop them as finely as possible with a sharp knife.

For flowers: 1 ounce per quart of water, let steep 2 hours, tightly covered. More fragile flowers require less time. Most flowers can be infused whole.

For seeds: 1 ounce per pint of water, let steep 30 minutes, tightly covered. More fragrant seeds such as fennel need less time (15 minutes), rose hips longer (3 to 4 hours). Most seeds possess very strong seed coats to protect them from the world until they sprout. You will need to break the seed coat in order for the solvent to work; the seeds should be powdered as finely as possible.

For barks and roots: 1 ounce per pint of water, let steep 8 hours, tightly covered. Some barks, such as slippery elm, need less time (1 to 2 hours). Most barks and roots are infused after being dried; powder them as finely as possible. If you are using fresh roots, mince them as finely as possible.

If you keep the containers tightly covered, the volatile components in the herb will remain in the liquid rather than evaporating into the air. The heat will vaporize the volatiles and they will rise up in the steam, then collect on the underside of the lid. As the mixture cools, the volatiles will condense and drip from the lid back into the infusion. This ensures that the essential oils, which are very volatile, will still be present. You can easily identify an herb that has a high volatiles content; it will have a strong essential oil or perfumey smell to it. These must always be covered when making a hot infusion.

When you are ready to use the infusion, pour off the water and squeeze out the marc as much as possible. The liquid in the saturated herbs is often much stronger than the infused liquid, so keep it if you can.

Measuring Herbal Medicines

It seems nearly everyone uses a different way to describe how much to take; some say milliliters (ml), some say drops, some say dropperful, some say teaspoon or tablespoon, so here is a conversion table for you. It may help.

A drop: A drop is not always a drop (see why there's confusion?). A drop of water and a drop of alcohol are about the same, but a drop of glycerine is bigger — about five times bigger than a drop of water — because it is so viscous. Nevertheless, pretty much everyone treats a drop as a drop. Now, is that clear or what?

Dropperful: A 1-ounce glass tincture bottle has a standard glass dropper that fits in it, and when it's full of tincture that is what I call a dropperful. It generally holds around 30 drops, so I consider a dropperful to be 30 drops, or 1.5 ml. Normally, a glass dropper will fill only halfway with one squeeze, so it takes two to get a full dropper.

A milliliter is, for water or alcohol, 20 drops, or two-thirds of a dropperful.

A teaspoon is 5 ml or 100 drops or three and one-third dropperfuls.

A tablespoon is $1/2$ ounce, 15 ml, 3 teaspoons, 300 drops.

An ounce is in the neighborhood of 600 drops.

COLD INFUSIONS

Cold infusions are preferable for some herbs. The bitter components of herbs tend to be less soluble in cold water. Yarrow, for instance, is much less bitter when prepared in cold water. Usually cold infusions need to steep for much longer periods of time, though each herb is different. The necessity for a cold infusion rarely arises; nevertheless, it may. If so, place the herb in room-temperature water, cover, and let steep overnight.

INFUSION EQUIPMENT

There are many kinds of infusion pitchers and mugs available; they are pretty common. Most of them have some form of basket in which to place the herbs (and a lid to cover them). The basket is suspended at the top of the mug or pitcher so that the herbs and the liquid do not mix together. It does make it a bit easier. (Avoid plastic if you can; use stainless steel, glass, or pottery infusers.) You can also buy (or make) small cloth bags to hold the herbs, which you then suspend in whatever container you are using. A tea ball will also work but I don't find them as effective; they don't usually hold enough herb.

The best infusers work by holding the herb in the upper part of the pot, so that only the upper portion of the liquid is in contact with the herb. As the water at the top of the infuser becomes saturated with the herbal constituents, it gets heavier and sinks to the bottom. This creates a circulating current in the water that brings the unsaturated water to the top of the jar where it can then infuse as well. This will make the strongest infusion. You can also just put the herb in a jar with hot water and cover it; it will work fine but it won't be quite as strong as this method.

A Hot Infusion for Parasites

INGREDIENTS:

2 ounces fresh ginger root, chopped finely

2 ounces dried sida leaf

2 ounces dried wormwood leaf (*Artemisia absinthium*)

2 quarts water

Place herbs in container, pour near-boiling water on top, cover tightly, and let sit overnight. Strain and press the marc to remove as much liquid as possible. Drink 1 cup four times per day. This recipe will make enough to last 2 days. Continue for 8 days (making the infusion again as necessary). This is a good infusion for treating intestinal worms (you can just use the wormwood and ginger if you wish). It will be very bitter, though the ginger will help that a bit.

Decoctions

Decoctions are much stronger than infusions. Basically, they are boiled infusions. There are two forms of decoctions: 1) simple decoctions, and 2) concentrated decoctions. A simple decoction is any water extract that is boiled for a short length of time. Concentrated decoctions are boiled until the water is reduced to some extent. Normally, herbs that are highly resinous or filled with volatile oils are not decocted. Only herbs whose constituents are not damaged by heat are boiled.

It is important to begin with cold water, not warm or hot, then add the herbs and bring it to a boil. The extraction will be more efficient if you begin with cold water because different constituents extract better at different temperatures.

Some herbs, such as isatis, are stronger if they are boiled for a few minutes simply because the higher heat is a better extractant. Herbs high in polysaccharides such as reishi are also often helped by boiling; polysaccharides tend to extract more efficiently when decocted. In essence, anytime an herb is boiled, no matter how short a time, it is considered to be a decoction. If you are just boiling the herb to better extract the constituents, you are making a simple decoction.

A Simple Decoction

1 oz herb   1 pint cold water

. . . .

Combine the herb and water. Bring to boil. Boil for at least 15 minutes (some herbs will need longer). Let cool enough that you can handle it. Strain the decoction to remove the herb.

Press the herb to remove all the liquid. Add enough water to bring the liquid back to 1 pint. Take as directed.

In a concentrated decoction, which is more common than simple decoctions, the herb is boiled in water long enough that the amount of water you began with is reduced to some extent, often by half, sometimes more. This acts to concentrate the constituents in less liquid, making the medicine stronger. Concentrated decoctions are not often drunk as a tea (reishi is an exception). However, they are sometimes used in smaller doses similarly to a tincture. Once the decoction is made it is allowed to cool, the liquid strained, then dispensed a tablespoon at a time—usually three or four times a day depending on the herb and the disease. The usual dosage range for concentrated decoctions, depending on the herb, is 1 to 4 fluid ounces a day.

The most common form of medicine made from concentrated decoctions is a cough syrup. They are also used to make fomentations — that is, very condensed water extracts that are soaked into a cloth and applied to the surface of the body (to treat pain and inflammation in a joint, for example). Decoctions are also used as enemas — should the need arise, which everyone hopes it won't. This gets a very strong concentrate into the bowel where it will, usually, rather easily move across the membranes of the colon into the bloodstream.

When you are making your concentrated decoctions, use porcelain, glass, or stainless steel pots if you can; iron and aluminum will often contaminate the mix. When the decoction is cool, prepare it as needed for whatever you are going to use it for. Concentrated decoctions will last longer than infusions, especially if kept cold. Syrups will often last a year in a refrigerator just fine.

A Concentrated Decoction for Sore Throat and Upper Respiratory Infection

INGREDIENTS:

1 ounce dried elderberries
Pinch of cayenne
3 cups cold water

Wildflower honey
Juice of 1 lemon

Combine elderberries and cayenne with water. Bring to a boil, then reduce heat and simmer, uncovered, until liquid is reduced by half. Let cool enough that you can work with it. Strain liquid and press elderberries to remove as much liquid as possible. Add wildflower honey to taste. Add juice of one lemon. Store in refrigerator. Take 1 tablespoon or more as often as needed at the onset of sore throat or upper respiratory infections.

Alcohol Extractions

Because alcohol extractions, i.e., tinctures, keep so well over time and because they are so easily dispensed, many herbalists prefer them over infusions. They are made by immersing a fresh plant in full-strength alcohol or a dried plant in an alcohol and water mixture.

I am a fan of using pure grain alcohol for tinctures. What that means in practice, however, is using an alcohol that is 190 proof, or 95 percent alcohol. (There is such a thing as 100 percent or 200-proof

The Origin of "Proof"

As an aside: In the eighteenth century the English navy paid sailors partly in rum. The watering of drinks has always been a problem. So to test their rum before accepting it as pay, the sailors would soak gunpowder with it. If the gunpowder would still burn, the rum was "proved." Hence 100 proof. The rum had to be a minimum of 57.5 percent alcohol for the gunpowder to burn, but that has since been watered down to a simple rule of thumb, 50 percent alcohol = 100 proof.

alcohol, but the only people who generally use it are scientists or large commercial enterprises; you will probably never see it.) Most people buy their 190-proof alcohol at their local liquor store; the most common brand in the United States is called Everclear.

Some states — some countries — will not allow their citizens to buy 190-proof alcohol (for their own good, of course). If you live in such a place, you will have to cross state (or country) lines and buy your alcohol from a more enlightened place or else make do with what they allow you buy. In such places, most people use a 40 to 50 percent alcohol-content vodka; that is, 80 to 100 proof. Get the highest proof you can — you will see why this is important as we go on.

In the United States, the amount you pay for liquor, regardless of what you are buying, is directly proportional to its alcohol content. The actual cost of a gallon of 190-proof alcohol is about US$1.00. The rest of the cost is federal and state taxes — which are then taxed again as sales tax when you buy the thing. So you may be tempted to buy a lower-proof vodka because it is cheaper. That is a bad idea. Your tinctures will be weak.

Fresh Plant Tinctures

Fresh plant tinctures, again, are made by putting the fresh herb in pure grain alcohol. These tinctures are nearly always made in a one-to-two ratio, which is written 1:2. (There are a few exceptions.) This ratio means you are using 1 part herb (dry weight measurement) to 2 parts liquid (liquid measurement). The amount of herb in such ratios is always indicated by the first number, the amount of liquid by the second number.

So, for example, if you have 3 ounces (dry weight measure) of fresh echinacea flower heads, you would place them in a jar with 6 ounces (liquid measure) of 190-proof alcohol. I generally use well-sealed Mason or Ball jars, stored out of the sun and shaken daily. At the end of 2 weeks the herb is decanted and squeezed through a cloth until as dry as possible (an herb or wine press is good for this), and the resulting liquid is then stored in labeled amber bottles.

Fresh plants naturally contain a certain percentage of water and alcohol is a very good extractor of water. (One of the main symptoms of a hangover comes from the alcohol extracting the water from your body — you get the same kind of headache from too much alcohol as you do from dehydration.) Alcohol will pull not only the medicinal constituents out of the plant but the plant's water as well.

The water in the fresh plant dilutes the alcohol; how much depends on the kind of plant it is. Peppermint has a lot of water in it, 50 percent or more by weight. So what you get when you tincture fresh peppermint leaves is a tincture that is about 50 percent alcohol and 50 percent water. Myrrh gum has virtually no water in it, so you end up with a tincture that is 95 percent alcohol and 5 percent water — and all that water was already in the alcohol, assuming you began with 95 percent alcohol.

Fresh leafy plants may be chopped or left whole before being placed into the alcohol or pureed with the alcohol in a blender. Fresh roots should be ground with the alcohol in a blender into a pulpy mush. (I generally think it better to make root tinctures from dry roots but there are a few exceptions; coral root is one.)

Pressing Herbal Tinctures

When your tinctures are done and you pour off the liquid, the marc will still have some, often a great deal of, liquid in it. The marc needs to be pressed to remove the remaining tincture. Most people do this by hand. The best thing to use is a good-quality cloth with a close weave to it — I use the same surgical cloths hospitals do; they hold up really well. An herb press facilitates this immensely, though a cider press, depending on the style, will work very well, too. You will get a lot more out of a press than doing it by hand, but they do tend to be expensive.

With fresh plants you can generally get out about as much liquid as you put in; with dried material, especially roots, you get out as much as you can. Sometimes this isn't much.

Dried Plant Tinctures

Plants, as they dry, lose their natural moisture content. When making a tincture of a dried plant, the amount of water you add to the menstruum is the amount that was present in the plant when it was fresh. This enables the extraction of the water-soluble constituents to occur.

Dried plants are usually tinctured at a one-to-five ratio, which is written 1:5. (There are, as always, exceptions.) That means 1 part dried herb to 5 parts liquid. Fresh *Echinacea angustifolia* root, for example, contains 30 percent water by weight. If you have 10 ounces of powdered root (dry weight), you would then add to it 50 ounces of liquid (liquid measurement). This gives you your 1:5 ratio. The tricky part for many people comes in figuring out how much of that liquid should be water and how much should be alcohol. In this instance you want your liquid to be 30 percent water (fresh echinacea root's water content), that is, 30 percent of 50 ounces, which would be 15 ounces of water. The rest of the liquid will be alcohol, that is, 35 ounces.

In a formulary or materia medica, the tincture instructions for this particular plant would look something like this:

Echinacea angustifolia, fresh root tincture 1:2; dried root tincture 1:5, 70% alcohol. 30–60 drops as needed. Acute conditions: 30 drops minimum each hour.

It is just *assumed* that you already know that all fresh plant tinctures at 1:2 will be using 95 percent alcohol. (Note: Everyone I know just assumes that the 95 percent alcohol they are using is 100 percent; no one I know takes that 5 percent into account in figuring this stuff out. Life is too short.)

Again, don't use tap water if you can avoid it. Powder the herbs you are tincturing as finely as possible — many people in the United States use a Vitamix for this. It is a pretty indestructible mixer/grinder, especially if you get a commercial-grade unit. (The demo video shows them grinding 2x4s into sawdust.)

Unless the herbs become tremendously hard when dried (as red root does), it is best to store herbs as whole as possible until they are needed. This reduces the cell surface area that is exposed to air. Oxygen degrades plant matter fairly quickly.

How Long Will Tinctures Last?

Tinctures should be kept out of the sun — a dark, cool room is good. Keeping them in dark or amber-colored glass jars is even better — though if they are in the dark you can leave them in clear jars as many of us do with our larger quantities of tincture. Tinctures will, in general, last many years. However, you should know about precipitation, a very neglected area of herbal medicine.

The constituents that you have extracted from the herbs are held in suspension in a liquid medium. Over time, some of these constituents will precipitate out and settle on the bottom of the tincture bottle. Some herbs such as *Echinacea angustifolia* root are heavy precipitators, while others, like elder flower, are such light precipitators that you will almost never see a precipitate in the bottle. Unfortunately, there has been little study on this, nor has a chart of herbal precipitation rates ever been prepared (as far as I know; intent searching has never turned one up). Technically, we need one that shows both rate of precipitation and the amount of precipitation for each plant.

Some herbalists will add 1 to 2 ounces of glycerine to every 16 ounces of tincture (10 to 15 percent of the total liquid) to help slow down or eliminate precipitation. It does help retard the precipitation of tannins; I am not sure how well it works for other constituents or over time but you might try it and see how it works if precipitation becomes a concern for you.

You will find that some herbs will produce an ever larger precipitate on the bottom of your storage bottles as time goes by. It is not possible to get that precipitate back into solution. Most herbalists simply shake the bottle prior to dispensing and suggest the user do the same before ingesting it. I do it this way and it seems to work fine, medicinally speaking.

There is, as yet, no data on whether the efficacy of a tincture is affected by precipitation. Certainly the ones that do not precipitate are good for decades if kept in a dark, cool location in well-sealed bottles.

Dried plant tinctures, like fresh, are left to macerate for 2 weeks, out of the light, before decanting.

Combination Tincture Formulas

In spite of our aversion in the United States toward the metric system, all scientific glassware in the United States is metric. Most herbalists use a *graduated cylinder* to measure the amount of tincture they are pouring out (available from any scientific glassware company). Most herbal bottles, of course, are in ounces, while the measuring cylinders are in milliliters. Roughly, 30 milliliters is equal to 1 ounce.

As an example, if you were going to make a combination tincture formula for the early onset of colds and flu, a good mix would be 10 ml each of echinacea, red root, and licorice tinctures mixed together. This would give you 1 fluid ounce total.

You can mix something like this in the graduated cylinder, as long as your hand is steady, then pour the mixture into a 1-ounce amber bottle with a dropper lid. Dosage would be one dropperful at least each hour during the onset of upper respiratory infections. This will usually prevent the onset of colds and flu if your immune system is relatively healthy.

Treatment of Children

Children's bodies are much smaller than adults', and if you are using herbal medicines with them, you need to adjust the dosages. You can determine the dosages for children through one of three approaches:

Clark's rule: Divide the weight in pounds by 150 to give an approximate fraction of an adult's dose. For a 75-pound child, the dose would be 75 divided by 150 or 1/2 the adult dose. (This is the rule I find most useful.)

Cowling's rule: The age of a child at his or her next birthday divided by 24. For a child coming 8 years of age, the dose would be 8 divided by 24 or 1/3 the adult dose.

Young's rule: The child's age divided by (12 + age of child). For a 3-year-old it would be 3 divided by (12 + 3; that is, 15) for a dose of $1/5$ the adult dose.

A Comment on Alcohol

There has been a tremendous resurgence of puritanitis in the United States and a few other parts of the globe (notably the UK) the past 20 years or so. One object of attention of this spasming of the puritan reflex has been the evils of alcohol. Many on the Right and on the Left seem to think it is some sort of inherently evil substance that is going to destroy Western civilization or at least make God really, really mad.

Alcohol existed long before human beings emerged out of the ecological matrix of this planet. It is a highly natural substance, both inside and outside of our bodies. *All* living beings partake of it, including trees, bees, and elephants. (Not kidding.) All of them enjoy it. It facilitates the functioning of the body, enhances organ function in many respects, and reduces the incidence of many diseases. It is not an evil substance.

One of the continual queries about tinctures concerns the alcohol content. Many people are afraid to take tinctures because of the evil alcohol in them.

To be really specific: The amount of alcohol in tinctures is incredibly tiny. Less than you will get from eating a few pieces of bread (yes, bread does have alcohol in it, enough to produce a breathalyzer reading of 0.05 just by itself). If you are taking 20 drops of a 60 percent alcohol tincture *every* hour for an acute condition, you will get about $1/17$ of an ounce of alcohol over the course of a day (less than 2 ml). If you are taking a general dose (20 drops three times daily), you will be getting about $1/30$ of an ounce over a day. Again, this is less than you will get from eating two slices of bread.

If this truly is a problem for you, you can make infusions or use glycerites — though the glycerites really aren't as effective and the water extractions won't extract some of the more important alcohol-soluble constituents. Some people heat their tinctures to remove the alcohol; it doesn't work very well and I suspect the heat alters the quality of the tincture. I don't recommend it.

Childhood Ear Infections

Most childhood ear infections can be treated successfully with herbs. Tinctures, glycerites, honeys, teas, and herbal steams are all effective approaches.

Children are most susceptible to ear infections from antibiotic-resistant strains of *Haemophilus influenzae, Staphylococcus aureus, Streptococcus pneumoniae,* and *Branhamella catarrhalis.* The following kinds of remedies have been found highly effective for treating them, individually or together. These kinds of ear infections often accompany flus and colds; this will help if they do.

Children's Ear Oil

INGREDIENTS:

5 cloves garlic

4 ounces olive oil

20 drops eucalyptus essential oil

Chop garlic finely, place in small baking dish with olive oil, cook over low heat overnight, and strain, pressing garlic cloves well. Add essential oil to garlic oil and mix well. Place in amber bottle for storage. To use: Hold glass eyedropper under hot water for 1 minute, dry well (quickly), and suction up ear oil from bottle. Place 2 drops in each ear every half hour or as often as needed for 2 to 7 days.

Brigitte Mars's Herbal Tea for Ear Infections

INGREDIENTS:

1 ounce elder flower (*Sambucus* spp.)

1 ounce licorice root

1 ounce Mormon tea (*Ephedra viridis*)

1 ounce peppermint leaf

1 ounce rose hips

1 quart water

Wildflower honey (optional)

Roughly crush all herbs. Bring water to a near boil, then pour over the herbs and allow to steep until cooled enough to drink. Consume as hot as is comfortable for drinking. Sweeten with honey if desired. As much as is wanted can be consumed. The Mormon tea is a decongestant, the rose hips are slightly astringent and anti-inflammatory and high in vitamin C, the elder flowers are slightly sedative and reduce fevers, the licorice root is anti-inflammatory and tastes good and is antiviral and antibacterial, and the peppermint helps reduce fevers and decongests and is calming. Catnip can be added to help lower fever.

Ear Infection Tincture Combination

INGREDIENTS:

1 ounce *Echinacea angustifolia* tincture

1 ounce ginger tincture of ginger

1 ounce licorice tincture

1 ounce red root tincture

Mix together the tinctures. Give one dropperful (30 drops) of the combination tincture each hour per 150 pounds of body weight until symptoms cease. Best administered in juice. Dosage should be altered for the child's weight. Eucalyptus and sage tinctures can also be used. You can also prepare this as a glycerite or a medicinal honey.

To Lower a Fever in a Child

The best herb for lowering seriously high fevers is coral root (*Corallorhiza maculata*), as either a tea or tincture. Tea: 1 teaspoon of the root steeped in 8 ounces water for 30 minutes and then drunk. Tincture: Up to 30 drops for a child of 60 pounds. Brigitte Mars's herbal tea for ear infections (page 325), with the addition of catnip, is also exceptionally effective in lowering fevers. Yarrow and peppermint teas are excellent too. Finally, bathing with cool water will also work very well.

Treating Diarrhea in Children

The use of a tea and tincture combination is usually effective. See the recipes that follow.

Rosemary Gladstar's Tea for Diarrhea

INGREDIENTS:

3 parts blackberry root

2 parts slippery elm bark

Mix the herbs together (for example 3 ounces blackberry root and 2 ounces slippery elm bark). Simmer 1 teaspoon of the herb mixture in 1 cup water for 20 minutes. Strain and cool. Take 2 to 4 tablespoons every hour or as often as needed.

Tincture Combination for Diarrhea

INGREDIENTS:

1 ounce acacia tincture

1 ounce berberine plant tincture

1 ounce cryptolepis tincture

1 ounce evergreen needle tincture

Combine the tinctures, and shake well. Give 1 dropperful (30 drops) for every 150 pounds of body weight every 1 to 2 hours in water or orange juice until symptoms cease.

A Final Note

You, more than anyone else ever will, know how you are feeling in your body. Pay close attention to how you respond to any medicines you take. If you don't feel right when you take an herbal medicine, stop taking it.

APPENDIX B

SOURCES OF SUPPLY

A weed is a plant that has mastered every survival skill except for learning how to grow in rows.

— Doug Larson

Many of the herbs I have talked about in this book — and, of course, a great many others — grow wild. Even if you live in a city you can find many of them cohabitating with you or only a short drive away. Since many of these herbs are invasives, most people will be glad for you to take them away.

If you need to buy your herbs, the Internet is a good way to seek them. I suggest running a web search for the herbs you are looking for to find the cheapest prices; if you are persistent you can often save half off normal retail.

If you are going to be buying a lot of herbs and you live in the United States it makes sense to buy a resale license from your state. The price is often minimal and it will allow you to buy wholesale; most wholesalers will want a resale certificate before they will sell to you.

And, of course, you can grow them yourself. Once established most of the herbs in this book will provide medicine for you and your family forever.

Here are some of the best sources I know of for the herbs in this book. All of them are in the United States.

1stChineseHerbs.com
5018 Viewridge Drive
Olympia, WA 98501
888-842-2049
www.1stchineseherbs.com
Wonderful people with a very large selection of Chinese herbs, including most of those discussed in this book. Most herbs by the pound.

Elk Mountain Herbs
214 Ord Street
Laramie, WY 82070
307-742-0404
www.elkmountainherbs.com
Wonderful tinctures from local wildcrafted Western plants.

Green Dragon Botanicals

48 Elliot Street, Suite D
Brattleboro, VT 05301
877-591-1874
www.greendragonbotanicals.com

A good source for Japanese
knotweed.

Healing Spirits Herb Farm and Education Center

61247 Route 415
Avoca, NY 14809
607-566-2701
www.healingspiritsherbfarm.com

Matthias and Andrea Reisen have
been growing wonderful medicinal
plants for years. The plants just jump
out of the bag and laugh when you
open it up.

Horizon Herbs, LLC

P. O. Box 69
Williams, OR 97544
541-846-6704
www.horizonherbs.com

Richo Cech has spent much of his
life learning how to grow common
and rare medicinals. He has seeds or
young stock for most of the plants in
this book as well as great information
on how to grow them.

Mountain Rose Herbs

P. O. Box 50220
Eugene, OR 97405
800-879-3337
www.mountainroseherbs.com

A nice selection, sustainably
produced.

Pacific Botanicals

4840 Fish Hatchery Road
Grants Pass, OR 97527
541-479-7777
www.pacificbotanicals.com

This is perhaps the best wholesaler
(they also sell retail) in the U.S. Their
herbs are magnificent. Normally, all
are sold by the pound.

Sage Woman Herbs, Ltd.

108 East Cheyenne Road
Colorado Springs, CO 80906
888-350-3911
www.sagewomanherbs.com

They have some herbs otherwise
hard to get, especially isatis tincture
(just the root though).

Woodland Essence

392 Teacup Street
Cold Brook, NY 13324
315-845-1515
www.woodlandessence.com

Kate and Don make wonderful tinctures and medicines and can sell
you many of the herbal tinctures that
I discuss in this book; if they don't
have them, they can probably point
you in the right direction.

Zack Woods Herb Farm

278 Mead Road
Hyde Park, VT 05655
802-888-7278
www.zackwoodsherbs.com

Melanie and Jeff are wonderful
people and grow tremendously
beautiful medicinal plants. Very, very
high-quality herbs. Usually sold by the
pound.

NOTES

Chapter 1

1. Although I don't look at treatments for chikungunya fever virus in this book, some herbs have been found effective against it (in vitro): *Trigonostemon cherrieri, Flacourtia ramontchi, Anacolosa pervilleana.*

2. Stuart Levy, *The Antibiotic Paradox* (N.Y.: Plenum Press, 1992), 3.

3. Levy, *The Antibiotic Paradox,* 3.

4. Frank Ryan, *Virus X: Tracking the New Killer Plagues* (Boston: Little, Brown, and Company, 1997), 9.

5. Lynn Margulis and Dorion Sagan, *What Is Life?* (N.Y.: Simon and Schuster, 1995), 88.

6. Richard Lewontin, *The Triple Helix* (Cambridge, Mass.: Harvard University Press, 2000), 102–3.

7. Lynn Margulis, *Symbiotic Planet* (N. Y.: Basic Books, 1998), 75.

8. Ryan, *Virus X,* 10.

9. Lewontin, *The Triple Helix,* 125–26.

10. Ryan, *Virus X,* 51.

11. Ryan, 52.

Chapter 2

1. In contrast, read the description of the Native American use of lomatium while treating the flu epidemic on page 242.

Chapter 5

1. If you look at the bibliography for this book you will notice that I use a large number of scientific journal papers as sources for information on the plants. I have a couple of comments about that:

In general, I tend to give highest credence to studies performed in Asia (primarily Japan), South America (of which there are too few) and Africa (the best). For antibacterials, African researchers are doing the best work. For antivirals, researchers in China, Korea, Japan, and India are doing the best work.

Unfortunately, U.S. researchers are too often biased against plant medicines, too influenced by pharmaceutical money, and too biased in favor of technological medicine to be completely reliable. The unreliability of Western science in this respect is a growing problem, one becoming commonly recognized throughout the world. In fact, our scientific tradition in the West risks becoming an unreliable joke throughout the world in the coming decades.

Marcia Angell, M.D., has commented on this in a number of articles. She comments:

> It is simply no longer possible to believe much of the clinical research that is published, or to rely on the judgment of trusted physicians or authoritative medical guidelines. I take no pleasure in this conclusion, which I reached slowly and reluctantly over my two decades as an editor of *The New England Journal of Medicine.* [M. Angell, "Drug companies and doctors: A story of corruption," *New York Review of Books,* January 15, 2009]

Angell observes, earlier in that same article:

> In view of this control and the conflicts of interest that permeate the enterprise, it is not surprising that industry-sponsored trials published in medical journals consistently favor sponsor's drugs — largely because negative results are not published, positive results are repeated in slightly different forms, and a positive spin is put on even negative results. A review of seventy-four clinical trials of antidepressants, for example, found that thirty-seven of thirty-eight positive studies were published. But of the thirty-six negative studies, thirty-three were either not published or published in a form that conveyed a positive outcome.

John Ioannidis, in a rather remarkable article published in *PLoS Medicine,* noted:

There is increasing concern that in modern research, false findings may be the majority of, even the vast majority of, published research claims. However, this should not be surprising. It can be proven that most claimed research findings are false. [J. P. A. Ioannidis, "Why most published research findings are false," *PLoS Medicine* 2, no. 8 (2005): e124]

And then he goes on to do just that.

The point of all this is to say that modern scientific research, while useful, is not the last word, nor are Western studies the most reliable. If we are to create a modern healing tradition in the West, in the true sense of that word "healing," then a very different paradigm than the one in use at the moment needs to be developed. So, while I do focus in some depth on journal papers and what are normally considered to be "scientific" studies, I take them with a large grain of salt.

It takes some time to really learn to read journal papers and I don't mean from this developing an understanding of the terminology. While all the journal papers tend to follow the same structural outline and most use the same type of authorial voice, there are huge differences in the papers. With time and experience it is possible to tell which of the papers' authors know what they are doing and which do not, which are truly deep-thinking and which are barely average researchers, which of them are doing it for the money and which are genuinely interested in understanding what they are studying, which allow their humanity to guide their work and which do not. These factors alter the outcomes of the work considerably, though there has been little study of their influences. However, most people *think* that the use of journal papers confers legitimacy — and to be fair, some of them really are very good.

2. Curiously enough, many of the strongest antibacterial and antiviral plants are invasives. The dynamics of this are complex, not nearly so simple as one might think. Yes, invasives are tremendously potent simply by virtue of their capacity to take over ecosystems into which they are introduced. But this ignores the homeodynamis factors and deeply interwoven feedback systems that exist in the Earth ecosystem. Plants move throughout ecosystems in response to multiple complex factors, not simply because a seed hitchhiked on someone's shoe. Their impacts as they move are extremely complex and often highly sophisticated. And the question must always be asked, "What are they *doing* here?"

To give a very simple view outside contemporary perspectives: Amur honeysuckle (*Lonicera maackii*) is a shrub native to Japan, Korea, China, and Russia. It is an escaped cultivar in the United States and is invasive nearly everywhere it gets established. It is labeled invasive/banned in Connecticut, prohibited in Massachusettes, a noxious weed in Vermont, and invasive in Wisconsin and Tennessee. According to contemporary orientations regarding invasive species, the plant is considered to be a serious threat to ecosystem diversity and health and it is to be eradicated with extreme prejudice. However, the plant strongly affects the numbers of eggs laid by the mosquito *Aedes triseriatus,* a primary vector of La Crosse encephalitis virus (named after La Crosse, Wisconsin), reducing egg numbers considerably. The more honeysuckle there is, the fewer mosquitoes, the less the incidence of the viral disease in those areas. The plant also contains compounds that are specific for reducing inflammation, especially in the brain, during infection. They protect neurons and microglial cells from damage. This particular mosquito is also a vector for dengue fever (and other viruses), which is an emerging virus in the southern United States in such states as Texas and Georgia. Amur honeysuckle is also invasive in both those states. After 30 years of this work, I have continually seen that invasives show up in the regions where they are needed for the exact diseases that are emerging there. I can no longer discount it just because the mechanism for that process can't be seen with reductionist eyes.

3. S. H. Song and Z. Z. Wang, "Analysis of essential oils from different organs of Scutellaria baicalensis," *Zhong Yao Cai* 33, no. 8 (2010): 1265–70.

4. American Botanical Council, *The ABC Clinical Guide to Elder Berry* (Austin, Tex.: American Botanical Council, 2004), 8.

5. L. Johnson, "Elderberry for Cold and Flu Relief," *Healthy Living* (blog), CBN.com, http//blogs.cbn.com/healthyliving/archive/2011/10/13/elderberry-for-cold-and-flu-relief.aspx, October 13, 2011.

6. E. Parziale, "Elderberry," part of the Backyard Herbalist site hosted at Tripod.com, http//earthnotes.tripod.com/elderberry.htm, 1999.

7. F. Vandenbussche et al., "Analysis of the in planta antiviral activity of elderberry ribosome-inactivating proteins," *European Journal of Biochemistry* 271 (2004): 1508–15.

8. Thanks, Adam.

9. S. Harada, "The broad anti-viral agent glycyrrhizin directly modulates the fluidity of plasma membrane and HIV-1 envelope," *Biochemical Journal* 392 (2005): 191–99.

10. M. Moore, *Medicinal Plants of the Pacific Northwest* (Santa Fe, N.M.: Red Crane Books, 1993), 167.

11. Moore, *Medicinal Plants of the Pacific Northwest,* 167–68.

12. P. S. Beauchamp et al., "Essential oil composition of six *Lomatium* species attractive to Indra swallowtail butterfly (*Papilio indra*): Principal component analysis against essential oil composition of *Lomatium dissectum* var. *multifidum*," *Journal of Essential Oil Research* 21 (2009): 535–42.

13. E. Krebs, *Bulletin of the Nevada State Board of Health,* no. 1 (Carson City, Nev., January 1920).

BIBLIOGRAPHY

The problem with digital books is that you can always find what you are looking for but you need to go into a bookstore to find what you weren't looking for.

— Paul Krugman

Books

Abascal, Kathy. *Herbs and Influenza: How Herbs Used in the 1918 Flu Pandemic Can Be Effective Today.* Vashon, Wash.: Tigana Press, 2006.

Buhner, Stephen Harrod. *Healing Lyme Disease Coinfections: Complementary and Holistic Treatments for Bartonella and Mycoplasma.* Rochester, Vt.: Inner Traditions, 2013.

——. *Herbal Antibiotics,* 2nd ed. North Adams, Mass.: Storey Publishing, 2012.

——. *The Lost Language of Plants: The Ecological Importance of Plant Medicines to Life on Earth.* White River Junction, Vt.: Chelsea Green, 2002.

Chang, Hson-Mou, and Paul Pui-Hay But. *Pharmacology and Applications of Chinese Materia Medica.* 2 vols. River Edge, N.J.: World Scientific, 1987.

Felter, Harvey Wickes, and John Uri Lloyd. *King's American Dispensatory.* 2 vols. Sandy, Ore.: Eclectic Medical Publications, 1983.

Foster, Steven, and Yue Chongxi. *Herbal Emissaries.* Rochester, Vt.: Healing Arts Press, 1992.

Gladstar, Rosemary, and Pamela Hirsch. *Planting the Future.* Rochester, Vt.: Healing Arts Press, 2000.

Grieve, Maude. *A Modern Herbal.* 2 vols. N.Y.: Dover, 1971.

Griggs, Barbara. *Green Pharmacy.* Rochester, Vt.: Healing Arts Press, 1991.

Hobbs, Christopher. *Medicinal Mushrooms,* Loveland, Colo.: Interweave Press, 1995.

Lappé, Marc. *When Antibiotics Fail.* Berkeley, Calif.: North Atlantic Books, 1986.

Levy, Stuart. *The Antibiotic Paradox.* N.Y.: Plenum Press, 1992.

Manandhar, Narayan P. *Plants and People of Nepal.* Portland, Ore.: Timber Press, 2002.

Miller, Orson K. *Mushrooms of North America.* N.Y.: E. P. Dutton, 1972.

Moerman, Daniel. *Native American Ethnobotany.* Portland, Ore.: Timber Press, 1998.

Moore, Michael. *Medicinal Plants of the Desert and Canyon West.* Sante Fe: Museum of New Mexico Press, 1989.

——. *Medicinal Plants of the Mountain West.* Sante Fe: Museum of New Mexico Press, 1979.

——. *Medicinal Plants of the Pacific West.* Sante Fe, N.M.: Red Crane Books, 1993.

Nadkarni, K. M., and A. K. Nadkarni. *Indian Materia Medica,* 3rd ed. Bombay: Popular Prakashan, 1954.

Scheld, W. Michael, Richard Whitley, and Christina M. Marra. *Infections of the Central Nervous System.* Philadelphia: Lippincott Williams and Wilkins, 2004.

Weiss, Rudolph. *Herbal Medicine.* Gothenburg, Sweden: AB Arcanum, 1988.

Wu, Jing-Nuan. *An Illustrated Chinese Materia Medica.* N.Y.: Oxford University Press, 2005.

Zhu, You-Ping. *Chinese Materia Medica.* Amsterdam: Harwood Academic Publishers, 1998.

Journal Papers and Other Publications

Comment: Many of the research papers that are published in the West, and a good number of those from the East and South, are easily found on the very useful Internet database PubMed. That has made this kind of research much easier; it is fostering the wide dispersal of the scientific study of plant medicines. At the same time, there is a powerful movement among many of the world's researchers to begin publishing their studies only in open-source Internet journals, which means that you can access the whole journal article, not just the abstract.

A substantial number of the journals that had been prominent in the past are now so exclusive, so expensive, that many universities are abandoning them. Some journals that originally cost $200 per year for a university subscription are now in the $20,000 range — and at the same time, the professors and researchers are still doing all the work on them without remuneration. Further, many of the formerly prominent journals are now owned by big corporations, sometimes pharmaceutical companies, and they do control what is printed. And finally, many of the non-open-source journals are now writing their abstracts in such a way as to eliminate any reasonable transfer of information. If you want *any* of the useful information from the study, you gotta pay. The normal fee range for a four-page article tends to be anywhere from $34 to $51 for 24-hour access. Some of the publishers even restrict users' ability to print the articles; they are read-only. As the Supreme Court of the United States once said (in its better days), "Well, there's no definition of piggish in the law, but we recognize it when we see it."

The open-source movement is altering things considerably, and it's about time.

As I have noted in this book and elsewhere, many of the Chinese studies have not been translated into English and are not available on PubMed. However, the Chinese National Knowledge Infrastructure (CNKI) database is developing into an Eastern form of PubMed. It is in its infancy but it is going to be a powerhouse eventually, especially when it comes to plant medicines. The Asian cultures are not caught up in the pharmaceutical-dominated prejudice of the Western medical system. They know plant medicines work; they just want to find out how to use them most effectively. So they are beginning to create a unique hybrid composed of traditional healing approaches and Western medicine, which we in the West would do well to emulate in our own fashion. (But you know, horses might make a comeback, so we keep putting our cultural money on the manufacture of buggy whips — the new ones we are making even have computer chips in them, a CD, *and* a GPS.)

Though the Chinese journal articles, for the most part, have not been translated into English, the abstracts for them *are* in English. This is opening up a tremendous amount of research that has, formerly, not been accessible. The best way to access this site, if you are interested, is to get on Google Scholar, then type in what you are looking for, like this: scutellaria cnki. Or: cordyceps cnki. This will open that world to you — it's worth it.

My bibliographical references for CNKI listings will look like this:

Wang, G., et al. Anti-tumor activity study of extract from Scutellaria barbata D. Don. *Modern Journal of Integrated Traditional Chinese and Western Medicine*, 2004-09, CNKI.

The first number after the journal title is the year of publication, and the second number is the issue. The paper above, for example, was published in issue 9 of 2004. Google's search engine does have a bit of trouble scanning the CNKI database at this point, so if you are trying to access that exact article you pretty much have to type the title in verbatim on Google Scholar with the appendage CNKI and then look over the entries that appear. It will be there somewhere. (Some of the abstract translations are challenging, so be prepared.)

Google Scholar, PubMed, and CNKI are much like bookstores — you will often find what you were not looking for. A lot of useful discoveries come from that, if you are willing to trust it.

The Viruses

Miscellaneous

Bennett, R. et al. La Crosse virus infectivity, pathogenesis, and immunogenicity in mice and monkeys. *Virology Journal* 5, no. 25 (2008): 525–40.

Cassidy, L., and J. Patterson. Mechanism of La Crosse virus inhibition by ribavirin. *Antimicrobial Agents and Chemotherapy* 33, no. 11 (1989): 2009–11, 1989.

Charrel, R., et al. Chikungunya outbreaks — the globalization of vectorborne diseases. *New England Journal of Medicine* 356, no. 8 (2007): 769–71.

Chen, Y., et al. Dengue virus infectivity depends on envelope protein binding to target cell heparan sulfate. *Nature Medicine* 3, no. 8 (1997): 866–71.

Deas, T., et al. Inhibition of flavivirus infections by antisense olidomers specifically suppressing viral translation and RNA replication. *Journal of Virology* 79, no. 5 (2005): 4599–609.

De Clerq, Eric. Antivirals and antiviral strategies. *Nature Reviews, Microbiology* 2 (2004): 704–20.

Epstein, Paul. Emerging diseases and ecosystem instability: New threats to public health. *American Journal of Public Health* 85, no. 2 (1995): 168–72.

Erwin, P., et al. La Crosse encephalitis in eastern Tennessee. *American Journal of Epidemiology* 155, no. 11 (2002): 1060–65.

Furr, Samantha, and Ian Marriott. Viral CNS infections: Role of glial pattern recognition receptors in neuroinflammation. *Frontiers in Microbiology* 3, article 201 (2012).

Gaggar, A., et al. Proline-glycine-proline (PGP) and high mobility group box 1 protein (HMGB1). *Open Respiratory Medicine Journal* 4 (2010): 32–38.

Halsey, E., et al. Correlation of serotype-specific dengue virus infection with clinical manifestations. *PLoS* 6, no. 5 (2012): e1638.

Kaushik, D., et al. Microglial responses to viral challenges. *Frontiers in Bioscience* 17 (2011): 2187–205.

Kuiken, T., et al. Emerging viral infections in a rapidly changing world. *Current Opinion in Biotechnology* 14, no. 6 (2003): 641–46.

Li, X. F., et al. Protective activity of the ethanol extract of Cynachum paniculatum (BUNGE) Kitagawa on treating herpes encephalitis. *International Journal of Immunopathological Pharmacology* 25, no. 1 (2012): 259–66.

Mackenzie, J. Emerging viral diseases: An Australian perspective. *Emerging Infectious Diseases* 5, no. 1 (1999): 1–8.

Mackenzie, J., et al. Emerging flaviviruses: The spread of and resurgence of Japanese encephalitis, West Nile, and dengue viruses. *Nature Medicine* 10, no. 12 (2004): S98–109.

Mackenzie, J., et al. Emerging viral diseases of Southeast Asia and the western Pacific. *Emerging Infectious Diseases* 7, no. 3, supplement (2001): 497–504.

Nichol, S., et al. Emerging viral diseases. *Proceedings of the National Academy of Sciences* 97, no. 23 (2000): 12411–12.

Pekosz, Andrew, and Gregory Glass. Emerging viral diseases. *Maryland Medicine* 9, no. 1 (2008): 11–16.

Pekosz, A., et al. Induction of apoptosis by La Crosse virus infection and role of neuronal differentiation and human Bcl-2 expression in its prevention. *Journal of Virology* 70, no. 8 (1996): 5329–35.

Pekosz, A., et al. Protection from La Crosse virus encephalitis with recombinant glycoproteins. *Journal of Virology* 69, no. 6 (1995): 3475–81.

Schwartz, R., and R. Pellicciari. Manipulation of brain kynurenines: Glial targets, neuronal effects, and clinical opportunities. *Journal of Pharmacology and Experimental Therapeutics* 303, no. 1 (2002): 1–10.

Steiner, I., et al. Viral encephalitis: A review of diagnostic methods and guidelines for management. *European Journal of Neurology* 12 (2005): 331–43.

Sun, S., and D. Wirtz. Mechanics of enveloped virus entry into host cells. *Biophysical Journal* 90, no. 1 (2006): L10–12.

Uchil, P., et al. Nuclear location of flavivirus RNA synthesis in infected cells. *Journal of Virology* 80, no. 11 (2006): 5451–64.

Villarreal, L. P., V. R. Defilippis, and K. A. Gottlieb. Acute and persistent viral life strategies and their relationship to emerging diseases. *Virology* 272, no. 1 (2000): 1–6.

Wang, H., et al. Novel HMGB1-inhibiting therapeutic agents for experimental sepsis. *Shock* 32, no. 4 (2009): 348–57.

Whitley, R., and J. Gnann. Viral encephalitis: Familiar infections and emerging pathogens. *Lancet* 359 (2002): 507–13.

Wu, S., et al. Antiviral effects of an iminosugar derivative on flavivirus infections. *Journal of Virology* 76, no. 8 (2002): 3596–604.

Influenza

Alleva, L., et al. Systemic release of high mobility group box 1 protein during severe murine influenza. *Journal of Immunology* 181 (2008): 1454–59.

Bermejo-Martin, J., et al. Host adaptive immunity deficiency in severe pandemic influenza. *Critical Care* 14, no. 5 (2010): R167.

Hagau, N., et al. Clinical aspects and cytokine response in severe H1N1 influenza A virus infection. *Critical Care* 14 (2010): R203.

Ito, Y., et al. Increased levels of cytokines and high-mobility group box 1 are associated with the development of severe pneumonia, but not acute encephalopathy, in 2009 H1N1 influenza-infected children. *Cytokine* 56, no. 2 (2011): 180–87.

Julkunen, I., et al. Inflammatory responses in influenza A virus infection. *Vaccine* 19, suppl. 1 (2000): S32–37.

Julkunen, I., et al. Molecular pathogenesis of influenza A virus infection and virus-induced regulation of cytokine gene expression. *Cytokine Growth Factor Rev* 12, no. 2–3 (2001): 171–80.

Kobasa, D., et al. Aberrant innate immune response in lethal infection of macaques with the 1918 influenza virus. *Nature* 445, no. 18 (2007): 319–23.

Kosai, K., et al. Elevated levels of high mobility group box chromosomal protein-1 (HMGB1) in sera from patients with severe bacterial pneumonia coinfected with influenza virus. *Scandinavian Journal of Infectious Diseases* 40, no. 4 (2008) :338–42.

Larsen, D., et al. Systemic and mucosal immune responses to H1N1 influenza virus infection in pigs. *Veterinary Microbiology* 74 (2000): 117–31.

Lee, N., et al. Cytokine response patterns in severe pandemic 2009 H1N1 and seasonal influenza among hospitalized adults. *PLoS One* 6, no. 10 (2011): e26050.

Lee, N., et al. Hypercytokinemia and hyperactivation of phospho-p38 mitogen-activated protein kinase in severe human influenza A virus infection. *Clinical Infectious Diseases* 45 (2007): 723–31.

Mauad, T., et al. Lung pathology in fatal novel human influenza A (N1N1) infection. *American Journal of Respiratory and Critical Care Medicine* 181 (2010): 72–79.

Ohta, T., et al. Serum concentrations of complement anaphylatoxins and proinflammatory mediators in patients with 2009 H1N1 influenza. *Microbiology and Immunology* 55, no. 3 (2011): 191–98.

Oslund, K., and N. Baumgarth. Influenza-induced innate immunity: Regulators of viral replication, respiratory tract pathology, and adaptive immunity. *Future Virology* 6, no. 8 (2011): 951–62.

Phung, T., et al. Key role of regulated upon activation normal T-cell expressed and secreted, nonstructural protein1 and myeloperoxidase in cytokine storm induced by influenza virus PR-8 (A/H1N1) infection in A549 bronchial epithelial cells. *Microbiology and Immunology* 55, no. 12 (2011): 874–84.

Sladkova, T., and F. Kostolansky. The role of cytokines in the immune response to influenza A infection. *Acta Virologica* 50, no. 3 (2006): 151–62.

Teijara, J., et al. Endothelial cells are central orchestrators of cytokine amplification during influenza virus infection. *Cell* 146, no. 6 (2011): 980–91.

Thompson, C., et al. Infection of human airway epithelium by human and avian strains of influenza A virus. *Journal of Virology* 80, no. 16 (2006): 8060–68.

Us, D. Cytokine storm in avian influenza. *Mikrobiyoloji Bülteni* 42, no. 2 (2008): 365–80.

Walsh, K., et al. Suppression of cytokine storm with a sphingosine analog provides protection against pathogenic influenza virus. *Proceedings of the National Academy of Sciences* 108, no. 29 (2011): 12018–23.

Xuelian, Y., et al. Intensive cytokine induction in pandemic H1N1 influenza virus infection accompanied by robust production of IL-10 and IL-6. *PLoS One* 6, no. 12 (2011): e28680.

Japanese Encephalitis

Aleyas, A., et al. Functional modulation of dendritic cells and macrophages by Japanese encephalitis virus through MyD88 adaptor molecule-dependent and -independent pathways. *Journal of Immunology* 183, no. 4 (2010): 2462–74.

Aleyas, A., et al. Multifront assault on antigen presentation by Japanese encephalitis virus subverts CD8+ T cell responses. *Journal of Immunology* 185, no. 3 (2010): 1429–41.

Biswas, S., et al. Immunomodulatory cytokines determine the outcome of Japanese encephalitis virus infection in mice. *Journal of Medical Virology* 82, no. 2 (2010): 304–10.

Cao, S., et al. Japanese encephalitis virus wild strain infection suppresses dendritic cells maturation and function, and causes the expansion of regulatory T cells. *Virology Journal* 8 (2011): 39.

Chen, C., et al. Astrocytic alteration induced by Japanese encephalitis virus infection. *Neuroreport* 11, no. 9 (2000): 1833–37.

Chen, C., et al. Glial activation involvement in neuronal death by Japanese encephalitis virus infection. *Journal of General Virology* 91 (2010): 1028–37.

Chen, C., et al. Glutamate released by Japanese encephalitis virus-infected microglia involves TNF-α signaling and contributes to neuronal death. *Glia* 60, no. 3 (2012): 487–501.

Chen, C., et al. Src signaling involvement in Japanese encephalitis virus-induced cytokine production in microglia. *Neurochemistry International* 58, no. 8 (2011): 924–33.

Chen, C., et al. TNF-α and IL-1ß mediate Japanese encephalitis virus-induced RANTES gene expression in astrocytes. *Neurochemistry International* 58, no. 2 (2011): 234–42.

Chen, C., et al. Upregulation of RANTES gene expression in neuroglia by Japanese encephalitis virus infection. *Journal of Virology* 78, no. 22 (2004): 12107–19.

Das, A., et al. Abrogated inflammatory response promotes neurogenesis in a murine model of Japanese encephalitis. *PLoS One* 6, no. 3 (2011): e17225.

Das, S., et al. Critical role of lipid rafts in virus entry and activation of phosphoinositide 3' kinase/Akt signaling during early stages of Japanese encephalitis virus infection in neural stem/progenitor cells. *Journal of Neurochemistry* 115, no. 2 (2010): 537–49.

Das, S., et al. Japanese encephalitis virus infection induces IL-18 and IL-1beta in microglia and astrocytes: Correlation with in vitro cytokine responsiveness of glial cells and subsequent neuronal death. *Journal of Neuroimmunology* 195, no. 1–2 (2008): 60–72.

Das, S., and A. Basu. Japanese encephalitis virus infects neural progenitor cells and decreases their proliferation. *Journal of Neurochemistry* 106, no. 4 (2008): 1624–36.

Ghosh, D., and A. Basu. Japanese encephalitis — a pathological and clinical perspective. *PLoS* 3, no. 9 (2009): e437.

Ghoshal, A., et al. Proinflammatory mediators released by activated microglia induces neuronal death in Japanese encephalitis. *Glia* 55, no. 5 (2007): 483–96.

Hong-Lin, S., et al. Japanese encephalitis virus infection initiates endoplasmic reticulum stress and unfolded protein response. *Journal of Virology* 76, no. 9 (2002): 4162–71.

Khanna, N., et al. Induction of hypoglycaemia in Japanese encephalitis virus infection: The role of T lymphocytes. *Clinical and Experimental Immunology* 107, no. 2 (1997): 282–87.

Kim, E., et al. Paradoxical effects of chondroitin sulfate-E on Japanese encephalitis viral infection. *Biochemical and Biophysical Research Communications* 409(4): 717-22, 2011.

Kumar, S., et al. Some observations on the tropism of Japanese encephalitis virus in rat brain. *Brain Research* 1268 (2009): 135–41.

Liao, S., et al. Japanese encephalitis virus stimulates superoxide dismutase activity in rat glial cultures. *Neuroscience Letters* 324, no. 2 (2002): 133–36.

Lin, C., et al. Interferon antagonist function of Japanese encephalitis virus NS4A and its interaction with DEAD-box RNA helicase DDX42. *Virus Research* 137, no. 1 (2008): 49–55.

Lin, R., et al. Blocking of the alpha interferon Jak-Stat signaling pathway by Japanese encephalitis virus infection. *Journal of Virology* 78, no. 17 (2004): 9285–94.

Lin, R., et al. Replication-incompetent virions of Japanese encephalitis virus trigger neuronal cell death by oxidative stress in a culture system. *Journal of General Virology* 85 (2004): 521–33.

Mathus, A., et al. Breakdown of blood-brain barrier by virus-induced cytokine during Japanese encephalitis virus infection. *International Journal of Experimental Pathology* 73, no. 5 (1992): 603–11.

Mishra, M., and A. Basu. Minocycling neuroprotects, reduces microglial activation, inhibits caspase 3 induction, and viral replication following Japanese encephalitis. *Journal of Neurochemistry* 105, no. 5 (2008): 1582–95.

Mori, Y., et al. Nuclear localization of Japanese encephalitis virus core protein enhances viral replication. *Journal of Virology* 79, no. 6 (2005): 3448–58.

Nazmi, A., et al. RIG-1 mediates innate immune response in mouse neurons following Japanese encephalitis virus infection. *PLoS One* 6, no. 6 (2011): e21761.

Ogata, A., et al. Japanese encephalitis virus neurotropism is dependent on the degree of neuronal maturity. *Journal of Virology* 65, no. 2 (1991): 880–86.

Raung, S., et al. Japanese encephalitis virus infection stimulates Src tyrosine kinase in neuron/glia. *Neuroscience Letters* 419, no. 3 (2007): 263–68.

Raung, S., et al. Tyrosine kinase inhibitors attenuate Japanese encephalitis virus-induced neurotoxicity. *Biochemical and Biophysical Research Communications* 327, no. 2 (2005): 399–406.

Saxena, S., et al. Induction of nitric oxide synthase during Japanese encephalitis virus infection. *Archives of Biochemistry and Biophysics* 391, no. 1 (2001): 1–7.

Saxena, S., et al. An insufficient anti-inflammatory cytokine response in mouse brain is associated with increased tissue pathology and viral load during Japanese encephalitis virus infection. *Archives of Virology* 153, no. 2 (2008): 283–92.

Saxena, V., et al. Kinetic of cytokine profile during intraperitoneal inoculation of Japanese encephalitis virus in BALB/c mice model. *Microbes and Infection* 10(10-11): 1210-7, 2008.

Srivastava, R., et al. Status of proinflammatory and anti-inflammatory cytokines in different brain regions of a rat model of Japanese encephalitis. *Inflammation Research* 61, no. 4 (2012): 381–89.

Swarup, V., et al. Tumor necrosis factor receptor-1-induced neuronal death by TRADD contributes to the pathogenesis of Japanese encephalitis. *Journal of Neurochemistry* 103, no. 2 (2007): 771–83.

Tandon, A., et al. Alteration in plasma glucose levels in Japanese encephalitis patients. *International Journal of Experimental Pathology* 83, no. 1 (2002): 39–46.

Tani, H., et al. Involvement of ceramide in the propagation of Japanese encephalitis virus. *Journal of Virology* 84, no. 6 (2010): 2798–807.

Thongtan, T., et al. Characterization of putative Japanese encephalitis virus receptor molecules on microglial cells. *Journal of Medical Virology* 84, no. 4 (2012): 615–23.

Thongtan, T., et al. Highly permissive infection of microglial cells by Japanese encephalitis virus: A possible role as a viral reservoir. *Microbes and Infection* 12, no. 1 (2010): 37-45.

Tsao, C., et al. Japanese encephalitis virus infection activates caspase-8 and -9 in a FADD-independent and mitochondrion-dependent manner. *Journal of General Virology* 89 (2008): 1930–41.

Yang, K., et al. A model to study neurotropism and persistency of Japanese encephalitis virus infection in human neuroblastoma cells and leukocytes. *Journal of General Virology* 85 (2004): 635–42.

Yang, T., et al. Japanese encephalitis virus NS2B-NS3 protease induces caspase 3 activation and mitochondria-mediated apoptosis in human medulloblastoma cells. *Virus Research* 143, no. 1 (2009): 77–85.

Yang, Y., et al. Japanese encephalitis virus infection induces changes of mRNA profile of mouse spleen and brain. *Virology Journal* 8 (2011): 80.

Yasui, K. Neuropathogenesis of Japanese encephalitis virus. *Journal of Neurovirology* 8, suppl. 2 (2002): 112–14.

SARS

Berger, A., et al. Severe acute respiratory syndrome (SARS) — paradigm of an emerging viral infection. *Journal of Clinical Virology* 29 (2004): 13–22.

Chen, J., et al. Cellular immune responses to severe acute respiratory syndrome coronavirus (SARS-CoV) infection in senescent BALB/c mice. *Journal of Virology* 84, no. 3 (2010): 1289–301.

Glass, W., et al. Mechanisms of host defense following severe acute respiratory syndrome-associated coronavirus (SARS-CoV) pulmonary infection of mice. *Journal of Immunology* 173, no. 6 (2004): 4030–39.

Hogan, R., et al. Resolution of primary severe acute respiratory syndrome-associated coronavirus infection requires Stat1. *Journal of Virology* 78, no. 20 (2004): 11416–21.

Jiang, Y., et al. Characterization of cytokine/chemokine profiles of severe acute respiratory syndrome. *American Journal of Respiratory and Critical Care Medicine* 171 (2005): 850–57.

Law, H., et al. Chemokine up-regulation in SARS-coronavirus-infected monocyte-derived human dendritic cells. *Blood* 106, no. 7 (2005): 2366–74.

Lee, C., et al. Altered p38 mitogen-activated protein kinase expression in different leukocytes with increment of immunosuppressive mediators in patients with SARS. *Journal of Immunology* 172 (2004): 7841–47.

Li, D., et al. Association of RANTES with the replication of severe acute respiratory syndrome coronavirus in THP-1 cells. *European Journal of Medical Research* 10, no. 3 (2005): 117–20.

Nagata, N., et al. Mouse-passaged severe acute respiratory syndrome-associated coronavirus leads to lethal pulmonary edema and diffuse alveolar damage in adult but not young mice. *Immunopathology and Infectious Disease* 172, no. 6 (2008): 1625–37.

Okabayashi, T., et al. Cytokine regulation in SARS coronavirus infection compared to other respiratory virus infections. *Journal of Medical Virology* 78, no. 4 (2006): 417–24.

Oudit, G., et al. The role of ACE2 in pulmonary diseases — relevance for the nephrologist. *Nephrology, Dialysis, Transplantation* 24 (2009): 136265.

Pyrc, K., et al. Antiviral strategies against human coronaviruses. *Infectious Disorders Drug Targets* 7, no. 1 (2007): 59–66.

Rockx, B., et al. Early upregulation of acute respiratory distress syndrome-associated cytokines promoted lethal disease in aged-mouse model of severe acute respiratory syndrome coronavirus infection. *Journal of Virology* 83, no. 14 (2009): 7062–74.

Sims, A., et al. SARS-CoV replication and pathogenesis in an in vitro model of the human conducting airway epithelium. *Virus Research* 133, no. 1 (2008): 33–44.

Sims, A., et al. Severe acute respiratory syndrome coronavirus infection of human ciliated airway epithelia. *Journal of Virology* 79, no. 24 (2005): 15511–24.

Spiegel, M., et al. Interaction of severe acute respiratory syndrome-associated coronavirus with dendritic cells. *Journal of General Virology* 87 (2006): 1953–60.

Theron, M., et al. A probable role for IFN-gamma in the development of a lung immunopathology in SARS. *Cytokine* 32, no. 1 (2005): 30–38.

Yang, Y. H., et al. Autoantibodies against human epithelial cells and endothelial cells after severe acute respiratory syndrome (SARS)-associated coronavirus infection. *Journal of Medical Virology* 77, no. 1 (2005): 1–7.

Yang, Z., et al. PH-dependent entry of severe acute respiratory syndrome coronavirus is mediated by the spike glycoprotein and enhanced by dendritic cell transfer through DC-SIGN. *Journal of Virology* 78, no. 11 (2004): 5642–50.

Yen, Y., et al. Modeling the early events of severe acute respiratory syndrome coronavirus infection in vitro. *Journal of Virology* 80, no. 6 (2006): 2684–93.

Yoshikawa, T., et al. Severe respiratory syndrome (SARS) coronavirus-induced lung epithelial cytokines exacerbate SARS pathogenesis by modulating intrinsic functions of monocyte-derived macrophages and dendritic cells. *Journal of Virology* 83, no. 7 (2009): 3039–48.

Tick-Borne Encephalitis

Atrasheuskaya, A., et al. Changes in immune parameters and their correction in human cases of tick-borne encephalitis. *Clinical and Experimental Immunology* 131 (2003): 148–54.

Dumpis, U., et al. Tick-borne encephalitis. *Clinical Infectious Diseases* 28 (1999): 882–90.

Kaiser, Richard. The clinical and epidemiological profile of tick-borne encephalitis in southern Germany 1994–98. *Brain* 122 (1999): 2067–78.

Lepej, S., et al. Chemokines CXCL10 and CXCL11 in the cerebrospinal fluid of patients with tick-borne encephalitis. *Acta Neurologica Scandanavica* 115, no. 2 (2007): 109–14.

Mansfield, K., et al. Tick-borne encephalitis virus — a review of an emerging zoonosis. *Journal of General Virology* 90 (2009): 1781–94.

Pancewicz, S., et al. Decreased antioxidant-defense mechanisms in cerebrospinal fluid (CSF) in patients with tick-borne encephalitis (TBE). *Neurologia i Neurochirurgia Polska* 36, no. 4 (202): 767–76.

Singh, S., and H. Girschick. Tick-host interactions and their immunological implications in tick-borne diseases. *Current Science* 85, no. 9 (2003): 1284–98.

Stadler, K., et al. Proteolytic activation of tick-borne encephalitis virus by furin. *Journal of Virology* 71, no. 11 (1997): 8475–81.

Stiasny, K. et al. Role of metastability and acidic pH in membrane fusion by tick-borne encephalitis virus. *Journal of Virology* 75, no. 16 (2001): 7392–98.

Zajkowska, J., et al. Evaluation of CXCL10, CXCL11, CXCL12, and CXCL13 chemokines in serum and cerebrospinal fluid in patients with tick-borne encephalitis (TBE). *Advances in Medical Sciences* 56, no. 2 (2011): 311–17.

West Nile Encephalitis

Ambrose, R., and J. Mackenzie. West Nile virus differentially modulates the unfolded protein response to facilitate replication and immune invasion. *Journal of Virology* 85, no. 6 (2011): 2723–32.

Arjona. A., et al. Abrogation of macrophage migration inhibitory factor decreases West Nile virus lethality by limiting viral neuro-invasion. *Journal of Clinical Investigation* 117, no. 10 (2007): 3059–66.

Bai, F., et al. IL-10 signaling blockade controls murine West Nile virus infection. *PLoS Pathology* 5, no. 10 (2009): e1000610.

Bai, F., et al. A paradoxical role for neutrophils in the pathogenesis of West Nile virus. *Journal of Infectious Diseases* 202, no. 12 (2010): 1804–12.

Bode, A., et al. West Nile virus disease: A descriptive study of 228 patients hospitalized in a 4-county region of Colorado in 2003. *Clinical Infectious Diseases* 42 (2006): 1234–40.

Bourgeois, M., et al. Gene expression analysis in the thalamus and cerebrum of horses experimentally infected with West Nile virus. *PLoS One* 6, no. 10 (2011): e24371.

Brien, J., et al. Key role of T cell defects in age-related vulnerability to West Nile virus. *Journal of Experimental Medicine* 206, no. 12 (2009): 2735–45.

Brien, J., et al. West Nile virus-specific CD4 T cells exhibit direct antiviral cytokine secretion and cytotoxicity and are sufficient for antiviral protection. *Journal of Immunology* 181, no. 12 (2008): 8568–75.

Cheeran, M., et al. Differential responses of human brain cells to West Nile virus infection. *Journal of Neurovirology* 11, no. 6 (2005): 512–24.

Cheng, Y., et al. Major histocompatibility complex class 1 (MHC-1) induction by West Nile virus. *Journal of Infectious Diseases* 189, no. 4 (2004): 658–68.

Cheng, Y., et al. The role of tumor necrosis factor in modulating responses of murine embryo fibroblasts by flavivirus West Nile. *Virology* 329, no. 2 (2004): 361–70.

Dai, J., et al. ICAM-1 participates in the entry of West Nile virus into the central nervous system. *Journal of Virology* 82, no. 8 (2008): 4164–68.

Diamond, M., et al. B cells and antibody play critical roles in the immediate defense of disseminated infection by West Nile encephalitis virus. *Journal of Virology* 77, no. 4 (2003): 2578–86.

Getts, D., et al. Ly6c+ "inflammatory monocytes" are microglial precursors recruited in a pathogenic manner in West Nile virus encephalitis. *Journal of Experimental Medicine* 205, no. 10 (2008): 2319–37. Accessed via the *Journal of Experimental Medicine* website at jem.rupress.org.

Glass, W., et al. CCR5 deficiency increases risk of symptomatic West Nile virus infection. *Journal of Experimental Medicine* 203 (2006): 35–40.

Glass, W., et al. Chemokine receptor CCR5 promotes leukocyte trafficking to the brain and survival in West Nile virus infection. *Journal of Experimental Medicine* 202, no. 8 (2006): 1087–98.

Jiminez-Clavero, M. A. Animal viral diseases and global change: Bluetongue and West Nile fever as paradigms. *Frontiers in Genetics* 3, no. 105 (2012). Published electronically ahead of print June 13, 2012.

Jordan, I., et al. Ribavirin inhibits West Nile virus replication and cytopathic effect in neural cells. *Journal of Infectious Diseases* 182 (2000): 1214–17.

Keller, B., et al. Innate immune evasion by hepatitis C and West Nile virus. *Cytokine Growth Factor Reviews* 18, no. 5–6 (2007): 535–44.

Klein, R., et al. Neuronal CXCL10 directs CD8+ T cell recruitment and control of West Nile virus encephalitis. *Journal of Virology* 79, no. 17 (2005): 11457–66.

Kong, K., et al. West Nile virus attenuates activation of primary human macrophages. *Viral Immunology* 21, no. 1 (2008): 78–82.

Kumar, M., et al. Pro-inflammatory cytokines derived from West Nile virus (WNV)-infected SK-N-SH cells mediate neuroinflammatory markers and neuronal death. *Journal of Neuroinflammation* 7 (2010): 73–87.

Lim, J., and P. Murphy. Chemokine control of West Nile virus infection. *Experimental Cell Research* 317, no. 5 (2011): 569–74.

Mackenzie, J., et al. Cholesterol manipulation by West Nile virus perturbs the cellular membrane response. *Cell Host & Microbe* 2, no. 4 (2007): 229–39.

McCandless, E., et al. CXCR4 antagonism increases T cell trafficking in the central nervous system and improves survival from West Nile virus encephalitis. *Proceedings of the National Academy of Sciences* 105, no. 32 (2008): 11270–75.

Medigeshi, G., et al. West Nile virus infection activates the unfolded protein response, leading to CHOP induction and apoptosis. *Journal of Virology* 81, no. 20 (2007): 10849–60.

Morrey, J., et al. Effect of interferon-alpha and interferon-inducers on West Nile virus in mouse and hamster animal models. *Antiviral Chemistry and Chemotherapy* 15 (2004): 67–75.

Munoz-Erazo, L., et al. Microarray analysis of gene expression in West Nile virus-infected human retinal pigment epithelium. *Molecular Vision* 18 (2012): 730–43.

Murray, K., et al. Risk factors for encephalitis and death from West Nile virus infection. *Epidemiology and Infection* 134 (2006): 1325–32.

Peterson, L., et al. West Nile virus: A primer for the clinician. *Annals of Internal Medicine* 137, no. 3 (2002): 173–79.

Puig-Basagoiti, F., et al. High-throughput assays using a luciferase-expressing replicon, virus-like particles, and full-length virus for West Nile virus drug discovery. *Antimicrobial Agents and Chemotherapy* 49, no. 12 (2005): 4980–88.

Qian, F., et al. Impaired interferon signaling in dendritic cells from older donors infected in vitro with West Nile virus. *Journal of Infectious Diseases* 203, no. 10 (2011): 1415–24.

Roe, K., et al. West Nile virus-induced disruption of the blood-brain barrier in mice is characterized by the degradation of the junctional complex proteins and increase in multiple matrix metalloproteinases. *Journal of General Virology* 93, pt. 6 (2012): 1193–203.

Samuel, M., et al. Alpha/beta interferon protects against lethal West Nile virus infection by restricting cellular tropism and enhancing neuronal survival. *Journal of Virology* 79, no. 21 (2005): 13350–61.

Samuel, M., et al. Caspase 3-dependent cell death of neurons contributes to the pathogenesis of West Nile virus encephalitis. *Journal of Virology* 81, no. 6 (2007): 2614–23.

Samuel, M., et al. Pathogenesis of West Nile virus infection: A balance between virulence, innate and adaptive immunity, and viral evasion. *Journal of Virology* 80, no. 19 (2006): 9349–60.

Sapkal, G., et al. Neutralization escape variant of West Nile virus associated with altered peripheral pathogenicity and differential cytokine profile. *Virus Research* 158, no. 1–2 (2011): 130–39.

Schneider, B., et al. Aedes aegypti saliva alters leukocyte recruitment and cytokine signaling by antigen-presenting cells during West Nile infection. *PLoS One* 5, no. 7 (2010): e11704.

Shen, J., et al. Early E-selectin, VCAM-1, ICAM-1, and late major histocompatibilty complex antigen induction on human endothelial cells by flavivirus and comodulation of adhesion molecule expression by immune cytokines. *Journal of Virology* 71, no. 12 (1997): 9323–32.

Shirato, K., et al. The kinetics of proinflammatory cytokines in murine peritoneal macrophages infected with envelope protein-glycosylated of non-glycosylated West Nile virus. *Virus Research* 121, no. 1 (2006): 11–16.

Shrestha, B., et al. CD8+ T cells require perforin to clear West Nile virus from infected neurons. *Journal of Virology* 80, no. 1 (2006): 119–29.

Shrestha, B., et al. Infection and injury of neurons by West Nile encephalitis virus. *Journal of Virology* 77, no. 24 (2003): 13203–13.

Sitati, E., et al. CD40-CD40 ligand interactions promote trafficking of CD8+ T cells into the brain and protection against West Nile virus encephalitis. *Journal of Virology* 81, no. 18 (2007): 9801–11.

Styer, L., et al. Mosquito saliva causes enhancement of West Nile virus infection in mice. *Journal of Virology* 85, no. 4 (2011): 1517–27.

Szretter, K., et al. The immune adaptor molecule SARM modulates tumor necrosis factor alpha production and microglia activation in the brainstem and restricts West Nile pathogenesis. *Journal of Virology* 83, no. 18 (2009): 9329–38.

Town, T. Toll-like receptor 7 mitigates lethal West Nile encephalitis via interleukin 23-dependent immune cell infiltration and homing. *Immunity* 30 (2009): 24253.

Venter, M., et al. Cytokine induction after laboratory-acquired West Nile virus infection. *New England Journal of Medicine* 360 (2009): 1260–62.

Verma, S., et al. Cyclooxygenase-2 inhibitor blocks the production of West Nile virus-induced neuroinflammatory markers in astrocytes. *Journal of General Virology* 92 (2011): 507–15.

Verma, S., et al. Reversal of West Nile virus-induced blood-brain barrier disruption and tight junction proteins degradation by matrix metalloproteinases inhibitor. *Virology* 397, no. 1 (2010): 130–38.

Wang, P., et al. Matrix metalloproteinase 9 facilitates West Nile virus entry into the brain. *Journal of Virology* 82, no. 18 (2008): 8978–85.

Wang, T., et al. Toll-like receptor 3 mediates West Nile virus entry into the brain causing lethal encephalitis. *Nature Medicine* 10, no. 12 (2004): 1366–73.

Wang, Y., et al. CD8+ T cells mediate recovery and immunopathology in West Nile virus encephalitis. *Journal of Virology* 77, no. 24 (2003): 13323–34.

Welte, T., et al. Immune responses to an attenuated West Nile virus NS4B-P38G mutant strain. *Vaccine* 29, no. 29–30 (2011): 4853–61.

Wen, J., et al. Inhibition of interferon signaling by the New York 99 strain and Kunjin subtype of West Nile virus involves blockage of STAT1 and STAT2 activation by nonstructural proteins. *Journal of Virology* 79, no. 3 (2005): 1934–42.

Xiao, S., et al. West Nile virus infection in the golden hamster (Mesocricetus auratus): A model for West Nile encephalitis. *Emerging Infectious Diseases* 7, no. 4 (2001): 714–21.

Zhang, B., et al. CXCR3 mediates region-specific antiviral T cell trafficking within the central nervous system during West Nile virus encephalitis. *Journal of Immunology* 180, no. 4 (2008): 2641–49.

Zhang, B., et al. TNF-alpha-dependent regulation of CXCR3 expression modulates neuronal survival during West Nile virus encephalitis. *Journal of Neuroimmunology* 224, no. 1–2 (2010): 28–38.

The Herbs

Miscellaneous

Ahmad, A., et al. Antiviral properties of extract of Opuntia streptacantha. *Antiviral Research* 30, no. 2–3 (1996): 75–85.

Allard, P., et al. Alkylated flavanones from the bark of Cryptocarya chartacea as dengue virus NS5 polymerase inhibitors. *Journal of Natural Products* 74, no. 11 (2011): 2446–53.

Alleva, L., et al. Using complementary and alternative medicines to target the host response during severe influenza. *Evidence-Based Complementary and Alternative Medicine* 7, no. 4 (2010): 501–10.

Arora, R. Potential of complementary and alternative medicine in preventive management of novel H1N1 flu (swine flu) pandemic. *Evidence-Based Complementary and Alternative Medicine* (2011). doi: 10.1155/2011/586506.

Bergner, P. Influenza prevention. *Medical Herbalism* 15, no. 4 (2008): 2–8.

Boon, A., et al. In vitro effect of bioactive compounds on influenza virus specific B- and T-cell responses. *Scandinavian Journal of Immunology* 55 (2002): 24–32.

Calderon-Montano, J., et al. A review on the dietary flavonoid kaempferol. *Mini Reviews in Medicinal Chemistry* 11, no. 4 (2011): 298–344.

Charuwichitratana, S., et al. Herpes zoster: Treatment with Clinacanthus nutans cream. *International Journal of Dermatology* 35, no. 9 (1996): 665–66.

Chen, F., et al. In vitro susceptibility of 10 clinical isolates of SARS coronavirus to selected antiviral compounds. *Journal of Clinical Virology* 31, no. 1 (2004): 69–75.

Chiu, Y., et al. Inhibition of Japanese encephalitis virus infection by the sulfated polysaccharide extracts from Ulva lactuca. *Marine Biotechnology* 14, no. 4 (2012): 468–78. Published electronically ahead of print December 23, 2011.

Choi, H., et al. Inhibitory effect on replication of enterovirus 71 of herb methanol extract. *Journal of Applied Biological Chemistry* 51, no. 3 (2008): 123–27.

Choi, H., et al. Inhibitory effect on replication of enterovirus 71 of herb plant water extracts. *Journal of Cosmetics and Public Health* 4, no. 1 (2008): 9–12.

Conley, A., et al. Invasive plant alters ability to predict disease vector distribution. *Ecological Applications* 21, no. 2 (2011): 329–34.

De Clercq, Eric. Potential antivirals and antiviral strategies against SARS coronavirus infections. *Expert Review of Anti-infective Therapy* 4, no. 2 (2006): 291–302.

Devi, B., and K. Manoharan. Antiviral medicinal plants — an ethnobotanical approach. *Journal of Phytology* 1, no. 6 (2009): 417–21.

Efferth, T., et al. The antiviral activities of artemisinin and artesunate. *Clinical Infectious Diseases* 47 (2008): 804–11.

Elsässer-Beile, U., et al. Cytokine production in leukocyte cultures during therapy with Echinacea extract. *Journal of Clinical Laboratory Analysis* 10, no. 6 (1996): 441–45.

Faral-Tello, P., et al. Cytotoxic, virucidal, and antiviral activity of South American plant and algae extracts. *Scientific World Journal* (2012). doi: 10.1100/2012/174837.

Fokina, G., et al. The antiviral action of medicinal plant extracts in experimental tick-borne encephalitis. *Voprosy Virusologii* 38 , no. 4 (1993): 170–73.

Gaby, A. Natural remedies for herpes simplex. *Alternative Medicine Review* 22, no. 2 (2006): 93–101.

Greenway, F., et al. Temporary relief of postherpetic neuralgia pain with topical geranium oil. *American Journal of Medicine* 115, no. 7 (2003): 586–87.

Gupta, P., et al. Antiviral profile of Nyctanthes arbortristis L. against encephalitis causing viruses. *Indian Journal of Experimental Biology* 43, no. 12 (2005): 1156–60.

Hafidh, R., et al. Asia is the mine of natural antiviral products for public health. *Open Complementary Medicine Journal* 1 (2009): 58–68.

Haidari, M., et al. Pomegranate (Punica granatum) purified polyphenol extract inhibits influenza virus and has a synergistic effect with oseltamivir. *Phytomedicine* 16, no. 12 (2009): 1127–36.

Hake, I., et al. Neuroprotection and enhanced neurogenesis by extract from the tropical plant Knema laurina after inflammatory damage in living brain tissue. *Journal of Neuroimmunology* 206, no. 1–2 (2009): 91–99.

Herrmann, F., et al. Diversity of pharmacological properties in Chinese and European medicinal plants: Cytotoxicity, antiviral, and anti-trypanosomal screening of 82 herbal drugs. *Diversity* 3 (2011): 547–80.

Ho, T., et al. Emodin blocks the SARS coronavirus spike protein and angiotensin-converting enzyme 2 interaction. *Antiviral Research* 74, no. 2 (2007): 92–101.

Hsu, C., et al. An evaluation of the additive effect of natural herbal medicine on SARS or SARS-like infectious diseases in 2003: A randomized, double-blind, and controlled pilot study. *Evidence-Based Complementary and Alternative Medicine* 5, no. 3 (2008): 355–62.

Hsu, H., et al. Anti-enterovirus 71 activity screening of Taiwanese folk medicinal plants and immune modulation of Ampelopsis brevipedunculata (Maxim.) Trautv against the virus. *African Journal of Microbiology Research* 5, no. 17 (2011): 2500–2511.

Jassim, S. A. A., and M. A. Naji. Novel antiviral agents: A medicinal plant perspective. *Journal of Applied Microbiology* 95 (2003): 412–27.

Jenny, M., et al. Crinum latifolium leaf extracts suppress immune activation cascades in peripheral blood mononuclear cells and proliferation of prostate tumor cells. *Scientia Pharmaceutica* 79 (2011): 323–35.

Jia, F., et al. Identification of palmatine as an inhibitor of West Nile virus. *Archives of Virology* 155, no. 8 (2010): 1325–29.

Jiao, F., et al. A randomized trial of Ligustrazini hydrochlorioi in the treatment of viral encephalitis in children. *Journal of Nepal Paediatric Society* 30, no. 2 (2010): 119–22.

Kalra, M., et al. Cold and flu: Conventional vs botanical and nutritional therapy. *International Journal of Drug Development and Research* 3, no. 1 (2011): 314–27.

Kang, Dae Gill, et al. Anti-hypertensive effect of water extract of danshen on renovascular hypertension through inhibition of renin angiotensin system. *American Journal of Chinese Medicine* 30, no. 1 (2002): 87–93.

Kimmel, E., et al. Oligomeric procyanidins stimulate innate antiviral immunity in dengue virus infected human PBMCs. *Antiviral Research* 90, no. 1 (2011): 80–86.

Kitazato, K., et al. Viral infectious disease and natural products with antiviral activity. *Drug*

Discoveries and Therapeutics 1, no. 1 (2007): 14–22.

Kongkaew, C., and N. Chaiyakunapruk. Efficacy of Clinacanthus nutans extracts in patients with herpes infection. *Complementary Therapies in Medicine* 19, no. 1 (2011): 47–53.

Krylova, N., et al. In vitro activity of luromarin against tick-borne encephalitis virus. *Antibiotiki i Khimioteripiia* 55, no. 7–8 (2010): 17–19.

Kurokawa, M., et al. Development of new antiviral agents from natural products. *Open Antimicrobial Agents Journal* 2 (2010): 49–57.

Kurokawa, M., and K. Shiraki. New antiviral agents from traditional medicines. *Journal of Traditional Medicie* 22, suppl. 1 (2005): 138–44.

Lee, R., and M. Balick. Flu for you? The common cold, influenza, and traditional medicine. *Ethnomedicine* 2, no. 3 (2006): 252–55.

Li, S., et al. Identification of natural compounds with antiviral activities against the SARS-associated coronavirus. *Antiviral Research* 67 (2005): 18–23.

Li, W., et al. A cardiovascular drug rescues mice from lethal sepsis by selectively attenuating a late-acting proinflammatory mediator, high mobility group box 1. *Journal of Immunology* 178, no. 6 (2007): 3856–64.

Li, Y., et al. Antiviral activities of medicinal herbs traditionally used in southern mainland China. *Phytotherapy Research* 18, no. 9 (2004): 718–22.

Martinez, C., et al. Research advances in plant-made flavivirus antigens. *Biotechnology Advances* 30, no. 6 (2012): 1493–505. Published electronically ahead of print March 28, 2012.

McNamara, M., et al. The treatment of an acute herpes zoster outbreak with an herbal, antiviral remedy in an immunocompromised individual. A case study from the Klearsen Corporation (Boulder, Colo.), hosted on the website of the retailer Nature's Rite. www. mynaturesrite.com/pdfs/casestudyshingles. pdf, accessed May 22, 2012.

Mori, K., et al. Nerve growth factor-inducing activity of Hericium erinaceus in 1321N1 human astrocytoma cells. *Biological & Pharmaceutical Bulletin* 31, no. 9 (2008): 1727–32.

Nawawi, A., et al. Anti-herpes simplex virus activity of alkaloids isolated from Stephania cepharantha. *Biological & Pharmaceutical Bulletin* 22, no. 3 (1999): 268–74.

Niu, L., et al. Evaluating the effect of herpes zoster treatment with three regimens. *Chinese Journal of Dermatovenereology*, 2007-08, CNKI.

Park, J., et al. Characteristic of alkylated chalcones from Angelica keiskei on influenza virus neuraminidase inhibition. *Bioorganic & Medicinal Chemistry Letters* 21, no. 18 (2011): 5602–4.

Reichling, J., et al. Essential oils of aromatic plants with antibacterial, antifungal, and cytotoxic properties – an overview.

Forschende Komplementärmedizin 16 (2009): 79–90.

Reis, S., et al. Immunomodulating and antiviral activities of Uncaria tomentosa on human monocytes infected with Dengue virus-2. *International Immunopharmacology* 8, no. 3 92008): 468–76.

Roner, M., et al. Antiviral activity obtained from aqueous extracts of the Chilean soapbark tree (Quillaja saponaria Molina). *Journal of General Virology* 88, pt. 1 (2007): 275–85.

Roxas, M. Herpes zoster and postherpetic neuralgia: Diagnosis and therapeutic considerations. *Alternative Medicine Review* 11, no. 2 (2006): 102–13.

Roxas, M., and Julie Jurenka. Colds and influenza: A review of diagnosis and conventional, botanical, and nutritional considerations. *Alternative Medicine Review* 12, no. 1 (2007): 25–48.

Sabini, M., et al. Evaluation of antiviral activity of aqueous extracts from Achyrocline satureioides against Western equine encephalitis. *Natural Products Research* 26, no. 5 (2012): 405–15.

Sang, S., et al. Treatment of herpes zoster with Clinacanthus nutans (bi phaya yaw) extract. *Journal of the Medical Association of Thailand* 78, no. 11 (1995): 624–27.

Shin, W., et al. Broad-spectrum antiviral effect of Agrimonia pilosa extract on influenza viruses. *Microbiology and Immunology* 54, no. 1 (2010): 11–19.

Simoes, L., et al. Antiviral activity of Distictella elongata (Vahl) Urb. (Bignoniaceae), a potentially useful source of anti-dengue drugs from the state of Minas Gerais, Brazil. *Letters in Applied Microbiology* 53, no. 6 (2011): 602–7.

Solanki, J., et al. Pharmacognostic and preliminary phytochemical evaluation of the leaves of Crinum latifolium L. *International Journal of Pharmaceutical Sciences and Research* 2, no. 12 (2011): 3219–23.

Souhail, M., et al. Plants as a source of natural antiviral agents. *Asian Journal of Animal and Veterinary Advances* 6, no. 12 (2011): 1125–52.

Su, F., et al. A water extract of Pueraria lobata inhibited cytotoxicity of enterovirus 71 in a human foreskin fibroblast cell line. *Kaohsiung Journal of Medical Sciences* 24, no. 10 (2008): 523–30.

Sun, X., et al. Observation of the efficacy of Ampelopsis brevipedunculata Trautv in the treatment of herpes zoster. *Journal of Traditional Chinese Medicine* 6, no. 1 (1986): 17–18.

Swarup, V., et al. Antiviral and anti-inflammatory effects of rosmarinic acid in an experimental murine model of Japanese encephalitis. *Antimicrobial Agents and Chemotherapy* 51, no. 9 (2007): 3367–70.

Tang, L., et al. Screening of anti-dengue activity in methanolic extracts of medicinal plants. *BMC Complementary and Alternative Medicine* 12 (2012): 3–13.

Thomas, S., et al. Micronutrient intake and the risk of herpes zoster. *International Journal of Epidemiology* 35 (2006): 307–14.

Tsai, F., et al. Kaempferol inhibits enterovirus 71 replication and internal ribosome entry site (IRES) activity through FUBP and HNRP proteins. *Food Chemistry* 128, no. 2 (2011): 312–22.

Wang, C., et al. Antiviral ability of Kalanchoe gracilis leaf extract against enterovirus 71 and coxsackie A16. *Evidence-Based Complementary and Alternative Medicine* (2012). doi: 10.1155/2012/503165.

Wang, H., et al. The aqueous extract of a popular herbal nutrient supplement, Angelica sinensis, protects mice against lethal endotoxemia and sepsis. *Journal of Nutrition* 136 (2006): 360–65.

Wang, W., et al. Effect of Salvia miltiorrhiza on renal pathological change and expression of ACE and ACE2 in rats with aristolochic acid induced nephropathy. *Chinese Journal of Integrated Traditional and Western Nephrology*, 2009-02, CNKI.

Weckesser, S., et al. Topical treatment of necrotising herpes zoster with betulin from birch bark. *Forschende Komplementärmedizin* 17, no. 5 (2010): 271–73.

Wen, C., et al. Traditional Chinese medicine herbal extracts of Cibotium barometz, Gentiana scabra, Dioscorea batas, Cassia tora, and Taxillus chinensis inhibit SARS-CoV replication. *Journal of Traditional and Complementary Medicine* 1, no. 1 (2011): 41–50.

Weon, J., et al. Neuroprotective compounds isolated from Cynanchum paniculatum. *Archives of Pharmaceutical Research* 35, no. 4 (2012): 617–21.

Yamaya, M., et al. Hochy-ekki-to inhibits rhinovirus infection in human tracheal epithelial cells. *British Journal of Pharmacology* 150 (2007): 702–10.

Yarmolinsky, L., et al. Antiviral activity of ethanol extracts of Ficus binjamina and Lilium candidum in vitro. *New Biotechnology* 26, no. 6 (2009): 307–13.

Ye, X., et al. Effect of puerarin injection on the mRNA expressions of AT1 and ACE2 in spontaneous hypertension rats. *Chinese Journal of Integrated Traditional and Western Medicine*, 2008-09, CNKI.

Yu, L., et al. Protection from H1N1 influenza virus infections in mice by supplementation with selenium. *Biological Trace Element Research* 141, no. 1–3 (2011): 254–61.

Yucharoen, R., et al. Anti-herpes simplex activity of extracts from the culinary herbs Ocimum sanctum L., Ocimum basilicum L., and Ocimum americanum L. *African Journal of Biotechnology* 10, no. 5 (2011): 860–66.

Yukawa, T., et al. Prophylactic treatment of cytomegalovirus infection with traditional herbs. *Antiviral Research* 32, no. 2 (1996): 63–70.

Zhang, M., et al. Effect of integrated traditional Chinese and Western medicine on SARS: A review of clinical evidence. *World Journal of Gastroenterology* 10, no. 23 (2004): 3500–3505.

Zhang, M., et al. A study of inhibiting effect of Flos Lonicerae-Radix astragali solution on varicella-zoster virus. *Medical Journal of Qilu*, 2003-2. CNKI.

Zhang, M., et al. The therapeutical effect of large dose of huang qi on elder patients with herpes zoster. *Chinese Journal of Dermatovenereology*, 2002-4, CNKI.

Zhang, T., et al. Anti-Japanese encephalitis-viral effects of kaempferol and daidzin and their RNA-binding characteristics. *PLoS One* 7, no. 1 (2012): e30259.

Zheng, M. An experimental study of the anti-HSV-II action of 500 herbal drugs. *Journal of Traditional Chinese Medicine* 9, no. 2 (1989): 113–16.

Zhu, S., et al. Caging a beast in the inflammation arena: Use of Chinese medicinal herbs to inhibit a late mediator of lethal sepsis, HMGB1. *International Journal of Clinical and Experimental Medicine* 1 (2008): 64–75.

Zhu, S., et al. Effects of EGb761 on renal tissue ACE2 protein and mRNA expression in adenine-induced renal interstitial fibrosis rats. *Chinese Traditional Patent Medicine*, 2011-11, CNKI.

Zhuang, M., et al. Procyandins and butanol extract of Cinnamomi cortex inhibit SARS-CoV infection. *Antiviral Research* 82, no. 1 (2009): 73–81.

Astragalus (*Astragalus membranaceus*)

Ai, P., et al. Aqueous extract of astragali radix induces human natriuresis through enhancement of renal response to arterial natriuretic peptide. *Journal of Ethnopharmacology* 116, no. 3 (2008): 413–21.

Anonymous. "Astragalus." Fact sheet in the *Herbs at a Glance* collection (U.S. Department of Health and Human Services National Center for Complementary and Alternative Medicine, updated 2008).

Anonymous. *Astragalus membranaceus.* Monograph, *Alternative Medicine Review* 8, no. 1 (2003): 72–77.

Batachandar, S., et al. Antimicrobial activity of Astragalus membranaceus against diarrheal bacterial pathogens. *International Journal of Ayurvedic Research*, January 2011.

Brush, J., et al. The effect of Echinacea purpurea, Astragalus membranaceus and Glycyrrhiza glabra on CD69 expression and immune cell activation in humans. *Phytotherapy Research* 20, no. 8 (2006): 687–95.

Burkhart, K. Astragalus membranaceus (Fisch ex Link) Bunge (astragalus), Fabaceae and related species. Paper, Bastyr University (Kenmore, Wash.), 2007, www.aaronsworld.com/Bastyr/Class%20Notes/Bot%20Med/Bot%20Med%20IV/Astragalus_membranaceus.pdf, accessed June 29, 2012.

Cho, J. H., et al. Myelophil, an extract mix of astragali radix and salviae radix, ameliorates chronic fatigue: A randomized, double-blind, controlled pilot study. *Complementary Therapies in Medicine* 17, no. 3 (2009): 141–46.

De-Hong, Y. U., et al. Studies of chemical constituents and their antioxidant activities from Astragalus mongholicus Bunge. *Biomedical and Environmental Sciences* 18 (2005): 297–301.

Dobrowolski, C., et al. In vitro rate of phagocytosis in macrophages stimulated by *Astragalus membranaceus*. *Journal of Research Across the Disciplines* (online at Jackson University, Jackson, Fla.), no. 1 (2009), www.ju.edu/jrad/documents/dobrowolski-am_research_paper.pdf.

Duan, P., et al. Clinical study on effect of astragalus in efficacy enhancing and toxicity reducing of chemotherapy in patients of malignant tumor. *Zhongguo Zhong Xi Yi Jie He Za Zhi* 22, no. 7 (2002): 515–17.

Feng, J., et al. The study of the efficacy of astragalus granule on neonatal hypoxic ischemic encephalopathy. *Journal of Pediatric Pharmacy*, 2009-01, CNKI.

Gao, X. P., et al. Effect of huangqi zengmian powder on interstitial response in patients with esophageal cancer at peri-operational period. *Zhongguo Zhong Xi Yi Jie He Za Zhi* 21, no. 3 (2001): 171–73.

Haixue, K., et al. Secocycloartane triterpenoidal saponins from the leaves of *Astragalus membranaceus* Bunge. *Helvetica Chimica Acta* 92, no. 5 (2009): 950–58.

Huang, X., et al. Effect of sulfated astragalus polysaccharide on cellular infectivity of infectious bursal disease virus. *International Journal of Biological Macromolecules* 42, no. 2 (2008): 166–71.

Huang, X., et al. Sulfated modification conditions optimization of astragalus polysaccharide by orthogonal test and anti IBDV activity determination of the modifiers. *Zhong Yao Cai* 31, no. 4 (2008): 588–92.

Huang, Z. Q., et al. Effect of Astragalus membranaceus on T-lymphocyte subsets in patients with viral myocarditis. *Zhongguo Zhong Xi Yi Jie He Za Zhi* 15, no. 6 (1995): 328–30.

Hyun-Jung, P., et al. The effects of *Astragalus membranaceus* on repeated restraint stress-induced biochemical and behavioral responses. *Korean Journal of Physiology & Pharmacology* 13, no. 4 (2009): 315–19.

Ka-Shun Ko, J., et al. Amelioration of experimental colitis by *Astragalus membranaceus* through anti-oxidation and inhibition of adhesion molecule synthesis. *World Journal of Gastroenterology* 11, no. 37 (2005): 5787–94.

Kemper, K. J., et al. Astragalus (*Astragalus membranaceus*). Longwood Herbal Task Force, September 3, 1999. http://longwoodherbal.org/astragalus/astragalus.PDF.

Kong, X. F., et al. Chinese herbal ingredients are effective immune stimulators for chickens infected with the Newcastle disease virus. *Poultry Science* 85, no. 12 (2006): 2169–75.

Li, M., et al. Effects of astragalus injection on expression of perforin in myocardial infiltrating cells and serum TNF-α in mice with acute myocarditis. *Chinese Journal of Contemporary Pediatrics*, 2003-06, CNKI.

Li, S. P., et al. Astragalus polysaccharides and astragalosides regulate cytokine secretion in LX-2 cell line. *Zhejiang Da Xue Bao Yi Xue Ban* 36, no. 6 (2007): 543–48.

Li, S. P., et al. Synergy of Astragalus polysaccharides and probiotics (Lactobacillus and Bacillus cereus) on immunity and intestinal microbiota in chicks. *Poultry Science* 88, no. 3 (2009): 519–25.

Li, Z. P., et al. Effect of mikvetch injection on immune function of children with tetralogy of Fallot after radical operation. *Zhongguo Zhong Xi Yi Jie He Za Zhi* 24, no. 7 (2004): 596–600.

Liu, K. Z., et al. Effects of Astragalus and saponins of Panax notoginseng on MMP-9 in patients with type 2 diabetic macroangiopathyl. *Zhongguo Zhong Yao Za Zhi* 29, no. 3 (2004): 264–66.

Liu, W., et al. Influence of ganciclovir and Astragalus membranaceus on proliferation of hematopoietic progenitor cells of cord blood after cytomegalovirus infection in vitro. *Zhonghua Er Ke Za Zhi* 42, no. 7 (2004): 490–94.

Liu, Z., et al. Effect of astragalus injection on immune function in patients with congestive heart failure. *Zhongguo Zhong Xi Yi Jie He Za Zhi* 23, no. 5 (2003): 351–53.

Lu, G., et al. Effect of astragalus polysaccharides on blood routine and antioxidant capacity of canine infected with CDV. *Journal of Anhui Agricultural Sciences*, 2010-12, CNKI.

Lu, M.-C., et al. Effect of Astragalus membranaceus in rats on peripheral nerve regeneration: In vitro and in vivo studies. *Journal of Trauma* 68, no. 2 (2010): 434–40.

Mao, S. P., et al. Modulatory effect of Astragalus membranaceus on Th1/Th2 cytokine in patients with herpes simplex keratitis. *Zhongguo Zhong Xi Yi Jie He Za Zhi* 24, no. 2 (2004): 121–23.

Mao, X. F., et al. Effects of beta-glucan obtained from the Chinese herb *Astragalus membranaceus* and lipopolysaccharide challenge on performance, immunological, adrenal, and somatotropic responses of weanling pigs. *Journal of Animal Science* 83 (2005): 2775–82.

Matkowski, A., et al. Flavonoids and phenol carboxylic acids in Oriental medicinal plant *Astragalus membranaceus* acclimated in Poland. *Zeitschrift für Naturforschung C* 58, no. 7–8 (2003): 602–4.

Meschino, J. Astragalus (Astragalus membranaceus Moench): A powerful daily supplement for the immune system. Paper for RenaiSanté Institute of Integrative Medicine, n. d. Accessed online at www.meschinohealth.com/ArticleDirectory/Astragalus_A_Powerful_Daily_Supplement_for_the_Immune_System.

Mikaeili, A., et al. Anti-candidal activity of Astragalus verus in the in vitro and in vivo guinea pig models of cutaneous and systemic candidiasis. *Revista Brasileira de Farmacognosia* [online] 22, no. 5 (2012): 1035–43.

Nalbantsoy, A., et al. Evaluation of the immuno-modulatory properties in mice and in vitro anti-inflammatory activity of cycloartane type saponins from Astragalus species. *Journal of Ethnopharmacology* 139, no. 2 (2011): 574–81.

Peng, A., et al. Herbal treatment for renal dis-eases. *Annals of the Academy of Medicine, Singapore* 34 (2005): 44–51.

Peng, T., et al. The inhibitory effect of Astragalus membranaceus on coxsackie B-3 virus RNA replication. *Chinese Medical Sciences Journal* 10, no. 3 (1995): 146–50.

Qu, Z., et al. Inhibition airway remodeling and transforming growth factor-ß1/Smad signal-ing pathway by astragalus extract in asth-matic mice. *International Journal of Molecular Medicine* 29, no. 4 (2012): 564–68.

Schafer, Peg. Astragalus membranaceus. Medicinal herb cultivation guide by Chinese Medicinal Herb Farm, 2009, http://chinesemedicinalherbfarm.com/Astragalus%20membran3.pdf.

Shabbir, M. Z., et al. Immunomodulatory effect of polyimmune (*Astragalus membranaceus*) extract on humoral response of layer birds vaccinated against Newcastle disease virus. *International Journal of Agriculture and Biology* 10 (2008): 585–87.

Shang, L., et al. Astragaloside IV inhibits adenovirus replication and apoptosis in A549 cells in vitro. *Journal of Pharmacy and Pharmacology* 63, no. 5 (2011): 688–94.

Shen, P., et al. Differential effects of isoflavones, from *Astragalus membranaceus* and *Pueraria thomsonii*, on the activation of PPARalpha, PPARgamma, and adipocyte differentia-tion in vitro. *Journal of Nutrition* 136 (2006): 899–905.

Sheng, B.-W., et al. Astragalus membranaceus reduces free radical-mediated injury to renal tubules in rabbits receiving high-energy shock waves. *Chinese Medical Journal* 118, no. 1 (2005): 43–49.

Shi, F. S., et al. Effect of astragalus saponin on vascular endothelial cell and its function in burn patients. *Zhongguo Zhong Xi Yi Jie He Za Zhi* 21, no. 10 (2001): 750–51.

Shi, J., et al. Therapeutic efficacy of astragalus in patients with chronic glomerulonephri-tis. *Acta Universitatis Medicinalis Secondae Shanghai*, 2001-01, CNKI.

Shu, L., et al. Empirical study in vitro of inhibit-ing action of membranaceus component A6 on influenza virus. *Modern Journal of Integrated Traditional Chinese and Western Medicine*, 2009-05, CNKI.

Su, L., et al. Effect of intravenous drip infusion of cyclophosphamide with high-dose astragalus injection in treating lupus nephritis. *Zhong Xi Yi Jie He Xue Bao* 5, no. 3 (2007): 272–75.

Sun, H., et al. Effect on exercise endurance capacity and antioxidant properties of Astragalus membranaceus polysaccharides (APS). *Journal of Medicinal Plants Research* 4, no. 10 (2010): 982–86.

Taixiang, W., et al. Chinese medical herbs for chemotherapy side effects in colorectal can-cer patients. *Cochrane Database of Systematic Reviews* 25, no. 1 (2005): CD004540.

Tang, L., et al. Phytochemical analysis of an antiviral fraction of radix astragali using HPCL-DAD-ESI-MS/MS. *Journal of Natural Medicine* 64, no. 2 (2010): 182–86.

Tin, M. Y. Study of the anticarcinogenic mecha-nisms of *Astragalus membranaceus* in colon cancer cells and tumor xenograft. Master's thesis, Hong Kong Baptist University, 2006.

Wang, F., et al. Effect of astragalus on cytokines in patients undergoing heart valve replace-ment. *Zhongguo Zhong Xi Yi Jie He Za Zhi* 28, no. 6 (2008): 495–98.

Wang, H., et al. Antifibrotic effect of the Chinese herbs, Astragalus mongholicus and Angelica sinensis, in a rat model of chronic puromycin aminonucleoside nephrosis. *Life Sciences* 13, no. 74 (2004): 1645–58.

Wang, H. F., et al. Effects of *Astragalus membra-naceus* on growth performance, carcass char-acteristics, and antioxidant status of broiler chickens. *Acta Agriculturae Scandinavica* 60, no. 3 (2010): 151–58.

Wang, M. S., et al. Clinical study on effect of astragalus injection and its immunoregula-tion action in treating chronic aplastic ane-mia. *Chinese Journal of Integrative Medicine* 13, no. 2 (2007): 98–102.

Wang, X., et al. Treatment of Astragalus mem-branaceus zhusheye for hemorrhagic fever with renal syndrome — a clinical observation of 91 cases. *Journal of Binzhou Medical College*, 2001-01, CNKI.

Wang, Z., et al. Antiviral action of combined use of rhizoma polygoni cuspidati and radix astragali on HSV-1 strain. *Zhongguo Zhong Yao Za Zhi* 24, no. 3 (1999): 176–80.

Wei, L., et al. Randomized double-blind con-trolled study of therapeutic effects of astraga-lus injection on children with cerebral palsy. *Applied Journal of General Practice*, 2008-03, CNKI.

Wojcikowski, K., et al. Effect of Astragalus mem-branaceus and Angelica sinensis combined with enalapril in rats with obstructive uropa-thy. *Phytotherapy Research* 24, no. 6 (2010): 875–84.

Wu, J., et al. Effect of astragalus injection on serious abdominal traumatic patients' cel-lular immunity. *Chinese Journal of Integrative Medicine* 12, no. 1 (2006): 29–31.

Wu, Y., et al. Inhibition of *Astragalus membra-naceus* polysaccharides against liver cancer cell HepG2. *African Journal of Microbiology Research* 4, no. 20 (2010): 2181–83.

Xian-qing, M., et al. Hypoglycemic effect of polysaccharide enriched extract of *Astragalus membranaceus* in diet induced insulin resistant C57BL/6J mice and its potential mechanism. *International Journal of Phytotherapy and Phytopharmacology* 16, no. 5 (2009): 416–25.

Xiaoyan, Z., et al. Effect of superfine pulverization on properties of *Astragalus membranaceus* powder. *Powder Technology* 203, no. 3 (2010): 620–25.

Yang, W. J., et al. Synergistic antioxidant activities of eight traditional Chinese herb pairs. *Biological & Pharmaceutical Bulletin* 32, no. 6 (2009): 1021–26.

Yao-Haur, K., et al. *Astragalus membranaceus* flavonoids (AMF) ameliorate chronic fatigue syndrome induced by food intake restriction plus forced swimming. *Journal of Ethnopharmacology* 122, no. 1 (2009): 28–34.

Ye, G., et al. Characterization of anti-Coxsackie virus B3 constituents of radix astragali by high-performance liquid chromatography coupled with electrospray ionization tandem mass spectrometry. *Biomedical Chromatography* 24, no. 11 (2010): 1147–51.

Zhang, C., et al. Effects of mixed Astragalus membranaceus and gentiana extracts on inhibiting influenza A virus. *Journal of YunYang Medical College*, 2010-03, CNKI.

Zhang, J., et al. Clinical study on effect of astragalus injection on left ventricular remodeling and left ventricular function in patients with acute myocardial infarction. *Zhongguo Zhong Xi Yi Jie He Za Zhi* 22, no. 5 (2002): 346–48.

Zhang, J. G., et al. Effect of astragalus injection on plasma levels of apoptosis-related factors in aged patients with chronic heart failure. *Chinese Journal of Integrative Medicine* 11, no. 3 (2005): 187–90.

Zhang, Y., et al. Effects of radix astragali on expression of transforming growth factor B1 and Smad 3 signal pathway in hypertrophic scar of rabbit. *Zhonghua Shao Shang Za Zhi* 26, no. 5 (2010): 366–70.

Zhang, Y., et al. Treatment of recurrent respiratory tract infections with astragalus particle. *Medical Journal of West China*, 2012-01, CNKI.

Zhang, Z., et al. Prevention of astragalus polysaccharides on poultry viral disease. *Journal of Animal Science and Veterinary Medicine*, 2010-04, CNKI.

Zhao, W., et al. Study on effects of Astragalus aksuensis against virus. *Chinese Pharmaceutical Journal*, 2001-01, CNKI.

Zhong, H., et al. Study on inhibitive effect of radix astragali and radix isatidis in vitro on procine parvovirus. *Journal of Northwest A and F University*, 2008-10, CNKI.

Zhu, H., et al. In vivo and in vitro antiviral activities of calycosin-7-O-beta-D-glycopyranoside against coxsackie virus B3. *Biological & Pharmaceutical Bulletin* 32, no. 1 (2009): 68–73.

Zou, Y., et al. Effect of astragalus injection combined with chemotherapy on quality of life in patients with advanced non-small cell lung cancer. *Zhongguo Zhong Xi Yi Jie He Za Zhi* 23, no. 10 (2003): 733–35.

Zuo, C., et al. Astragalus mongholicus ameliorates renal fibrosis by modulating HGF and TGF-beta in rats with unilateral ureteral obstruction. *Journal of Zhejiang University, Science, B* 10, no. 5 (2009): 380–90.

Zuo, L., et al. The preventative and curative effects of Astragalus membranaceus Bungo A6 on the mice infected with influenza virus. *Virologica Sinica* 12, no. 4 (1997): 342–47.

Zwickey, H., et al. The effect of Echinacea purpurea, Astragalus membranaceus and Glycyrrhiza glabra on CD25 expression in humans: A pilot study. *Phytotherapy Research* 21, no. 11 (2007): 1109–12.

Boneset *(Eupatorium perfoliatum)*

Abad, M., et al. Antiviral activity of some South American medicinal plants. *Phytotherapy Research* 13, no. 2 (1999): 142–46.

Bergner, P. Boneset and influenza: Historical notes and commentary. *Medical Herbalism* 13, no. 4 (2003): 16–20.

Daucus, S., and P. Bergner. Eupatorium: Clinical correspondence and commentary. *Medical Herbalism* 7, no. 4 (1996): 10–12.

de Souza Nunes, L. A. Contribution of homeopathy to the control of an outbreak of dengue in Macaé, Rio de Janeiro. *International Journal of High Dilution Research* 7, no. 25 (2008): 186–92.

Dubey, R. K., et al. Evaluation of *Eupatorium cannabinum* Linn. oil in enhancement of shelf life of mango fruits from fungal rotting. *World Journal of Microbiology and Biotechnology* 23 (2007): 467–73.

Duke, James A. Chemicals in: *Eupatorium perfoliatum* L. (Asteraceae). Entry in Dr. Duke's Phytochemical and Ethnobotanical Databases. www.ars-grin.gov/duke/ (accessed December 9, 2010).

Edgar, J. A., et al. Pyrrolizidine alkaloid composition of three Chinese medicinal herbs, Eupatorium cannabinum, E. japonicum and Crotalaria. *American Journal of Chinese Medicine* 20, no. 3–4 (1992): 281–88.

Elema, E. T., et al. Flavones and flavonol glycosides from Eupatorium cannabinum L. *Pharmaceutisch Weekblad, Scientific Edition* 11, no. 5 (1989): 161–64.

Garcia, C., et al. Virucidal activity of essential oils from aromatic plants of San Luis, Argentina. *Phytotherapy Research* 17 (2003): 1073–75.

Garcia, G., et al. Antiherpetic activity of some Argentine medicinal plants. *Fitoterapia* 41, no. 6 (1990): 542–46.

Gassinger, C. A. A controlled clinical trial for testing of efficacy of the homeopathic drug eupatorium perfoliatum D2 in the treatment of common cold (author's transl).

Arzneimittel-Forschung 31, no. 4 (1981): 732–36.

Habtemariam, S., and A. Macpherson. Cytotoxicity and antibacterial activity of ethanol extract from leaves of a herbal drug, boneset (Eupatorium perfoliatum). *Phytotherapy Research* 14, no. 7 (2000): 575–77.

Hensel, A., et al. Eupatorium perfoliatium L: Phytochemistry, traditional use, and current applications. *Journal of Ethnopharmacology* 138, no. 3 (2011): 641–51.

Herz, W., et al. Sesquiterpene lactones of Eupatorium perfoliatum. *Journal of Organic Chemistry* 42, no. 13 (1977): 2264–71.

Jacobs, J., et al. The use of homeopathic combination remedy for dengue fever symptoms: A pilot RCT in Honduras. *Homeopathy* 96, no. 1 (2007): 22–26.

Jaric, S., et al. An ethnobotanical study on the usage of wild medicinal herbs from Kopaonik Mountain (Central Serbia). *Journal of Ethnopharmacology* 111, no. 1 (2007): 160–75.

Kumar, S., et al. Molecular herbal inhibitors of Dengue virus: An update. *International Journal of Medicinal and Aromatic Plants* 2(1): 1-21, 2012.

Lang, G., et al. Antiplasmodial activities of sesquiterpene lactones from Eupatorium semialatum. *Zeitschrift für Naturforschung C* 57 (2002): 282–86.

Lexa, A., et al. Choleretic and hepatoprotective properties of Eupatorium cannabinum in the rat. *Planta Medica* 55, no. 2 (1989): 127–32.

Lira-Salazar, G., et al. Effects of homeopathic medications Eupatorium perfoliatum and Arsenicum album on parasitemia of Plasmodium berghei-infected mice. *Homeopathy* 95, no. 4 (2006): 223–28.

Maas, M., et al. Antiinflammatory activity of Eupatorium perfoliatum L. extracts, eupafolin, and dimeric guaianolide via iNOS inhibitory activity and modulation of inflammation-related cytokines and chemokines. *Journal of Ethnopharmacology* 137, no. 1 (2011): 371–81.

Maas, M., et al. Caffeic acid derivatives from Eupatorium perfoliatum L. *Molecules* 14, no. 1 (2008): 36–45.

Maas, M. Eupatorium perfoliatum L: Phytochemical characterization and functional in vitro investigations — antiinflammatory, antiprotozoal, and antiviral activities. Ph.D. thesis (summary), University of Münster, 2011, www.uni-muenster.de/imperia/md/content/pharmazeutische_biologie/prof_hensel/summary_mareike_maasaktuellx.pdf.

Maas, M., et al. An unusual dimeric guaianolide with antiprotozoal activity and further sesquiterpene lactones from Eupatorium perfoliatum. *Phytochemistry* 72, no. 7 (2011): 635–44.

Paolini, J., et al. Analysis of the essential oil from aerial parts of Eupatorium cannabinum subsp. corsicum (L.) by gas chromatography with electron impact and chemical ionization mass spectrometry. *Journal of Chromatography A* 1076, no. 1-2 (2005): 170–78.

Pengelly, A., et al. Eupatorium perfoliatum L.: Boneset. Appalachian Plant Monograph prepared by Tai Sophia Institute for Appalachian Center for Ethnobotanical Studies, September 2011, www.frostburg.edu/fsu/assets/File/ACES/eupatorium%20perfoliatum-final(1).pdf.

Robinson, G., et al. Medical attributes of Eupatorium perfoliatum — boneset. Paper developed as part of a medical botany course at Wilkes University (Wilkes-Barre, Penn.), July 2007. http://klemow.wilkes.edu/Eupatorium.html.

Rücker, G., et al. Allergenic sesquiterpene lactones from Eupatorium cannabinum L. and Kaunia rufescens (Lund ex de Candolle). *Natural Toxins* 5, no. 6 (1997): 223–27.

Tabanca, N., et al. Eupatorium capillifolium essential oil: Chemical composition, antifungal activity, and insecticidal activity. *Natural Product Communications* 5, no. 9 (2010): 1409–15.

Wagner, H., et al. Immunological studies of plant combination preparations. In-vitro and in-vivo studies on the stimulation of phagocytosis. *Arzneimittel-Forschung* 41, no. 10 (1991): 1072–76.

Wagner, H., et al. Immunostimulating action of polysaccharides (heteroglycans) from higher plants. *Arzneimittel-Forschung* 35, no. 7 (1985): 1069–75.

Woerdenbag, H. J. Enhanced cytostatic of the sesquiterpene lactone eupatoriopicrin by glutathione depletion. *British Journal of Cancer* 59, no. 1 (1989): 68–75.

Woerdenbag, H. J. Eupatorium cannabinum L. A review emphasizing the sesquiterpene lactones and their biological activity, *Pharmaceutisch Weekblad, Scientific Edition* 8 (1986): 245–51.

Yarnell, E. Eupatorium perfoliatum L. (boneset), Asteraceae. Paper, Bastyr University (Kenmore, Wash.), 2007, www.aaronsworld.com/Bastyr/Class%20Notes/Bot%20Med/Bot%20Med%20IV/Eupatorium_perfoliatum.pdf.

Zanon, S., et al. Search for antiviral activity of certain medicinal plants from Cordoba, Argentina. *Revista Latinoamericana de Microbiologia* 41 (1999): 59–62.

Chinese Skullcap (*Scutellaria baicalensis*)

7Song. The skullcaps — a Scutellaria monograph. Blog, Northeast School of Herbal Medicine, updated February 12, 2012. http://7song.com/blog/2012/02/the-skullcaps-a-scutellaria-monograph.

Akao, T., Y. Sakashita, M. Hanada, et al. Enteric excretion of baicalein, a flavone of scutellariae radix, via glucuronidation in rat:

involvement of multi drug resistance-associated protein2. *Pharmaceutical Research* 21, no. 11 (2004): 2120–26.

Arweiler, N. B., G. Pergola, J. Kuenz, et al. Clinical and antibacterial effect of an anti-inflammatory toothpaste formulation with Scutellaria baicalensis extract on experimental gingivitis. *Clinical Oral Investigation* 15, no. 6 (2011): 909–13.

Baikal skullcap. Landscaping Revolution, 2009. http://landscapingrevolution.com/ingrid_garden/herbs/baikal_skullcap.html (accessed March 29, 2012).

Baikal skullcap (Scutellaria baicalensis). Sigma-Aldrich Plant Profiler, 2010. www.sigmaaldrich.com/life-science/nutrition-research/learning-center/plant-profiler (accessed March 29, 2012).

Baylor, N., et al. Inhibition of human T cell leukemia virus by the plant flavonoid baicalin (7-glucronic acid, 5, 6-dihydroxyflavone). *Journal of Infectious Diseases* 165, no. 3 (1992): 433–37.

Ben-Nathan, D., et al. Protective effects of melatonin in mice infected with encephalitis viruses. *Archives of Virology* 149, no. 2 (1995): 223–30.

Bhandari, M., A. Bhandari, R. Prakesh, et al. Scutellaria baicalensis Georgi: A rising paradigm of herbal remedies. WebmedCentral 1, no. 11 (2010): WMC001105.

Blach-Olszewska, Z., B. Jatczak, A. Rak, et al. Production of cytokines and stimulation of resistance to viral infection in human leukocytes by Scutellaria baicalensis flavones. *Journal of Interferon & Cytokine Research* 28, no. 9 (2008): 571–81.

Bonham, M., J. Posakony, I. Coleman, et al. Characterization of chemical constituents in Scutellaria baicalensis with antiandrogenic and growth-inhibitory activities toward prostate carcinoma. *Clinical Cancer Research* 11, no. 10 (2005): 3905–14.

Bonilla, E., et al. Melatonin and viral infections. *Journal of Pineal Research* 36, no. 2 (2004): 73–79.

Broncel, M. Antiatherosclerotic properties of flavones from the roots of Scutellaria baicalensis Georgi. *Wiadomości Lekarskie* 60, no. 5–6 (2007): 294–97.

Chan, B. C., M. Ip, C. B. Lau, et al. Synergistic effects of baicalein with ciprofloxacin against NorA over-expressed methicillin of MRSA pyruvate kinase. *Journal of Ethnopharmacology* 137, no. 1 (2011): 767–73.

Chen, C.-M., L.-F. Wang, and K.-T. Cheng. Maternal baicalin treatment increases fetal lung surfactant phospholipids in rats. *Evidence-Based Complementary and Alternative Medicine* (2011). doi: 10.1093/ecam/nep073.

Chen, G., et al. Effect of baicalin and tetramethylpyrazine on intracranial hypertension of infectious brain edema in rabbits. *Zhongguo Zhong Xi Yi Jie He Za Zhi* 19, no. 4 (1999): 224–26.

Chen, L., J. Dou, Z. Su, et al. Synergistic activity of baicalein with ribavirin against influenza A (H1N1) virus infections in cell culture and in mice. *Antiviral Research* 91, no. 3 (2011): 314–20.

Chen, X., H. Nishida, and T. Konishi. Baicalin promoted the repair of DNA single strand breakage caused by H(2)O(2) in cultured NIH3T3 fibroblasts. *Biological and Pharmaceutical Bulletin* 26, no. 2 (2003): 282–84.

Choi, J. H., A. Y. Choi, H. Yoon, et al. Baicalein protects HT22 murine hippocampal neuronal cells against endoplasmic reticulum stress-induced apoptosis through inhibition of reactive oxygen species production and CHOP induction. *Experimental and Molecular Medicine* 42, no. 12 (2010): 811–22.

Chu, Z. Y., M. Chu, and Y. Teng. Effect of baicalin on in vivo anti-virus. *Zhongguo Zhong Yao Za Zhi* 32, no. 22 (2007): 2413–15.

Cole, I. B., J. Cao, A. R. Alan, et al. Comparisons of Scutellaria baicalensis, Scutellaria lateriflora and Scutellaria racemosa: Genome size, antioxidant potential and phytochemistry. *Planta Medica* 74, no. 4 (2008): 474–81.

Dai, Z. J., X. J. Wang, Q. Xue, et al. Effects of Scutellaria barbata drug-containing serum on apoptosis and mitochondrial transmembrane potential of hepatoma H22 cells. *Zhong Xi Yi Jie He Xue Bao* 6, no. 8 (2008): 821–26.

Dou, J., L. Chen, G. Xu, et al. Effects of baicalin and its inhibition of hemagglutinin-neuraminidase. *Archives of Virology* 156, no. 5 (2011): 793–801.

Du, Y., X. Y. Chen, H. Y. Yang, et al. Determination of wogonin in rat plasma by liquid chromatography-tandem mass spectrometry. *Yao Xue Xue Bao* 37, no. 5 (2002): 362–66.

Dygai, A. M., N. I. Suslov, E. G. Skurikhin, et al. The modulating effects of preparations of Baikal skullcap (Scutellaria baicalensis) on erythron reactions under conditions of neurotic exposures. *Eksperimental'naia i Klinicheskaia Farmakologiia* 61, no. 1 (1998): 37–39.

Fong, Y. K., C. R. Li, S. K. Wo, et al. In vitro and in situ evaluation of herb-drug interactions during intestinal metabolism and absorption of baicalein. *Journal of Ethnopharmacology* 141, no. 2 (2012): 742–43. Published electronically ahead of print August 26, 2011.

Franzblau, S. G., and C. Cross. Comparative in vitro antimicrobial activity of Chinese medicinal herbs. *Journal of Ethnopharmacology* 15, no. 3 (1986): 279–88.

Fu, Z., H. Lu, Z. Zhu, et al. Combination of baicalein and amphotericin B accelerates Candida albicans apoptosis. *Biological and Pharmaceutical Bulletin* 34, no. 2 (2011): 214–18.

Gao, H. M., Z. M. Wang, and J. Tian. Pharmacokinetics and metabolites of scutellarin in normal and model rats. *Yao Xue Xue Bao* 40, no. 11 (2005): 1024–27.

Gao, L., et al. Inhibiting effect of baicalin on influenza, herpes simplex and CoxB-3 virus infections in cultured cells. *Chinese Journal of New Drugs*, 2008-06, CNKI.

Gasiorowski, K., E. Lamer-Zarawska, J. Leszek, et al. Flavones from root of Scutellaria baicalensis Georgi: Drugs of the future in neurodegeneration? *CNS and Neurological Disorders Drug Targets* 10, no. 2 (2011): 184–91.

Go, W. J., J. H. Ryu, F. Qiang, and H. K. Han. Evaluation of the flavonoid oroxylin A as an inhibitor of P-glycoprotein-mediated cellular efflux. *Journal of Natural Products* 72, no. 9 (2009): 1616–19.

Goldberg, V. E., V. M. Ryzhakov, M. G. Matiash, et al. Dry extract of Scutellaria baicalensis as a hemostimulant in antineoplastic chemotherapy in patients with lung cancer. *Eksperimental'naia i Klinicheskaia Farmakologiia* 60, no. 6 (1997): 28–30.

Guo, S. S., et al. The cytology mechanism of antiparainfluenza virus infection of total flavone of Scutellaria barbata. *Acta Pharmaceutica Sinica* 44, no. 12 (2009): 1348–52.

Guo, X. Y., L. Yang, Y. Chen, et al. Identification of the metabolites of baicalein in human plasma. *Journal of Asian Natural Products* 13, no. 9 (2011): 861–68.

Hamada, H., M. Hiramatsu, R. Edamatsu, et al. Free radical scavenging action of baicalein. *Archives of Biochemistry and Biophysics* 306, no. 1 (1993): 261–66.

Han, Y., et al. The inhibition effects of baicalin on neurotoxic action induced by kainic acid. *Acta Academiae Medicinae Jiangxi*, 1995-01, CNKI.

Hao, H., Y. Aixia, L. Dan, et al. Baicalin suppresses expression of chlamydia protease-like activity factor in Hep-2 cells infected by Chlamydia trachomatis. *Fitoterapia* 80, no. 7 (2009): 448–52.

Hao, H., Y. Aixia, F. Lei, et al. Effects of baicalin on Chlamydia trachomatis infection in vitro. *Planta Medica* 76, no. 1 (2010): 76–78.

Hattori, A., H. Migitaka, M. Ligo, et al. Identification of melatonin in plants and its effects on plasma melatonin levels and binding to melatonin receptors in vertebrates. *Biochemistry and Molecular Biology International* 35, no. 3 (1995): 627–34.

He, H. J., Z. Y. Lv, Z. Y. Li, et al. Efficacy of combined treatment with albendazole and baicalein against eosinophilic meningitis induced by Angiostrongylus cantonensis in mice. *Journal of Helminthology* 85, no. 1 (2011): 92–99.

Hou, Y. C., S. P. Lin, S. Y. Tsai, et al. Flavonoid pharmacokinetics and tissue distribution after repeated dosing of the roots of Scutellaria barbata in rats. *Planta Medica* 77, no. 5 (2011): 455–60.

Hsieh, C.-J., K. Hall, T. Ha, et al. Baicalein inhibits IL-1β- and TNF-α-induced inflammatory cytokine production from human mast cells via regulation of the NF-κB pathway. *Clinical and Molecular Allergy* 5, no. 5 (2007): 1–10.

Huang, W.-H., A.-R. Lee, and C.-H. Yang. Antioxidative and anti-inflammatory activities of polyhydroxyflavonoids of Scutellaria baicalensis Georgi. *Bioscience, Biotechnology, and Biochemistry* 70, no. 10 (2006): 2371–80.

Huang, Y., S. Y. Tsang, X. Yao, et al. Biological properties of baicalein in cardiovascular system. *Current Drug Targets — Cardiovascular & Haematological Disorders* 5, no. 2 (2005): 177–84.

Hwang, Y. K., M. Jinhua, B. R. Choi, et al. Effects of Scutellaria baicalensis on chronic cerebral hypoperfusion-induced memory impairments and chronic lipopolysaccharide infusion-induced memory impairments. *Journal of Ethnopharmacology* 371, no. 1 (2011): 681–89.

Jeong, K., Y.-C. Shin, S. Park, et al. Ethanol extract of Scutellaria baicalensis Georgi prevents oxidative damage and neuroinflammation and memorial impairments in artificial senescense mice. *Journal of Biomedical Science* 18, no. 14 (2011): 1–12.

Ju, W. Z., F. Liu, T. Wu, et al. Simultaneous determination of baicalin and chlorogenic acid in human plasma by UPLC-MS/MS. *Yao Xue Xue Bao* 42, no. 10 (2007): 1074–77.

Jung, H. S., M. H. Kim, N. G. Gwak, et al. Antiallergic effect of Scutellaria baicalensis on inflammation in vivo and in vitro. *Journal of Ethnopharmacology* 141, no. 1 (2012): 345–49. Published electronically ahead of print March 3, 2012.

Kim, E. H., B. Shim, S. Kang, et al. Anti-inflammatory effects of Scutellaria baicalensis extract via suppression of immune modulators and MAP kinase signaling molecules. *Journal of Ethnopharmacology* 126, no. 2 (2009): 320–31.

Kim, H. M., E. J. Moon, E. Li, et al. The nitric oxide-producing activities of Scutellaria baicalensis. *Toxicology* 135, no. 2–3 (1999): 109–15.

Kim, Y. H., D. W. Jeong, Y. C. Kim, et al. Pharmacokinetics of baicalein, baicalin and wogonin after oral administration of a standardized extract of Scutellaria baicalensis, PF-2405 in rats. *Archives of Pharmaceutical Research* 30, no. 2 (2007): 260–65.

Kim, Y. H., D. W. Jeong, I. B. Paek, et al. Liquid chromatography with tandem mass spectrometry for the simultaneous determination of baicalein, baicalin, oroxylin A and wogonin in rat plasma. *Journal of Chromatography B Analytical Technologies in the Biomedical and Life Sciences* 844, no. 2 (2006): 261–67.

Kimura, Y., and M. Sumiyoshi. Effects of baicalein and wogonin isolated from Scutellaria baicalensis roots on skin damage in acute UVB-irradiated hairless mice. *European Journal of Pharmacology* 661, no. 1–3 (2011): 124–32.

Kolar, J., and I. Machackova. Melatonin in higher plants: Occurrence and possible functions. *Journal of Pineal Research* 39 (2005): 333–41.

Kong, B., J. Wang, and Y. L. Xiong. Antimicrobial activity of several herb and spice extracts in culture medium and in vacuum-packaged pork. *Journal of Food Protection* 70, no. 3 (2007): 641–47.

Konoshima, T., et al. Studies on inhibitors of skin tumor promotion. XI. Inhibitory effects of flavonoids from Scutellaria baicalensis on Epstein-Barr virus activation and their anti-tumor-promoting activities *Chemical and Pharmaceutical Bulletin* (Tokyo) 40, no. 2 (1992): 531–33.

Kowalczyk, E., P. Krzesinski, M. Kura, et al. Pharmacological effects of flavonoids from Scutellaria baicalensis. *Przegląd Lekarski* 63, no. 2 (2006): 95–96.

Kuroda, M., et al. Chemical constituents of the aerial parts of Scutellaria lateriflora and their alpha-glycosidase inhibitory activities. *Natural Products Communications* 7, no. 4 (2012): 471–74.

Lai, M.-Y., S.-L. Hsiu, C.-C. Chen, et al. Urinary pharmacokinetics of baicalein, wogonin and their glycosides after oral administration of scutellariae radix in humans. *Biological and Pharmaceutical Bulletin* 26, no. 1 (2003): 79–83.

Lai, M. Y., S. L. Hsiu, Y. C. Hou, et al. Significant decrease of cyclosporine bioavailability in rats caused by a decoction of the roots of Scutellaria baicalensis. *Planta Medica* 70, no. 2 (2004): 132–37.

Latella, G., et al. Prevention of colonic fibrosis by Boswellia and Scutellaria extracts in rats with colitis induced by 2,4,5-trinitrobenzene sulphonic acid. *European Journal of Clinical Investigation* 38, no. 6 (2008): 410–20.

Lee, A., et al. Synthesis and structure-activity relationships of flavonoids derived from Scutellaria baicalensis Georgi as potent anti-flu agents against Tamiflu-resistant H1N1 virus and H3N2 virus. *Journal of Chinese Medicine Research and Development* 1, no. 1 (2012): 28–36.

Lee, H., Y. O. Kim, H. Kim, et al. Flavonoid wogonin from medicinal herb is neuroprotective by inhibiting inflammatory activation of microglia. *FASEB Journal* 17, no. 13 (2003): 1943–44.

Lee, J. H., and S. R. Lee. The effect of baicalein on hippocampal neuronal damage and metalloproteinase activity following transient global cerebral ischaemia. *Phytotherapy Research* 26, no. 11 (2012): 1614–19. Published electronically ahead of print February 17, 2012.

Levy, R. M., R. Saikovsky, E. Schmidt, et al. Flavocoxid is as effective as naproxen for managing the signs and symptoms of osteoarthritis of the knee in humans: A short-term randomized, double-blind pilot study. *Nutrition Research* 29, no. 5 (2009): 298–304.

Li, B. Inhibition of HIV infection by baicalin — a flavonoid compound purified from Chinese herbal medicine. *Cellular & Molecular Biology Research* 39, no. 2 (1993): 119–24.

Li, B. Q., T. Fu, Y. Dongyan, et al. Flavonoid baicalin inhibits HIV-1 infection at the level of viral entry. *Biochemical and Biophysical Research Communications* 276, no. 2 (2000): 534–38.

Li, C., G. Lin, and Z. Zuo. Pharmacological effects and pharmacokinetics properties of radix scutellaria and its bioactive flavones. *Biopharmaceutics & Drug Disposition* 32, no. 8 (2011): 427–45.

Li, C., L. Zhang, Z. Zuo, et al. Identification and quantification of baicalein, wogonin, oroxylin A and their major glucoronide conjugated metabolites in rat plasma after oral administration of radix scutellariae. *Journal of Pharmaceutical and Biomedical Analysis* 54, no. 4 (2011): 750–58.

Li, Y., P. Zhuang, B. Shen, et al. Baicalin promotes neuronal differentiation of neural stem/progenitor cells through modulating p-stat3 and bHLH family protein expression. *Brain Research* 6, no. 1429 (2012): 36–42.

Lim, B. O., R. W. Choue, H. Y. Lee, et al. Effect of the flavonoid components obtained from Scutellaria radix on the histamine, immunoglobulin e and lipid peroxidation of spleen lymphocytes of Sprague-Dawley rats. *Bioscience, Biotechnology, and Biochemistry* 67, no. 5 (2003): 1126–29.

Lin, A. M., Y. H. Ping, G. F. Chang, et al. Neuroprotective effect of oral S/B remedy (Scutellaria baicalensis Georgi and Bupleurum scorzonerifolium Willd.) on iron-induced neurodegeneration in the nigrostriatal dopaminergic system of rat brain. *Journal of Ethnopharmacology* 134, no. 3 (2011): 884–91.

Lin, B. Polyphenols and neuroprotection against ischemia and neurodegeneration. *Mini Reviews in Medicinal Chemistry* 11, no. 14 (2011): 1222–38.

Lin, W., et al. Study on the prevention effect of extracts from several medicinal plants on mosaic virus disease of Momordica grosvenori Swingle. *Journal of Anhui Agricultural Sciences*, 2009-04, CNKI.

Lin, Y. Study on the inhibitory effect of Scutellaria baicalensis Georgi on neuraminidase of influenza A virus. Paper for Asia University, 2010, http://asiair.asia.edu.tw/ir/handle/310904400/10902 (accessed May 19, 2012).

Liu, G., N. Rajesh, X. Wang, et al. Identification of flavonoids in the stems and leaves of Scutellaria baicalensis Georgi. *Journal of Chromatography B Analytical Technologies in the Biomedical and Life Sciences* 879, no. 13–14 (2011): 1023–28.

Liu, L., Y. X. Deng, Y. Liang, et al. Increased oral AUC of baicalin in streptozotocin-induced beta-glucuronidase. *Planta Medica* 76, no. 1 (2010): 70–75.

Liu, T. M., and X. H. Jiang. Studies on the absorption kinetics of baicalin and baicalein in rats' stomachs and intestines. *Zhongguo Zhong Yao Za Zhi* 31, no. 12 (2006): 999–1001.

Lixuan, Z., D. Jingcheng, Y. Wenqin, et al. Baicalin attenuates inflammation by inhibiting NF-kappaB activation in cigarette smoke induced inflammatory models. *Pulmonary Pharmacology & Therapeutics* 23, no. 5 (2010): 411–19.

Lu, T., J. Song, F. Huang, et al. Comparative pharmacokinetics of baicalin after oral administration of pure baicalin, radix scutellariae extract and huang-lian-jie-du-tang to rats. *Journal of Ethnopharmacology* 110, no. 3 (2007): 412–18.

Lu, Y., R., Joerger, and C. Wu. Study of the chemical composition and antimicrobial activities of ethanol extracts from roots of Scutellaria baicalensis Georgi. *Journal of Agricultural and Food Chemistry* 59, no. 20 (2011): 10934–42.

Lu, Z. Clinical comparative study of intravenous piperacillin sodium or injection of scutellaria compound in patients with pulmonary infection. *Zhong Xi Yi Jie He Za Zhi* 10, no. 7 (1990): 413–15, 389.

Luo, J., et al. Effect of glucoside of root of Scutellaria baicalensis against Ureaplasma urealyticum in vitro. *Journal of Microbiology*, 2006-05, CNKI.

Luo, X., X. Zhou, P. Su, et al. Effects of Scutellaria baicalensis stem-leaf total flavonoid on proliferation of vassal smooth muscle cells stimulated by high triglyceride blood serum. *Zhongguo Zhong Yao Za Zhi* 34, no. 21 (2009): 2803–7.

Ma, S. C., J. Du, P. P. But, et al. Antiviral Chinese medicinal herbs against respiratory syncytial virus. *Journal of Ethnopharmacology* 79, no. 2 (2002): 205–11.

Mai, S., et al. Clinical observation of baicalin used in treatment of bacterial meningitis. *Maternal and Child Health Care of China*, 2006-04, CNKI.

Makino, T., A. Hishida, Y. Goda, et al. Comparison of the major flavonoid content of S. baicalensis, S. lateriflora, and their commercial products. *Journal of Natural Medicines* 62, no. 3 (2008): 294–99.

Martin, J., and J. Dusek. The baikal scullcap (Scutellaria baicalensis Georgi) — a potential source of new drugs. *Ceská a Slovenská Farmacie* 51, no. 6 (2002): 277–83.

Morgan, S. L., J. E. Baggott, L. Moreland, et al. The safety of flavocoxid, a medical food, in the dietary management of knee osteoarthritis. *Journal of Medicinal Food* 12, no. 5 (2009): 1143–48.

Murch, S. J., H. P. Rupasinghe, D. Goodenowe, et al. A metabolic analysis of medicinal diversity in huang-qin (Scutellaria baicalensis Georgi) genotypes: Discovery of novel compounds. *Plant Cell Reports* 23, no. 6 (2004): 419–25.

Nagai, T., et al. Inhibition of influenza virus sialidase and anti-influenza virus activity by plant flavonoids. *Chemical and Pharmaceutical Bulletin* (Tokyo) 38, no. 5 (1990): 1329–32.

Nagai, T., Y. Miyaichi, T. Tomimori, et al. In vivo anti-influenza virus activity of plant flavonoids possessing inhibitory activity for influenza virus sialidase. *Antiviral Research* 19, no. 3 (1992): 207–17.

Nagai, T., R. Moriguchi, Y. Suzuki, et al. Mode of action of the anti-influenza virus activity of plant flavonoid, 5,7,4'-trihydroxy-8-methoxyflavone, from the roots of Scutellaria baicalensis. *Antiviral Research* 26, no. 1 (1995): 11–25.

Nagai, T., Y. Suzuki, T. Tomimori, et al. Antiviral activity of plant flavonoid, 5,7,4'-trihydroxyl-8-methoxyflavone, from the roots of Scutellaria baicalensis against influenza A (H3N2) and B viruses. *Biological and Pharmaceutical Bulletin* 18, no. 2 (1995): 295–99.

Ozmen, A., S. Madlener, S. Bauer, et al. In vitro anti-leukemic activity of the ethno-pharmacological plant Scutellaria orientalis ssp. carica endemic to western Turkey. *Phytomedicine* 17, no. 1 (2010): 55–62.

Pant, C. C., A. B. Melkani, L. Mohan, et al. Composition and antibacterial activity of essential oil from Scutellaria grossa Wall ex Benth. *Natural Product Research* 26, no. 2 (2012): 190–92.

Peng, J., Q. Qi, Q. You, et al. Subchronic toxicity and plasma pharmacokinetic studies on wogonin, a natural flavonoid, in Beagle dogs. *Journal of Ethnopharmacology* 124, no. 2 (2009): 257–62.

Perez, A. T., B. Arun, D. Tripathy, et al. A phase 1B dose escalation trial of Scutellaria barbata (BZL101) for patients with metastatic breast cancer. *Breast Cancer Research and Treatment* 120, no. 1 (2010): 111–18.

Piao, H. Z., I. Y. Choi, J. S. Park, et al. Wogonin inhibits microglial cell migration via suppression of nuclear factor-kappa B activity. *International Immunopharmacology* 8, no. 12 (2008): 1658–62.

Reiter, R. J., D. X. Tan, S. Burkhardt, et al. Melatonin in Plants. *Nutrition Reviews* 59, no. 9 (2001): 286–90.

Scute root (Scutellaria baicalensis). Entry in *Important Herbs from Around the World* of the Tillotson Institute of Natural Health, www.tillotsoninstitute.com/important-herbs/scute-root-scutellaria-baicalensis-.html (accessed March 29, 2012).

Scutellaria baicalensis Georgi. Entry in the Germplasm Resources Information Network (GRIN) database of the USDA Agricultural Research Service National Genetic Resources Program, www.ars-grin.gov/cgi-bin/npgs/html/taxon.pl?33424 (accessed March 29, 2012).

Shang, X., X. He, X. He, et al. The genus Scutellaria: An ethnopharmacological and phytochemical review. *Journal of Ethnopharmacology* 128, no. 2 (2010): 279–313.

Shang, Y.-Z., H. Miao, J.-J. Cheng, et al. Effects of amelioration of total flavonoids from stems and leaves of Scutellaria baicalensis Georgi on deficits, neuronal damage and free radicals disorder induced by cerebral ischemia in rats. *Biological and Pharmaceutical Bulletin* 29, no. 4 (2006): 805–10.

Sheng, J. P., H. R. Chen, and L. Shen. Comparative study on selenium and amino acids content in leaves of planted and wild Scutellaria baicalensis. *Guang Pu Xue Yu Guang Pu Fen Xi* 29, no. 1 (2009): 211–13.

Sheng, J. P., H. R. Chen, and L. Shen. Determination of six mineral elements in roots, stems, leaves, flowers and seeds of Scutellaria baicalensis by FAAS. *Guang Pu Xue Yu Guang Pu Fen Xi* 29, no. 2 (2009): 519–21.

Sherwood, K., and C. Idso. The pharmacological activity of Scutellaria plants. *CO2 Science* 12, no. 24 (2009): 17.

Shi, R., S. Qiqo, D. Yu, et al. Simultaneous determination of five flavonoids from Scutellaria barbata extract in rat plasma by LC-MS/MS and its application to pharmacokinetic study. *Journal of Chromatography B Analytical Technologies in the Biomedical and Life Sciences* 879, no. 19 (2011): 1625–32.

Shih, Y. T., I. J. Chen, Y. C. Wu, et al. San-huang-xie-xin-tang protects against activated microglia and 6-OHDA-induced toxicity in neuronal SH-SY5Y cells. *Evidence-Based Complementary and Alternative Medicine* (2011). doi: 10.1093/ecam/nep025.

Smol'ianinov, E. S., V. E. Gol'dberg, M. G. Matiash, et al. Effect of Scutellaria baicalensis extract on the immunological status of patients with lung cancer receiving antineoplastic chemotherapy. *Eksperimental'naia i Klinicheskaia Farmakologiia* 60, no. 6 (1997): 49–51.

Song, L. Study development on pharmacodynamics effect of Scutellaria. *Chinese Archives of Traditional Chinese Medicine*, 2008-08, CNKI.

Song, S. H., and Z. Z. Wang. Analysis of essential oils from different organs of Scutellaria baicalensis. *Zhong Yao Cai* 33, no. 8 (2010): 1265–70.

Suk, K., H. Lee, S. S. Kang, et al. Flavonoid baicalein attenuates activation-induced cell death of brain microglia. *Journal of Pharmacology and Experimental Therapeutics* 305, no. 2 (2003): 638–45.

Tang, Z. M., M. Peng, and C. J. Zhan. Screening 20 Chinese herbs often used for clearing heat and dissipating toxin with nude mice model of hepatitis C viral infection. *Zhongguo Zhong Xi Yi He Za Zhi* 23, no. 6 (2003): 447–48.

Tian, S., G. He, J. Song, et al. Pharmacokinetic study of baicalein after oral administration in monkeys. *Fitoterapia* 83, no. 3 (2012): 532–40. Published electronically ahead of print January 8, 2012.

Trinh, H. T., E. H. Joh, H. Y. Kwak, et al. Antipruritic effect of baicalin and its metabolites, baicalein and oroxylin A, in mice. *Acta Pharmacologica Sinica* 31, no. 6 (2010): 718–24.

Tsai, P. L., and T. H. Tsai. Pharmacokinetics of baicalin in rats and its interactions with cyclosporin A, quinine and SKF-525A: A microdialysis study. *Planta Medica* 70, no. 11 (2004): 1069–74.

Tsai, T. H., S. C. Liu, P. L. Tsai, et al. The effects of the cyclosporin A, a P-glycoprotein inhibitor, on the pharmacokinetics of baicalein in the rat: A microdialysis study. *British Journal of Pharmacology* 137, no. 8 (2002): 1314–20.

Tsao, T. F., M. G. Newman, Y. Y. Kwok, et al. Effect of Chinese and Western antimicrobial agents on selected oral bacteria. *Journal of Dental Research* 61, no. 9 (1982): 1103–6.

Tseng, Y. P., Y. C. Wu, Y. L. Ley, et al. Scutellaria radix suppresses hepatitis B virus production in human hepatoma cells. *Frontiers in Bioscience (Elite Edition)* 1, no. 2 (2010): 1538–47.

Udut, E. V., V. V. Zhdanov, L. A. Gur'iantseva, et al. Mechanisms of the erythropoiesis-stimulating effect of skullcap (Scutellaria baicalensis) extract. *Eksperimental'naia i Klinicheskaia Farmakologiia* 68, no. 4 (2005): 43–45.

Wang, G. F., Z. F. Wu, L. Wan, et al. Influence of baicalin on the expression of receptor activator of nuclear factor-kappaB ligand in cultured human periodontal ligament cells. *Pharmacology* 77, no. 2 (2006): 71–77.

Wang, H., et al. Studies on chemical constituents of the roots of Scutellaria viscidula Bge. *Journal of Shenyang Pharmaceutical University*, 2003-05, CNKI.

Wang, X., et al. Antivirus effects of Scutellaria baicalensis root preparations by two different extraction methods on coxsackie B_(3m) and its cell protection function in vitro. *Chinese Pharmaceutical*, 2006, CNKI.

Wolfson, P., and D. L. Hoffmann. An investigation into the efficacy of Scutellaria lateriflora in healthy volunteers. *Alternative Therapies in Health and Medicine* 9, no. 2 (2003): 74–78.

Wu, J., D. Hu, and K. X. Wang. Study of Scutellaria baicalensis and baicalin against antimicrobial susceptibility of Helicobacter pylori strains in vitro. *Zhong Yao Cai* 31, no. 5 (2008): 707–10.

Xiao, L., et al. Comparative study on HPLC-FPS of radix scutellariae of various sources. *Journal of Shenyang Pharmaceutical University*, 2004-01, CNKI.

Xiao, L., et al. Isolation and identification of the chemical constituents of roots of Scutellaria amoena C.H. Wright. *Journal of Shenyang Pharmaceutical University*, 2003-09, CNKI.

Xie, L. H., X. Wang, P. Basnet, et al. Evaluation of variation of acteoside and three major flavonoids in wild and cultivated Scutellaria baicalensis roots by micellar electrokinetic chromatography. *Chemical & Pharmaceutical Bulletin* (Tokyo) 50, no. 7 (2002): 896–99.

Xiong, Z., B. Jiang, P. F. Wu, et al. Antidepressant effects of a plant-derived flavonoid baicalein involving extracellular signal-regulated kinases cascade. *Biological and Pharmaceutical Bulletin* 34, no. 2 (2011): 253–59.

Xu, G., J. Dou, L. Zhang, et al. Inhibitory effects of baicalein on the influenza virus in vivo is determined by baicalin in the serum. *Biological and Pharmaceutical Bulletin* 33, no. 2 (2010): 238–43.

Xu, S., et al. Antiviral effect and mechanism of Scutellaria baicalensis Georgi. *Chinese Archives of Traditional Chinese Medicine,* 2007-07, CNKI.

Yan, X., et al. Therapeutic effects of baicalin on encephaledema followed by the laboratory brain blood swelling in neonatal rats. *Pediatric Emergency Medicine,* 2004-04, CNKI.

Yang, D., H. Hu, S. Huang, et al. Study of the inhibitory activity, in vitro, of baicalein and baicalin against skin fungi and bacteria. *Zhong Yao Cai* 23, no. 5 (2000): 272–74.

Yang, J., et al. Experimental research on the antivirus function in vitro Scutellaria baicalensis Georgi extractant. *Science Technology and Engineering,* 2007-12, CNKI.

Yang, L., X. L. Zheng, H. Sun, et al. Catalase suppression-mediated H(2)O(2) accumulation in cancer cells by wogonin effectively blocks tumor necrosis factor-induced NF-κB activation and sensitizes apoptosis. *Cancer Science* 102, no. 4 (2011): 870–76.

Yang, X., B. Huang, J. Chen, et al. In vitro effects of aqueous extracts of Astragalus membranaceus and Scutellaria baicalensis Georgi on Toxoplasma gondii. *Parasitology Research* 110, no. 6 (2012): 2221–27. Published electronically ahead of print December 17, 2011.

Yang, Y., et al. The protective effects of baicalin on pertussis bacilli-induced brain edema in rats. *Zhonghua Yi Xue Za Zhi* 78, no. 8 (1988): 630–32.

Yang, Z. C., B. C. Wang, X. S. Yang, et al. The synergistic activity of antibiotics combined with eight traditional Chinese medicines against two different strains of Staphylococcus aureus. *Colloids and Surface B Biointerfaces* 41, no. 2–3 (2005): 79–81.

Yoon, S. B., Y. J. Lee, S. K. Park, et al. Anti-inflammatory effects of Scutellaria baicalensis water extract on LPS-activated RAW 264.7 macrophages. *Journal of Ethnopharmacology* 125, no. 2 (2009): 286–90.

You, C. L., P. Q. Su, and X. X. Zhou. Study on effect and mechanism of Scutellaria baicalensis stem-leaf total flavonoid in regulating lipid metabolism. *Zhongguo Zhong Yao Za Zhi* 33, no. 9 (2008): 1064–66.

Yu, C., et al. Oren-gedoku-to and its constituents with therapeutic potential in Alzheimer's disease inhibit indoleamine 2, 3-dioxygenase activity in vitro. *Journal of Alzheimer's Disease* 22, no. 1 (2010): 257–66.

Yu, J., J. Lei, H. Yu, et al. Chemical composition and antimicrobial activity of the essential oil of Scutellaria barbata. *Phytochemistry* 65, no. 7 (2004): 881–84.

Yu, L. Z., J. Y. Wu, J. B. Luo, et al. Effects of different compositions of gegenqinlian decoction on experimental shigellosis in rabbits. *Di Yi Jun Yi Da Xue Xue Bao* 25, no. 9 (2005): 1132–34.

Yue, G. G., B. C. Chan, H. F. Kwok, et al. Screening for anti-inflammatory and bronchorelaxant activities of 12 commonly used Chinese herbal medicines. *Phytotherapy Research* 26, no. 6 (2012): 915–25. Published electronically ahead of print November 22, 2011.

Zeng, Y., C. Song, X. Ding, et al. Baicalin reduces the severity of experimental autoimmune encephalomyelitis. *Brazilian Journal of Medical and Biological Research* 40 (2007): 1003–10.

Zhang, D. Y., J. Wu, F. Ye, et al. Inhibition of cancer cell proliferation and prostaglandin E2 synthesis by Scutellaria baicalensis. *Cancer Research* 63, no. 14 (2003): 4037–43.

Zhang, H., and J. Huang. Preliminary study of traditional Chinese medicine treatment of minimal brain dysfunction: Analysis of 100 cases. *Zhong Xi Yi Jie He Za Zhi* 10, no. 5 (1990): 278–79, 260.

Zhang, J., et al. Content determination of baicalin in root of Scutellaria viscidula Bge by HPCL. *Lishizhen Medicine and Materia Medica Research,* 2008-03, CNKI.

Zhang, J. L., Q. M. Che, S. Z. Li, et al. Study on metabolism of scutellarin in rats by HPLC-MS and HPLC-NMR. *Journal of Asian Natural Products Research* 5, no. 4 (2003): 249–56.

Zhang, L., et al. In vitro study of baicalin on infection of respiratory syncytial virus. *Zhejiang Clinical Medical Journal,* 2008-12, CNKI.

Zhang, L., A. S. Ravipati, S. R. Koyyalamudi, et al. Antioxidant and anti-inflammatory activities of selected medicinal plants containing phenolic and flavonoid compounds. *Journal of Agricultural and Food Chemistry* 59, no. 23 (2011): 12361–67.

Zhang, L., D. Xing, Y. Ding, et al. A chromatographic method for baicalin quantification in rat thalamus. *Biomedical Chromatography* 19, no. 7 (2005): 494–97.

Zhang, L., D. Xing, W. Wang, et al. Kinetic difference of baicalin in rat blood and cerebral nuclei after intravenous administration of scutellariae radix extract. *Journal of Ethnopharmacology* 103, no. 1 (2006): 120–25.

Zhang, X., et al. An experimental study in bacteriostatic effect of decoction of Scutellaria baicalensis baicalin and debaicalin. *Journal of Heilonghang Commercial College,* 1997-04, CNKI.

Zhang, X. W., W. F. Li, W. W. Li, et al. Protective effects of the aqueous extract of Scutellaria baicalensis against acrolein-induced oxidative stress in cultured human umbilical vein endothelial cells. *Pharmaceutical Biology* 49, no. 3 (2011): 256–61.

Zhang, Y. Y., H. Y. Don, Y. Z. Guo, et al. Comparative study of Scutellaria planipes and Scutellaria baicalensis. *Biomedical Chromatography* 12, no. 1 (1998): 31–33.

Zhao, T., et al. Antiviral effects of active fraction from stems and leaves of Scutellaria baicalensis. *Journal of China Pharmaceutical University,* 2006-06, CNKI.

Zhao, T., et al. Study of antibacterial activity of active fraction from stems and leaves of Scutellaria baicalensis Georgi. *Chinese Pharmaceutical Bulletin*, 2007-07, CNKI.

Zheljazkov, V. D., C. L. Cantrell, M. W. Ebelhar, et al. Quality assessment and yield of baikal skullcap (Scutellaria baicalensis) grown at multiple locations. *Horticultural Science* 42, no. 5 (2007): 1183–87.

Zhou, J., F. Qu, H.-J. Zhang, et al. Comparison of anti-inflammatory and anti-nociceptive activities of Curcuma wenyujin Y.H. Chen et C. Ling and Scutellaria baicalensis Georgi. *Indian Journal of Medical Research* 7, no. 4 (2010): 339–49.

Zhou, X., et al. An in vitro study on the effects of radix scutellariae on three strains of cariogenic bacteria. *Journal of West China University of Medical Sciences*, 2002-03, CNKI.

Zhou, X. Q., H. Liang, X. H. Lu, et al. Flavonoids from Scutellaria baicalensis and their bio-activities. *Beijing Da Xue Xue Bao* 41, no. 5 (2009): 578–84.

Zhu, Y. X., X. Luo, D. P. Zhao, et al. Analysis of the content of mineral elements in Scutellaria baicalensis, skullcap tea and its solution. *Guang Pu Xue Yu Guang Pu Fen* 31, no. 11 (2011): 3112–14.

Zhu, Z., L. Zhao, X. Liu, et al. Comparative pharmacokinetics of baicalin and wogonoside by liquid chromatography-mass spectrometry after oral administration of xiaochaihu tang and radix scutellariae extract to rats. *Journal of Chromatography B Analytical Technologies in the Biomedical and Life Sciences* 878, no. 24 (2010): 2184–90.

Cordyceps (*Cordyceps sinensis*)

Ahn, Y. J., S. J. Park, S. G. Lee, et al. Cordycepin: Selective growth inhibitors derived from liquid culture of Cordyceps militaris against Clostridium spp. *Journal of Agricultural and Food Chemistry* 48, no. 7 (2000): 2744–48.

Bao, Z. D., Z. G. Wu, and F. Zheng. Amelioration of aminoglycoside nephrotoxicity by Cordyceps sinensis in old patients. *Zhongguo Zhong Xi Yi Jie He Za Zhi* 14, no. 5 (1994): 271–73, 259.

Boesi, Alessandro, and Francesca Cardi. Cordyceps sinensis medicinal fungus: Traditional use among Tibetan people, harvesting techniques, and modern uses. *HerbalGram* (American Botanical Council) 83 (2009): 52–61, http://cms.herbalgram.org/herbalgram/issue83/article3433.html.

Byeon, S. E., S. Y. Lee, A. R. Kim, et al. Inhibition of cytokine expression by butanol extract from Cordyceps bassiana. *Pharmazie* 66, no. 1 (2011): 58–62.

Byeon, S. E., J. Lee, B. C. Yoo, et al. p-38-targeted inhibition of interleukin-12 expression by ethanol extract from Cordyceps bassiana in lypopolysaccharide-activated macrophages. *Immunopharmacology and Immunotoxicology* 33, no. 1 (2011): 90–96.

Chang, Y., K. C. Jeng, K. F. Huang, et al. Effect of Cordyceps militaris supplementation on sperm production, sperm motility and hormones in Sprague-Dawley rats. *American Journal of Chinese Medicine* 36, no. 5 (2008): 849–59.

Chen, S., Z. Li, R. Krochmal, et al. Effect of Cs-4 (Cordyceps sinensis) on exercise performance in healthy older subjects: A double-blind, placebo-controlled trial. *Journal of Alternative and Complementary Medicine* 16, no. 5 (2010): 585–90.

Cheng, Z., W. He, X. Zhou, et al. Cordycepin protects against cerebral ischemia/reperfusion injury in vivo and in vitro. *European Journal of Pharmacology* 664, no. 1–3 (2011): 20–28.

Chiou, Y.-L., and C.-Y. Lin. The extract of Cordyceps sinensis inhibited airway inflammation by blocking NF-κB activity. *Inflammation* 35, no. 3 (2011): 985–93.

Cho, H. J., J. Y. Cho, M. H. Rhee, et al. Cordycepin (3'-deoxyadenosine) inhibits human platelet aggregation in a cyclic AMP- and cyclic GMP-dependent manner. *European Journal of Pharmacology* 558, no. 1–3 (2007): 43–51.

Cho, H. J., J. Y. Cho, M. H. Rhee, et al. Inhibitory effects of cordycepin (3'-deoxyadenosine), a component of Cordyceps militaris, on human platelet aggregation induced by thapsigargin. *Journal of Microbiology and Biotechnology* 17, no. 7 (2007): 1134–38.

Colson, S. N., F. B. Wyatt, D. L. Johnston, et al. Cordyceps sinensis- and Rhodiola rosea-based supplementation in male cyclists and its effect on muscle tissue oxygen saturation. *Journal of Strength & Conditioning Research* 19, no. 2 (2005): 358–63.

Ding, C., P. X. Tian, W. Xue, et al. Efficacy of Cordyceps sinensis in long term treatment of renal transplant patients. *Frontiers in Bioscience (Elite Edition)* 1, no. 3 (2011): 301–7.

El Ashry Fel, Z., M. F. Mahmoud, N. N. El Maraghy, and A. F. Ahmed. Effects of Cordyceps sinensis and taurine either alone or in combination on streptozotocin induced diabetes. *Food and Chemical Toxicology* 50, no. 3–4 (2012): 1159–65.

Gong, M. F., J. P. Xu, Z. Y. Chu, et al. Effect of Cordyceps sinensis sporocarp on learning-memory in mice. *Zhong Yao Cai* 34, no. 9 (2011): 1403–5.

Guo, P., Q. Kai, J. Gao, et al. Cordycepin prevents hyperlipidemia in hamsters fed a high-fat diet via activation of AMP-activated protein kinase. *Journal of Pharmacological Sciences* 113, no. 4 (2010): 395–403.

Han, E. S., J. Y. Oh, and H. J. Park. Cordyceps militaris extract suppresses dextran sodium sulfate-induced acute colitis in mice and production of inflammatory mediators from macrophages and mast cells. *Journal of Ethnopharmacology* 134, no. 3 (2011): 703–10.

Haritakun, R., M. Sappan, R. Suvannakad, et al. An antimycobacterial cyclodepsipeptide from the entomopathogenic fungus Ophiocordyceps communis BCC 16475. *Journal of Natural Products* 73, no. 1 (2010): 75–78.

Holliday, J., and M. Cleaver. Medicinal value of the caterpillar fungi species of the genus Cordyceps (Fr) Link (Ascomycetes). A review. *International Journal of Medicinal Mushrooms* 10, no. 3 (2008): 219–34.

Holliday, J., and M. Cleaver. On the trail of the yak: Ancient cordyceps in the modern world. June 2004. www.earthpulse.com/cordyceps_inc/cordyceps_story.pdf.

Holliday, J., M. Cleaver, and S. P. Wasser. Cordyceps. *Encyclopedia of Dietary Supplements* 1 (2005): 1–13.

Hsu, C. H., H. L. Sun, J. N. Sheu, et al. Effects of the immunomodulatory agent Cordyceps militaris on airway inflammation in a mouse asthma model. *Pediatrics & Neonatology* 49, no. 5 (2008): 171–78.

Huang, J. C., J. H. Li, T. X. Liu, et al. Effect of combined therapy with hypha cordyceps and ginkgo leaf tablet on micro-inflammation in patients undergoing maintenance hemodialysis. *Zhongguo Zhong Xi Yi Jie He Za Zhi* 28, no. 6 (2008): 502–4.

Hwang, I. K., S. S. Lim, K. Y. Yoo, et al. A phytochemically characterized extract of Cordyceps militaris and cordycepin protect hippocampal neurons from ischemic injury in gerbils. *Planta Medica* 74, no. 2 (2008): 114–19.

Jeong, J. W., C. Y. Jin, G. Y. Kim, et al. Anti-inflammatory effects of cordycepin via suppression of inflammatory mediators in BV2 microglial cells. *International Immunopharmacology* 10, no. 12 (2010): 1580–86.

Jeong, J. W., C. Y. Jin, C. Park, et al. Inhibition of migration and invasion of LNCaP human prostate carcinoma cells by cordycepin through inactivation of Akt. *International Journal of Oncology* 40, no. 5 (2012): 1697–704.

Jiang, Y., J. H. Wong, M. Fu, et al. Isolation of adenosine, iso-sinensetin and dimethyl-guanosine with antioxidant and HIV-1 protease inhibiting activities from fruiting bodies of Cordyceps militaris. *Phytomedicine* 18, no. 2–3 (2011): 189–93.

Jones, I. L., F. K. Moore, and C. L. Chai. Total synthesis of (+/-)-cordypyridones A and B and related epimers. *Organic Letters* 11, no. 23 (2009): 5526–29.

Jung, S. M., S. S. Park, W. J. Kim, et al. Ras/ERK1 pathway regulation of p27KIP1-mediated G1-phase cell-cycle arrest in cordycepin-induced inhibition of the proliferation of vascular smooth muscle cells. *European Journal of Pharmacology* 681, no. 1–3 (2012): 15–22.

Khan, A., et al. Cordyceps mushroom: A potent anticancer nutraceutical. *Open Nutraceuticals Journal* 3 (2010): 179–83.

Kim, H. G., B. Shrestha, S. Y. Lim, et al. Cordycepin inhibits lipopolysaccharide-induced inflammation by the suppression of NF-kappaB through Akt and p38 inhibition in RAW 264.7 macrophage cells. *European Journal of Pharmacology* 545, no. 2–3 (2006): 192–99.

Kim, J. H., D. K. Park, C. H. Lee, et al. A new isoflavone glycitein 7-o-beta-d-glucoside 4″-O-methylate, isolated from Cordyceps militaris grown on mucus hypersecretion in the human lung mucoepidermoid cells. *Phytotherapy Research* 26, no. 12 (2012): 1807–12. Published electronically ahead of print March 9, 2012.

Kim, K. M., Y. G. Kwon, H. T. Chung, et al. Methanol extract of Cordyceps pruinosa inhibits in vitro and in vivo inflammatory mediators by suppressing NF-kappaB activation. *Toxicology and Applied Pharmacology* 190, no. 1 (2003): 1–8.

King, B. Species diversity and production of antimicrobial compounds by Pacific Northwestern clavicipitalean entomogenous fungi (Cordyceps spp.). Master's thesis, University of British Columbia, 2006, http://circle.ubc.ca/handle/2429/18403.

Ko, K. M., and H. Y. Leung. Enhancement of ATP generation capacity, antioxidant activity and immunomodulatory activities by Chinese yang and yin tonifying herbs. *Chinese Medicine* 2, no. 3 (2007): 1–10.

Kuo, C.-F., C.-C. Chen, Y.-H. Luo, et al. Cordyceps sinensis mycelium protects mice from group A streptococcal infection. *Journal of Medical Microbiology* 54 (2005): 795–802.

Kuo, Y. C., W. J. Tsai, J. Y. Wang, et al. Regulation of bronchoalveolar lavage fluids cell function by the immunomodulatory agents from Cordyceps sinensis. *Life Sciences* 68, no. 9 (2001): 1067–82.

Lee, E. J., W. J. Kim, and S. K. Moon. Cordycepin suppresses TNF-alpha-induced invasion, migration and matrix metalloproteinase-9 expression in human bladder cancer cells. *Phytotherapy Research* 24, no. 12 (2010): 1755–61.

Lee, S. J., S. K. Kim, W. S. Choi, et al. Cordycepin causes p21WAF1-mediated G2/M cell-cycle arrest by regulating c-Jun N-terminal kinase activation in human bladder cancer cells. *Archives of Biochemistry and Biophysics* 490, no. 2 (2009): 103–9.

Lei, J., J. Chen, and C. Guo. Pharmacological study on Cordyceps sinensis (Berk.) Sacc. and ze-e Cordyceps. *Zhongguo Zhong Yao Za Zhi* 17, no. 6 (1992): 364–66.

Leu, S. F., S. L. Poon, H. Y. Pao, et al. The in vivo and in vitro stimulatory effects of cordycepin on mouse Leydig cell steroidogenesis. *Bioscience, Biotechnology, and Biochemistry* 75, no. 4 (2011): 723–31.

Li, C.-Y., C.-S. Chiang, and M.-L. Tsai. Two-sided effect of Cordyceps sinensis on dendritic cells in different physiological stages. *Journal of Leukocyte Biology* 85 (2009): 987–95.

Li, Y., W. J. Xue, P. X. Tian, et al. Clinical application of Cordyceps sinensis on immunosuppressive therapy in renal transplantation. *Transplant Proceedings* 41, no. 5 (2009): 1565–69.

Lin, X. X., Q. M. Xie, W. H. Shen, et al. Effects of fermented cordyceps powder on pulmonary function in sensitized guinea pigs and airway inflammation in sensitized rats. *Zhongguo Zhong Yao Za Zhi* 26, no. 9 (2001): 622–25.

Liu, Q., I. P. Hong, M. J. Ahn, et al. Anti-adipogenic activity of Cordyceps militaris in 3T3-L1 cells. *Natural Product Communications* 6, no. 12 (2011): 1839–41.

Liu, Y., et al. Effects of water extract from Cordyceps sinensis mycelium on anti-Newcastle disease virus. *Journal of Hebei University of Engineering*, 2011-02, CNKI.

Liu, Z., P. Li, D. Zhao, et al. Anti-inflammation effects of Cordyceps sinensis mycelium in focal cerebral ischemic injury in rats. *Inflammation* 34, no. 6 (2011): 639–44.

Liu, Z., P. Li, D. Zhao, et al. Protective effect of extract of Cordyceps sinensis in middle cerebral ischemia in rats. *Behavioral and Brain Functions* 6, no. 61 (2010): 1–6.

Lu, L. Study on effect of Cordyceps sinensis and artemisinin in preventing recurrence of lupus nephritis. *Zhongguo Zhong Xi Yi Jie He Za Zhi* 22, no. 3 (2002): 169–71.

Manabe, N., M. Sugimoto, Y. Azuma, et al. Effects of the mycelial extract of cultured Cordyceps sinensis on in vivo hepatic energy metabolism in the mouse. *Japanese Journal of Pharmacology* 70, no. 1 (1996): 85-88.

Muslim, N., and H. Rahman. A possible new record of Cordyceps species from Ginseng Camp, Maliau Basin, Sabah, Malaysia. *Journal of Tropical Biology and Conservation* 6 (2010): 39–41.

Ng, T. B., and H. X. Wang. Pharmacological actions of cordyceps, a prized folk medicine. *Journal of Pharmacy and Pharmacology* 57, no. 12 (2005): 1509–19.

Noh, E.-M., J.-S. Kim, H. Hur, et al. Cordycepin inhibits IL-1β-induced MMP-1 and MMP-3 expression in rheumatoid arthritis synovial fibroblasts. *Rheumatology* 48 (2009): 45–48.

Ohta, Y., et al. In vivo anti-influenza virus activity of an immunomodulatory acidic polysaccharide isolated from Cordyceps militaris grown on germinated soybeans. *Journal of Agriciculture and Food Chemistry* 55, no. 25 (2007): 10194–99.

Pan, B. S., C. Y. Lin, and B. M. Huang. The effect of cordycepin on steroidogenesis and apoptosis in MA-10 mouse Leydig tumor cells. *Evidence-Based Complementary and Alternative Medicine* (2011). doi: 10.1155/2011/750468.

Panda, A. K., and K. C. Swain. Traditional uses and medicinal potential of Cordyceps sinensis of Sikkim. *Journal of Ayurveda and Integrative Medicine* 2, no. 1 (2011): 9–13.

Parcell, A. C., J. M. Smith, S. S. Schulthies, et al. Cordyceps sinensis (CordyMax Cs-4) supplementation does not improve endurance exercise performance. *International Journal of Sport Nutrition and Exercise Metabolism* 14, no. 2 (2004): 236–42.

Park, D. K., W. S. Choi, and H. J. Park. Antiallergic activity of novel isofalvone methyl-glycosides from Cordyceps militaris grown on germinated soybeans in

antigen-stimulated mast cells. *Journal of Agricultural and Food Chemistry* 60, no. 9 (2012): 2309–15.

Park, D. K., W. S. Choi, P. J. Park, et al. Immunoglobulin and cytokine production from mesenteric lymph node lymphocytes is regulated by extracts of Cordyceps sinensis in C57BI/6N mice. *Journal of Medicinal Food* 11, no. 4 (2008): 784–88.

Paterson, R. M. Cordyceps: A traditional Chinese medicine and another fungal therapeutic biofactory? *Phytochemistry* 69 (2008): 1469–95.

Qi, W., Y. B. Yan, W. Lei, et al. Prevention of disuse osteoporosis in rats by Cordyceps sinensis extract. *Osteoporosis International* 23, no. 9 (2012): 2347–57. Published electronically ahead of print December 13, 2011.

Qian, G. M., G. F. Pan, and J. Y. Guo. Anti-inflammatory and antinociceptive effects of cordymin, a peptide purified from the medicinal mushroom Cordyceps sinensis. *Natural Product Research* 26, no. 24 (2012): 2358–62. Published electronically ahead of print February 21, 2012.

Rao, Y. K., S. H. Fang, and Y. M. Tzeng. Evaluation of the anti-inflammatory and anti-proliferation tumoral cells activities of Antrodia camphorate, Cordyceps sinensis, and Cinnamomum osmophloeum bark extracts. *Journal of Ethnopharmacology* 114, no. 1 (2007): 78–85.

Rao, Y. K., S. H. Fang, W. S. Wu, et al. Constituents isolated form Cordyceps militaris suppress enhanced inflammatory mediator's production and human cancer cell proliferation. *Journal of Ethnopharmacology* 131, no. 2 (2010): 363–67.

Shahed, A. R., S. I. Kim, and D. A. Shoskes. Down-regulation of apoptic and inflammatory genes by Cordyceps sinensis extract in rat kidney following ischemia/reperfusion. *Transplant Proceedings* 33, no. 6 (2001): 2986–87.

Shao, G. Treatment of hyperlipidemia with cultivated cordyceps — a double-blind, randomized placebo control trial. *Zhong Xi Yi Jie He Za Zhi* 5, no. 11 (1985): 652–54, 642.

Sheng, L., J. Chen, J. Li, et al. An exopolysaccharide from cultivated Cordyceps sinensis and its effects on cytokine expressions of immunocytes. *Applied Biochemistry and Biotechnology* 163, no. 5 (2011): 669–78.

Shin, S., S. Lee, and J. Kwon. Cordycepin suppresses expression of diabetes regulating genes by inhibition of lypopolysaccharide-induced inflammation in microphages. *Immune Network* 9, no. 3 (2009): 98–105.

Shin, S., S. Moon, Y. Park, et al. Role of cordycepin and adenosine on the phenotypic switch of macrophages via induced anti-inflammatory cytokines. *Immune Network* 9, no. 6 (2009): 255–64.

Siu, K. M., D. H. Mak, P. Y. Chiu, et al. Pharmacological basis of "yin-nourishing" and "yang-invigorating" actions of cordyceps, a Chinese tonifying herb. *Life Sciences* 76, no. 4 (2004): 385–95.

Sun, W., J. Yu, Y. M. Shi, et al. Effects of cordyceps extract on cytokines and transcription factors in peripheral blood mononuclear cells of asthmatic children during remission stage. *Zhong Xi Yi He Xue Bao* 8, no. 4 (2010): 341–46.

Sung, G.-H., N. L. Hywel-Jones, J.-M. Sung, et al. Phylogenic classification of cordyceps and the clavicipitaceous fungi. *Studies in Mycology* 57 (2007): 5–59.

Sung, G.-H., and J. W. Spatafora. Cordyceps cardinalis sp. nov., a new species of cordyceps with an east Asian-eastern North American distribution. *Mycologia* 96, no. 3 (2004): 658–66.

Thakur, A., R. Hui, Z. Hongyan, et al. Pro-apoptotic effects of Paecilomyces hepiali, a Cordyceps sinensis extract on human lung adenocarcinoma A549 cells in vitro. *Journal of Cancer Research and Therapeutics* 7, no. 4 (2011): 421–26.

Tsai, Y. J., L. C. Lin, and T. H. Tsai. Pharmacokinetics of adenosine and cordycepin, a bioactive constituent of Cordyceps sinensis in rat. *Journal of Agricultural and Food Chemistry* 58, no. 8 (2010): 4638–43.

Tu, S., Q. Zhou, R. Tang, et al. Proapoptotic effect of angiotensin II on renal tubular epithelial cells and protective effect of Cordyceps sinensis. *Zhong Nan Da Xue Xue Bao Yi Xue Ban* 37, no. 1 (2012): 67–72.

Wang, J., Y. M. Liu, W. Cao, et al. Anti-inflammation and antioxidant effect of cordymin, a peptide purified from the medicinal mushroom Cordyceps sinensis, in middle cerebral artery occlusion-induced focal cerebral ischemia in rats. *Metabolic Brain Disease* 27, no. 2 (2012): 159–65. Published electronically ahead of print February 12, 2012.

Wang, N. Q., L. D. Jiang, X. M. Zhang, et al. Effect of dongchong xiacao capsule on airway inflammation of asthmatic patients. *Zhongguo Zhong Yao Za Zhi* 32, no. 15 (2007): 1566–68.

Wang, S., F. Q. Wang, K. Feng, et al. Simultaneous determination of nucleosides, myriocin, and carbohydrates in cordyceps by HPLC coupled with diode array detection and evaporative light scattering detection. *Journal of Separation Science* 32, no. 23–24 (2009): 4069–76.

Wang, S.-H., W.-B. Yang, Y.-C. Liu, et al. A potent sphingomyelinase inhibitor from cordyceps mycelia contributes its cytoprotective effect against oxidative stress in macrophages. *Journal of Lipid Research* 52, no. 3 (2011): 471–79.

Wang, Y., M. Wang, Y. Ling, et al. Structural determination and antioxidant activity of a polysaccharide from the fruiting bodies of cultured Cordyceps sinensis. *American Journal of Chinese Medicine* 37, no. 5 (2009): 977–89.

Won, K. J., S. C. Lee, C. K. Lee, et al. Cordycepin attenuates neointimal formation by inhibiting reactive oxygen species-mediated responses in vascular smooth muscle cells in rats. *Journal of Pharmacological Sciences* 109, no. 3 (2009): 403–12.

Wong, H. S., H. Y. Leung, and K. M. Ko. "Yang-invigorating" Chinese tonic herbs enhance mitochondrial ATP generation in H9c2 cardiomyocytes. *Chinese Medicine* 2 (2011): 1–5.

Wong, J., et al. Cordymin, an antifungal peptide from the medicinal fungus Cordyceps militaris. *Phytomedicine* 18, no. 5 (2011): 387–92.

Wu, G., L. Li, G. H. Sung, et al. Inhibition of 2, 4-dinitrofluorobenzene-induced atopic dermatitis by tropical application of the butanol extract of Cordyceps bassiana in NC/Nga mice. *Journal of Ethnopharmacology* 134, no. 2 (2011): 504–9.

Xie, J. W., L. F. Huang, W. Hu, et al. Analysis of the main nucleosides in Cordyceps sinensis by LC/ESI-MS. *Molecules* 15, no. 1 (2010): 305–14.

Xu, F., J. B. Huang, L. Jiang, et al. Amelioration of cyclosporin nephrotoxicity by Cordyceps sinensis in kidney-transplanted recipients. *Nephrology Dialysis Transplantation* 10, no. 1 (1995): 142–43.

Yan, W., et al. Antiviral activity of Cordyceps guangdongensis against influenza virus infections in mice. *Acta Edulis Fungi* 17, no. 3 (2010): 68–70.

Yang, M. L., P. C. Kuo, T. L. Hwang, et al. Anti-inflammatory principles from Cordyceps sinensis. *Journal of Natural Products* 74, no. 9 (2011): 1996–2000.

Yu, H. M, S. Wang, and S. C. Huang. Comparison of the protective effects between cultured Cordyceps militaris and natural Cordyceps sinensis against oxidative damage. *Journal of Agricultural and Food Chemistry* 54, no. 8 (2006): 3132–38.

Yu, T., J. Shim, Y. Yang, et al. 3-(4-(tert-octyl) phenoxy)propane-1,2-diol suppresses inflammatory responses via inhibition of multiple kinases. *Biochemical Pharmacology* 83, no. 11 (2012): 1540–51.

Yue, G. G., C. B. Lau, K. P. Fung, et al. Effects of Cordyceps sinensis, Cordyceps militaris and their isolated compounds on ion transport in Calu-3 human airway epithelial cells. *Journal of Ethnopharmacology* 117, no. 1 (2008): 92–101.

Zhang, J., Y. Yu, Z. Zhang, et al. Effect of polysaccharide from cultured Cordyceps sinensis on immune function and anti-oxidation activity of mice exposed to 60Co. *International Immunopharmacology* 11, no. 12 (2011): 2251–57.

Zhong, S., et al. Advances in research of polysaccharides in Cordyceps species. *Food Technology and Biotechnology* 47, no. 3 (2009): 304–12.

Zhou, X., Z. Gong, Y. Su, et al. Cordyceps fungi: Natural products, pharmacological functions and developmental products. *Pharmacy and Pharmacology* 61 (2009): 279–91.

Zhou, X., L. Luo, W. Dressel, et al. Cordycepin is an immunoregulatory active ingredient of Cordyceps sinensis. *American Journal of Chinese Medicine* 36, no. 5 (2008): 967–80.

Zhu, J.-S., G. M. Halpern, and K. Jones. The scientific rediscovery of a precious ancient Chinese herbal regimen: Cordyceps sinensis. Part II. *Journal of Alternative and Complementary Medicine* 4, no. 4 (1998): 429–57.

Zhu, R., Y.-P. Chen, Y.-Y. Deng, et al. Cordyceps cicadae extracts ameliorate renal malfunction in a remnant kidney model. *Journal of Zhejiang University Science B (Biomedicine and Biotechnology)* 12, no. 12 (2011): 1024–33.

Zhu, Z. Y., Q. Yao, Y. Liu, et al. Highly efficient synthesis and anti tumor activity of monosaccharide saponins mimicking components of Chinese folk medicine Cordyceps sinensis. *Journal of Asian Natural Products Research* 14, no. 5 (2012): 429–35. Published electronically ahead of print March 20, 2012.

Zu, H., Q. Zhou, R. Huang, et al. Effect of Cordyceps sinensis on the expression of HIF-1α and NGAL in rats with renal ischemia-reperfusion injury. *Zhong Nan Da Xue Bao Yi Xue Ban* 37, no. 1 (2012): 57–66.

Elder (*Sambucus* spp.)

Akbulut, M., et al. Physiochemical characteristics of some wild grown European elderberry (Sambucus nigra L) genotypes. *Pharmacognosy Magazine* 5 (2009): 320–23.

American Botanical Council. *The ABC Clinical Guide to Elder Berry.* (Austin, TX: ABC, 2004).

Anonymous. Sambucus nigra. Monograph, *Alternative Medicine Review* 10, no. 1 (2005): 51–55.

Barak, V., et al. The effect of herbal remedies on the production of human inflammatory and anti-inflammatory cytokines. *Israel Medical Association Journal* 4, suppl. (2002): 919–22.

Barak, V., et al. The effect of Sambucol, a black elderberry-based, natural product on the production of human cytokines: I. Inflammatory cytokines. *European Cytokine Network* 12, no. 2 (2001): 290–96.

Bitsch, I., et al. Bioavailability of anthocyanidin-3-glycosides following consumption of elderberry extract and blackcurrant juice. *International Journal of Clinical Pharmacology and Therapeutics* 42, no. 5 (2004): 293–400.

Bitsch, R., et al. Urinary excretion of cyanidin glucosides and glucuronides in healthy humans after elderberry juice ingestion. *Journal of Biomedicine and Biotechnology* 5 (2004): 343–45.

Caceres, A., et al. Plant used in Guatemala for the treatment of gastrointestinal disorders. 1. Screening of 84 plants against enterobacteria. *Journal of Ethnopharmacology* 30, no. 1 (1990): 55–73.

Cao, G., et al. Anthocyanins are absorbed in glycated forms in elderly women: A pharmacokinetic study. *American Journal of Clinical Nutrition* 73, no. 5 (2001): 920–26.

Charlebois, D. Elderberry as a medicinal plant. In *Issues in New Crops and New Uses,* ed. J. Janick and A. Whipkey, 284–92. Alexandria, Va.: ASHS Press, 2007.

Chen, Y., et al. The Sambucus nigra type-2 ribosome-inactivating protein SNA-1′ exhibits in plant antiviral activity in transgenic tobacco. *FEBS Letters* 516, no. 1–3 (2002): 27–30.

Christensen, K., et al. Identification of bioactive compounds from flowers of black elder (Sambucus nigra L) that activate the human peroxisome proliferator-activated receptor (PPAR) gamma. *Phytotherapy Research* 24, suppl. 2 (2010): S129–32.

de Benito, F., et al. Constitutive and inducible type 1 ribosome-inactivating proteins (RIPs) in elderberry (Sambucus nigra L). *FEBS Letters* 428 (1998): 75–79.

de Benito, F., et al. Ebulitins: A new family of type 1 ribosome-inactivating proteins (rRNA N-glycosidases) from the leaves of Sambucus ebulus L that coexist with the type 2 ribosome-inactivating protein ebulin 1. *FEBS Letters* 360, no. 3 (1995): 299–302.

Elrod, S. Sambucus nigra agglutinin II and related lectins and their potential contribution to medicinal benefits of the elder tree. Paper prepared for a graduate course in advanced biochemistry and molecular biology at the University of Georgia, online at http://susanme.myweb.uga.edu/bcmb8010/report.pdf, accessed June 5, 2012.

Fink, R. HIV type-1 entry inhibitors with a new mode of action. *Antiviral Chemistry & Chemotherapy* 19, no. 6 (2009): 243–55.

Frank, T., et al. Absorption and excretion of elderberry (Sambucus nigra L) anthocyanins in healthy humans. *Methods and Findings in Experimental and Clinical Pharmacology* 29, no. 8 (2007): 525–33.

Frank, T., et al. Urinary pharmacokinetics of cyanidin glycosides in healthy young men following consumption of elderberry juice. *International Journal of Clinical Pharmacological Research* 25, no. 2 (2005): 47–56.

Furusawa, E., et al. Activity of Sambucus sieboldiana on Columbia SK and LGM virus infection in mice. *Experimental Biology and Medicine* 128, no. 4 (1968): 1196–99.

Girbes, T., et al. Ebulin 1, a nontoxic novel type 2 ribosome-inactivating protein from Sambucus ebulus leaves. *Journal of Biological Chemistry* 268, no. 24 (1993): 18196–99.

Glatthaar, B., et al. Antiviral activity of a composition of Gentiana lutea L, Primula veris L, Sambucus nigra L, Rumex spp and Verbena officinalis L (Sinupret) against viruses causing respiratory infections. *European Journal of Integrative Medicine* 1, no. 4 (2009): 258.

Hearst, C., et al. Antibacterial activity of elder (Sambucus nigra L) flower or berry against hospital pathogens. *Journal of Medicinal Plants Research* 4, no. 17 (2010): 1805-9.

Hwang, B., et al. Antifungal effect of (+)-pinoresinol isolated from Sambucus williamsii. *Molecules* 15 (2010): 3507–35.

Kaack, K., and T. Austed. Interaction of vitamin C and flavonoids in elderberry (Sambucus nigra L) during juice processing. *Plant Foods in Human Nutrition* 52, no. 3 (1998): 187–98.

Kabuce, N., and N. Priede. Sambucus nigra. NOBANIS — Invasive Alien Species Fact Sheet. From the Online Database of the North European and Baltic Network on Invasive Alien Species (NOBANIS; www.nobanis.org), www.nobanis.org/files/factsheets/sambucus_nigra.pdf, accessed March 12, 2012.

Kay, C., et al. Anthocyanins exist in the circulation primarily as metabolites in adult men. *Journal of Nutrition* 135, no. 11 (2005): 2582–88. Accessed online via http://jn.nutrition.org.

Ko'odziejl, B., et al. Effect of traffic pollution on chemical composition of raw elderberry (Sambucus nigra L). *Journal of Elementology* 17, no. 1 (2012): 67–78. Accessed online via www.uwm.edu.pl.

Krawitz, C., et al. Inhibitory activity of a standardized elderberry liquid extract against clinically-relevant human respiratory bacterial pathogens and influenza A and B viruses. *BMC Complementary and Alternative Medicine* 11 (2011): 16–22.

Lak, E., et al. Protective effect of Sambucus elbus extract on teratogenicity of albendazole. *Middle-East Journal of Scientific Research* 8, no. 3 (2011): 606–10.

Lee, J., and C. Finn. Anthocyanins and other polyphenolics in American elderberry (Sambucus canadensis) and European elderberry (S. nigra) cultivars. *Journal of the Science of Food and Agriculture* 87, no. 14 (2007): 2665–75.

Li, H., et al. Antiosteoporotic activity of the stems of Sambucus sieboldiana. *Biological & Pharmaceutical Bulletin* 21, no. 6 (1998): 594–98.

Liao, Q., et al. LC-MS determination and pharmacokinetic studies of ursolic acid in rat plasma after administration of the traditional Chinese medicinal preparation lu-ying extract. *Yakugaku Zasshi* 125, no. 6 (2005): 509–15.

Marczylo, T., et al. Pharmacokinetics and metabolism of the putative cancer chemopreventive agent cyanidin-3-glucoside in mice. *Cancer Chemotherapy and Pharmacology* 64, no. 6 (2009): 1261–68.

Martin, C. O., and S. P. Mott. American elder (Sambucus canadensis). Section 7.5.7 of the *U.S. Army Corps of Engineers Wildlife Resources Management Manual* (Vicksburg, Miss.: U.S. Army Engineer Waterways Experiment Station Environmental Lab, 1997).

McCutcheon, A. R., et al. Antibiotic screening of medicinal plants of the British Columbian native peoples. *Journal of Ethnopharmacology* 37, no. 3 (1992): 213–23.

McCutcheon, A. R., et al. Anti-mycobacterial screening of British Columbian medicinal plants. *Pharmaceutical Biology* 35, no. 2 (1997): 77–83.

McCutcheon, A. R., et al. Antiviral screening of British Columbian medicinal plants. *Journal of Ethnopharmacology* 49 (1995): 101–10.

Milbury, P., et al. Bioavailability of elderberry anthocyanins. *Mechanisms of Ageing and Development* 123, no. 8 (2002): 997–1006.

Mulleder, U., et al. Urinary excretion of cyanidin glycosides. *Journal of Biochemical and Biophysical Methods* 53, no. 1–3 (2002): 61–66.

Murcovic, M., et al. Effects of elderberry juice on fasting and postprandial serum lipids and low-density lipoprotein oxidatoin in healthy volunteers: A randomized, double-blind, placebo-controlled study. *European Journal of Clinical Nutrition* 58, no. 2 (2004): 244–49.

Quave, C., et al. Quorum sensing inhibitors of Staphylococcus aureus from Italian medicinal plants. *Planta Medica* 77, no. 2 (2011): 188–95.

Roschek, B., et al. Elderberry flavonoids bind to and prevent N1N1 infection in vitro. *Phytochemistry* 70, no. 10 (2009): 1255–61.

Schwaiger, S., et al. Identification and pharmacological characterization of the anti-inflammatory principal of the leaves of dwarf elder (Sambucus ebulis L). *Journal of Ethnopharmacology* 133 (2011): 704–9.

Serkedjieva, J., et al. Antiviral activity of the infusion (SHS-174) from flowers of Sambucus nigra L, aerial parts of Hypericum perforatum L, and roots of Saponaria officinalis L against influenza and herpes simplex viruses. *Phytotherapy Research* 4, no. 3 (1990): 97–100.

Shokrzadeh, M., and S. Saravi. The chemistry, pharmacology and clinical properties of Sambucus ebulus: A review. *Journal of Medicinal Plants Research* 4, no. 2 (2010): 95–103.

Smee, D., et al. Effects of Theramax on influenza virus infections in cell culture and mice. *Antiviral Chemistry & Chemotherapy* 21, no. 6 (2011): 231–37.

Suntar, I., et al. Wound healing potential of Sambucus ebulus L leaves and isolation of an active component, quercetin 3-O-glucoside. *Journal of Ethnopharmacology* 129, no. 10 (2010): 106–14.

Talavera, S., et al. Anthocyanins are efficiently absorbed from the small intestine in rats. *Journal of Nutrition* 134, no. 9 (2004): 2275–79.

Thole, J., et al. A comparative evaluation of the anticancer properties of European and American elderberry fruits. *Journal of Medicinal Food* 9, no. 4 (2006): 498–504.

Uncini Manganelli, R., et al. Antiviral activity in vitro of Urtica dioica L, Parietaria diffusa M et K and Sambucus nigra L. *Journal of Ethnopharmacology* 98, no. 3 (2005): 323–27.

Vandenbussche, F., et al. Analysis of the in planta antiviral activity of elderberry ribosome-inactivating proteins. *European Journal of Biochemistry* 271 (2004): 1508–15.

Waknine-Grinberg, J., et al. The immunomodulatory effect of Sambucol on leishmanial and malarial infections. *Planta Medica* 75, no. 6 (2009): 581–86.

Wu, X., et al. Absorption and metabolism of anthocyanins in elderly women after consumption of elderberry or blueberry. *Journal of Nutrition* 132, no. 7 (2002): 1865–71. Accessed online via http://jn.nutrition.org.

Zakay-Rones, Z., et al. Inhibition of several strains of influenza virus in vitro and reduction of symptoms by an elderberry extract (Sambucus nigra L) during an outbreak of influenza B in Panama. *Journal of Alternative and Complementary Medicine* 1, no. 4 (1995): 361–69.

Zakay-Rones, Z., et al. Randomized study of the efficacy and safety of oral elderberry extract in the treatment of influenza A and B virus infections. *Journal of International Medical Research* 32, no. 2 (2004): 132–40.

Zhang, T., et al. Simultaneous analysis of seven bioactive compounds in Sambucus chinensis Lindl by HPLC. *Analytical Letters* 43, no. 16 (2010): 2525–33.

Zhang, Y., et al. Study of the mechanisms by which Sambucus williamsii HANCE extract exerts protective effects against ocariectomy-induced osteoporosis in vivo. *Osteoporos International* 22, no. 2 (2011): 703–9.

Ginger (*Zingiber officinale*)

Ahui, M. L., et al. Ginger prevents Th2-mediated immune responses in a mouse model of airway inflammation. *International Immunopharmacology* 8, no. 12 (2008): 1626–32.

Ajith, T. A., et al. Zingiber officinale Roscoe prevents acetaminophen-induced acute hepatotoxicity by enhancing hepatic antioxidant status. *Food and Chemical Toxicology* 45, no. 11 (2007): 2267–72.

Altman, R. D., et al. Effects of a ginger extract on knee pain in patients with osteoarthritis. *Arthritis and Rheumatism* 44, no. 11 (2001): 2531–38.

Anonymous. Ginger. Entry in the Herbs at a Glance database of the National Center for Complementary and Alternative Medicine (NCCAM), http://nccam.nih.gov/health/ginger/, accessed February 1, 2013.

Anonymous. Ginger. Entry in *Wikipedia*, http://en.wikipedia.org/wiki/Ginger, accessed February 9, 2011.

Anonymous. Ginger: Zingiber officinale. Entry in the Herbs2000.com database, www.herbs2000.com/herbs/herbs_ginger.htm, accessed February 9, 2011.

Backon, J. Implication of thromboxane in the pathogenesis of Kawasaki disease and a suggestion for using novel thromboxane

synthetase inhibitors in its treatment. *Medical Hypotheses* 34, no. 3 (1991): 230–31.

Bajpai, D., and K. Chandra. Studies on the antiviral properties of plants with special reference to Zingiber capitatum. *Fitoterapia* 6, no. 1 (1990): 3–8.

Benchaluk, T., et al. Effects of *Zingiber officinale* Roscoe on methyl parathion intoxication in rats. *Chiang Mai Medical Journal* 49, no. 3 (2010): 81–88.

Bensch, K., et al. Investigations into the anti-adhesive activity of herbal extracts against Campylobacter jejuni. *Phytotherapy Research* 25, no. 8 (2011): 1125–32. Published electronically ahead of print January 31, 2011.

Betoni, J. E., et al. Synergism between plant extract and antimicrobial drugs used on Staphylococcus aureus diseases. *Memórias do Instituto Oswaldo Cruz* 101, no. 4 (2006): 387–90.

Betz, O., et al. Is ginger a clinically relevant antiemetic? A systematic review of randomized controlled trials. *Forschende Komplementärmedizin und Klassische Naturheilkunde* 12, no. 1 (2005): 14–23.

Bhat, J., et al. In vivo enhancement of natural killer cell activity through tea fortified with Ayurvedic herbs. *Phytotherapy Research* 24, no. 1 (2010): 129–35.

Black, C. D., et al. Ginger (Zingiber officinale) reduces muscle pain caused by eccentric exercise. *Journal of Pain* 11, no. 9 (2010): 894–903.

Borrelli, F., et al. Effectiveness and safety of ginger in the treatment of pregnancy-induced nausea and vomiting. *Obstetrics and Gynecology* 105, no. 4 (2005): 849–56.

Carrasco, F. R., et al. Immunomodulatory activity of Zingiber officinale Roscoe, Salvia officinalis L. and Syzygium aromaticum L. essential oils: Evidence for humor- and cell-mediated responses. *Journal of Pharmacy and Pharmacology* 61, no. 7 (2009): 961–67.

Chen, I. N., et al. Antioxidant and antimicrobial activity of Zingiberaceae plants in Taiwan. *Plant Foods for Human Nutrition* 63, no. 1 (2008): 15–20.

Choi, W., et al. Antiparasitic effects of Zingiber officinale (ginger) extract against Toxoplasma gondii. *Journal of Applied Biomedicine* 11, no. 1 (2013): 15–26. Published electronically ahead of print March 1, 2012. Accessed online via www.zsf.jcu.cz/jab19_ms.pdf.

Chrubasik, S., et al. Zingiber rhizoma: A comprehensive review on the ginger effect and efficacy profiles. *Phytomedicine* 12, no. 9 (2005): 684–701.

Chung, S. Y., et al. Potent modulation of P-glycoprotein activity by naturally occurring phenylbutenoids from Zingiber cassumunar. *Phytotherapy Research* 23, 4 (2009): 472–76.

Chung, S. Y., et al. Potent modulation of P-glycoprotein-mediated resistance by kaempferol derivatives isolated from Zingiber zerumbet. *Phytotherapy Research* 21, no. 6 (2007): 565–69.

Cwikla, C., et al. Investigations into the antibacterial activities of phytotherapeutics against Helicobacter pylori and Campylobacter jejuni. *Phytotherapy Research* 24, no. 5 (2010): 649–56.

Daswani, P. G., et al. Antidiarrhoeal activity of Zingiber officinale (Rosc.). *Current Science* 98, no. 2 (2010): 222–29.

Datta, A., et al. Antifilarial effect of Zingiber officinale on Dirofilaria immitis. *Journal of Helminthology* 61, no. 3 (1987): 268–70.

Demin, G., et al. Comparative antibacterial activities of crude polysaccharides and flavonoids from *Zingiber officinale* and their extraction. *Asian Journal of Traditional Medicines* 5, no. 6 (2010): 1.

Denyer, C. V., et al. Isolation of antirhinoviral sesquiterpenes from ginger (Zingiber officinale). *Journal of Natural Products* 57, no. 5 (1994)): 658–62.

Dügenci, S. K., et al. Some medicinal plants as immunostimulant for fish. *Journal of Ethnopharmacology* 88, no. 1 (2003): 99–106.

Egwurugwa, J. N., et al. Effects of ginger (Zingiber officinale) on cadmium toxicity. *African Journal of Biotechnology* 6, no. 18 (2007): 2078–82.

Fischer-Rasmussen, W., et al. Ginger treatment of hyperemesis gravidarum. *European Journal of Obstetrics, Gynecology and Reproductive Biology* 38, no. 1 (1991): 19–24.

Foster, Steven. Ginger *Zingiber officinale* — your food is your medicine. Monograph, Steven Foster Group, Inc., www.stevenfoster.com/education/monograph/ginger.html, accessed February 9, 2011.

Gato, C., et al. Lethal efficacy of extract from Zingiber officinale (traditional Chinese medicine) or [6]-shogaol and [6]-gingerol in Anisakis larvae in vitro. *Parasitology Research* 76, no. 8 (1990): 653–56.

Gaus, K., et al. Standardized ginger (Zingiber officinale) extract reduces bacterial load and suppresses acute and chronic inflammation in Mongolian gerbils infected with cagAHelicobacter pylori. *Pharmaceutical Biology* 47, no. 1 (2009): 92–98.

Habib, S., et al. Ginger extract (Zingiber officinale) has anti-cancer and anti-inflammatory effects on ethionine-induced hepatoma rats. *Clinics* 63, no. 6 (2008): 807–13.

Haghighi, M., et al. Comparing the effects of ginger (Zingiber officinale) extract and ibuprofen on patients with osteoarthritis. *Archives of Iranian Medicine* 8, no. 4 (2005): 267–71.

Heeba, G. H., et al. Effect of combined administration of ginger (Zingiber officinale Roscoe) and atorvastatin on the liver of rats. *Phytomedicine* 17, no. 14 (2010): 1076–81.

Imanishi, N., et al. Macrophage-mediated inhibitory effect of Zingiber officinale Rosc, a traditional Oriental herbal medicine, on the growth of influenza A/Aichi/2/68 virus. *American Journal of Chinese Medicine* 34, no. 1 (2006): 157–69.

Immanuel, G., et al. Dietary medicinal plant extracts improve growth, immune activity and survival of tilapia Oreochromis mossambicus. *Journal of Fish Biology* 74, no. 7 (2009): 1462–75.

Iqbal, Z., et al. In vivo anthelminic activity of *Allium sativum, Zingiber officinale, Cucurbita mexicana* and *Ficus religiosa. International Journal of Agriculture and Biology* 3, no. 4 (2001): 454–57.

Iqbal, Z., et al. In vivo anthelmintic activity of ginger against gastrointestinal nematodes of sheep. *Journal of Ethnopharmacology* 106, no. 2 (2006): 285–87.

Iwami, M., et al. Inhibitory effects of zingerone, a pungent component of Zingiber officinale Roscoe, on colonic motility in rats. *Journal of Natural Medicines* 65, no. 1 (2011): 89–94.

Jagetia, G. C., et al. Influence of ginger rhizome (Zingiber officinale Rosc) on survival, glutathione and lipid peroxidation in mice after whole-body exposure to gamma radiation. *Radiation Research* 160, no. 5 (2003): 584–92.

Khan, R., et al. Activity of solvent extracts of Prosopis spicigera, Zingiber officinale and Trachyspermum ammi against multidrug resistant bacterial and fungal. *Journal of Infection in Developing Countries* 4, no. 5 (2010): 292–300.

Koch, C., et al. Inhibitory effect of essential oils against herpes simplex virus type 2. *Phytomedicine* 15, no. 102 (2007): 71–78.

Koh, E. M., et al. Modulation of macrophage functions by compounds isolated from Zingiber officinale. *Planta Medica* 75, no. 2 (2009): 148–51.

Lakshmi, B. V., et al. Attenuation of acute and chronic restraint stress-induced perturbations in experimental animals by Zingiber officinale Roscoe. *Food and Chemical Toxicology* 48, no. 2 (2010): 530–35.

Lans, C., et al. Ethnoveterinary medicines used to treat endoparasites and stomach problems in pigs and pets in British Columbia, Canada. *Veterinary Parasitology* 148, no. 3–4 (2007): 325–40.

Lee, S., et al. Liquid chromatographic determination of 6-, 8-, 10-gingerol, and 6-shogaol in ginger (Zingiber officinale) as the raw herb and dried aqueous extract. *Journal of AOAC International* 90, no. 5 (2007): 1219–26.

Lin, R. J., et al. Larvicidal activities of ginger (Zingiber officinale) against Angiostrongylus cantonensis. *Acta Tropica* 115, no. 1–2 (2010): 69–76.

Lin, R. J., et al. Larvicidal constituents of Zingiber officinale (ginger) against Anisakis simplex. *Planta Medica* 76, no. 16 (2010): 1852–58.

Lopez, P., et al. Solid- and vapor-phase antimicrobial activities of six essential oils: Susceptibility of selected foodborne bacterial and fungal strains. *Journal of Agricultural and Food Chemistry* 53, no. 17 (2005): 6939–46.

Maghsoudi, S., et al. Preventive effect of ginger (Zingiber officinale) pretreatment on renal ischemia-reperfusion in rats. *European Surgical Research* 46, no. 1 (2011): 45–51.

Mahady, G. B., et al. Ginger (Zingiber officinale Roscoe) and the gingerols inhibit the growth of Cag A+ strains of Helicobacter pylori. *Anticancer Research* 23, no. 5A (2003): 3699–702.

Malu, S. P., et al. Antibacterial activity and medicinal properties of ginger (*Zingiber officinale*). *Global Journal of Pure and Applied Sciences* 15, no. 3 (2009): 365–68.

Masoud, H., et al. Comparing the effects of ginger (Zingiber officinale) extract and ibuprofen on patients with osteoarthritis. *Archives of Iranian Medicine* 8, no. 4 (2005): 267–71.

Merawin, L. T., et al. Screening of microfilaricidal effects of plant extracts against Dirofilaria immitis. *Research in Veterinary Science* 88, no. 1 (2010): 142–47.

Nagoshi, C., et al. Synergistic effect of [10]-gingerol and aminoglycosides against vancomycin-resistant enterococci (VRE). *Biological & Pharmaceutical Bulletin* 29, no. 3 (2006): 443–47.

Nanjundaiah, S. M., et al. Gastroprotective effect of ginger rhizome (Zingiber officinale) extract: Role of gallic acid and cinnamic acid in H+, K+-ATPase/H. pylori inhibition and anti-oxidative mechanism. *Evidence-Based Complementary and Alternative Medicine* (2011). doi: 10.1093/ecam/nep060.

Nogueira de Melo, G. A., et al. Inhibitory effects of ginger (Zingiber officinale Roscoe) essential oil on leukocyte migration in vivo and in vitro. *Journal of Natural Medicines* 65, no. 1 (2011): 241–46.

Nya, E. J., et al. Use of dietary ginger, Zingiber officinale Roscoe, as an immunostimulant to control Aeromonas hydrophila infections in rainbow trout, Oncorhynchus mykiss (Walbaum). *Journal of Fish Diseases* 32, no. 11 (2009): 971–77.

Park, K. J., et al. In vitro antiviral activity of aqueous extracts from Korean medicinal plants against influenza virus type A. *Journal of Microbiology and Biotechnology* 15, no. 5 (2005): 924–29.

Park, M., et al. Antibacterial activity of [10]-gingerol and [12]-gingerol isolated from ginger rhizome against periodontal bacteria. *Phytotherapy Research* 22, no. 11 (2008): 1446–49.

Presser, Art. Ginger (*Zingiber officinale*). Part of the Smart Supplementation series by the Huntington College of Health Sciences (Knoxville, Tenn.), 2001, www.hchs.edu/literature/Ginger.pdf.

Raji, Y., et al. Anti-inflammatory and analgesic properties of the rhizome extract of Zingiber officinale. *African Journal of Biomedical Research* 5 (2002): 121–24.

Reinhard, G., et al. Ginger — an herbal medicinal product with broad anti-inflammatory actions. *Journal of Medicinal Food* 8, no. 2 (2005): 125.

Sabul, B., et al. Caryophyllene-rich rhizome oil of Zingiber nimmonii from South India: Chemical characterization and antimicrobial activity. *Phytochemistry* 67, no. 22 (2006): 2469–73.

Sasikumar, B., C. Thankamani, V. Srinivasan, et al. *Ginger*. Calicut, Kerala, India: Indian Institute of Spices Research, October 2008. Accessed online via www.spices.res.in/pdf/package/ginger.pdf.

Schnitzler, P., et al. Susceptibility of drug-resistant clinical herpes simplex virus type 1 strains to essential oils of ginger, thyme, hyssop, and sandalwood. *Antimicrobial Agents and Chemotherapy* 51, no. 5 (2007): 1859–62.

Sephavand, R., et al. Ginger (Zingiber officinale Roscoe) elicits antinociceptive properties and potentiates morphone-induced analgesia in the rat radiant heat tail-flick test. *Journal of Medicinal Food* 13, no. 6 (2010): 1397–401.

Shaba, P., et al. In vitro trypanocidal activity of methanolic extracts of Quercus borealis leaves and Zingiber officinale roots against Trypanosoma evansi. *Greener Journal of Agricultural Sciences* 1, no. 1 (2011): 41–47.

Sharma, A., et al. Antibacterial activity of medicinal plants against pathogens causing complicated urinary tract infections. *Indian Journal of Pharmaceutical Sciences* 71, no. 2 (2009): 136–39.

Shivanand, D. J., et al. Fresh organically grown ginger (Zingiber officinale): Composition and effects on LPS-induced PGE_2 production. *Phytochemistry* 65 (2004): 1937–54.

Shukla, Y., et al. Cancer preventive properties of ginger: A brief review. *Food and Chemical Toxicology* 45, no. 5 (2007): 683–90.

Singh, A., et al. Experimental advances in pharmacology of gingerol and analogues. *Pharmacie Globale: International Journal of Comprehensive Pharmacy* 2, no. 4 (2010): 1–5.

Singh, G., et al. Chemistry, antioxidant and antimicrobial investigations on essential oil and oleoresins of Zingiber officinale. *Food and Chemical Toxicology* 46, no. 10 (2008): 3295–302.

Sookkongwaree, K., et al. Inhibition of viral proteases by Zingiberaceae extracts and flavones isolated from Kaempferia parviflora. *Pharmazie* 61, no. 8 (2006): 717–21.

Srivastava, K. C., et al. Ginger (Zingiber officinale) in rheumatism and musculoskeletal disorders. *Medical Hypotheses* 39, no. 4 (1992): 342–48.

Tan, B. K., et al. Immunomodulatory and antimicrobial effects of some traditional Chinese medicinal herbs: A review. *Current Medicinal Chemistry* 11, no. 11 (2004): 1423–30.

Thongson, C., et al. Antimicrobial effect of Thai spices against Listeria monocytogenes and Salmonella typhimurium CT104. *Journal of Food Protection* 68, no. 10 (2005): 2054–58.

Ueda, H., et al. Repeated oral administration of a squeezed ginger (Zingiber officinale) extract augmented the serum corticosterone level and had anti-inflammatory properties.

Bioscience, Biotechnology, and Biochemistry 74, no. 11 (2010): 2248–52.

van Breemen, R. B., et al. Cyclooxygenase-2 inhibitors in ginger (Zingiber officinale). *Fitoterapia* 82, no. 1 (2011): 38–43.

Wang, H. M., et al. Zingiber officinale (ginger) compounds have tetracycline-resistance modifying effects against clinical extensively drug-resistant Acinetobacter baumannii. *Phytotherapy Research* 24, no. 12 (2010): 1825–30.

Wang, X., et al. Anti-influenza agents from plants and traditional Chinese medicine. *Phytotherapy Research* 20, no. 5 (2006): 335–41.

Wattanathorn, J., et al. Zingiber officinale mitigates brain damage and improves memory impairment in focal cerebral ischemic rat. *Evidence-Based Complementary and Alternative Medicine* (2011). doi: 10.1155/2011/429505.

Yip, Y. B., et al. An experimental study on the effectiveness of massage with aromatic ginger and orange essential oil for moderate-to-severe knee pain among the elderly in Hong Kong. *Complementary Therapies in Medicine* 16, no. 3 (2008): 131–38.

Zhou, H. L., et al. The modulatory effects of the volatile oil of ginger on the cellular immune response in vitro and in vivo in mice. *Journal of Ethnopharmacology* 105, no. 1–2 (2006): 301–5.

Zick, S. M., et al. Quantitation of 6-, 8- and 10-gingerols and 6-shogaol in human plasma by high-performance liquid chromatography with electrochemical detection. *International Journal of Biomedical Science* 6, no. 3 (2010): 233–40.

Houttuynia (*Houttuynia cordata*)

Anonymous. Ecology of Houttuynia cordata. Entry in the Global Invasive Species Database of the IUCN/SSC Invasive Species Specialist Group (ISSG), www.issg.org/database/species/ecology.asp?si=854, accessed March 29, 2012.

Anonymous. Houttuynia cordata. Entry in the MedLibrary.org online encyclopedia, http://medlibrary.org/medwiki/Houttuynia_cordata, accessed April 16, 2012.

Anonymous, Houttuynia cordata. Entry in *Wikipedia,* http://en.wikipedia.org/wiki/Houttuynia_cordata, accessed October 29, 2012.

Baishakhee. Houttuynia cordata. Description on Only Foods website, www.onlyfoods.net/houttuynia-cordata.html, accessed March 29, 2012.

Banjerdpongchai, R., and P. Kongtawelert. Ethanolic extract of fermented Houttuynia cordata Thunb induces human Leukemic HL-60 and Molt-4 cell apoptosis via oxidative stress and a mitochondrial pathway. *Asian Pacific Journal of Cancer Prevention* 12 (2011): 2871–74.

Bhattacharyya, N., and S. Sarma. Assessment of availability, ecological feature, and habitat preference of the medicinal herb Houttuynia cordata Thunb in the Brahmaputra Valley of Assam, India. *Environmental Monitoring and Assessment* 160, no. 1–4 (2010): 277–87.

Blanke, K. Chameleon plant. Plant Fact Sheet from the University of Wisconsin Cooperative Extension,2009.

Chakraborti, S., S. Sangram, and R. Sinha. High frequency induction of multiple shoots and clonal propagation from rhizomatous nodal segments of Houttuynia cordata Thunb. — an ethnomedicinal herb of India. *InVitro Cellular and Development Biology — Plant* 42, no. 5 (2006): 394–98.

Chang, J. S., L. C. Chiang, C. C. Chen, et al. Antileukemic activity of Bidens pilosa L. var. minor (Blume) Sherff and Houttuynia cordata Thunb. *American Journal of Chinese Medicine* 29, no. 2 (2001): 303–12.

Chen, S. D., H. Gao, Q. C. Zhu, et al. Houttuynoids A–E, anti-herpes simplex virus active flavonoids with novel skeletons from Houttuynia cordata. *Organic Letters* 14, no. 7 (2012): 1772–75.

Chen, X., Z. Wang, Z. Yang, et al. Houttuynia cordata blocks HSV infection through inhibition of NF-κB activation. *Antiviral Research* 92, no. 2 (2011): 341–45.

Chen, Y. Y., J. F. Liu, C. M. Chen, et al. A study of the antioxidative and antimutagenic effects of Houttuynia cordata Thunb. using an oxidized frying oil-fed model. *Journal of Nutritional Science and Vitaminology* (Tokyo) 49, no. 5 (2003): 327–33.

Chiang, L. C., J. S. Chang, C. C. Chen, et al. Anti-herpes simplex virus activity of Bidens pilosa and Houttuynia cordata. *American Journal of Chinese Medicine* 31, no. 3 (2003): 355–62.

Cho, E. J., T. Yokozawa, D. Y. Rhyu, et al. The inhibitory effects of 12 medicinal plants and their component compounds on lipid peroxidation. *American Journal of Chinese Medicine* 31, no. 6 (2003): 907–17.

Cho, E. J., T. Yokozawa, D. Y. Rhyu, et al. Study on the inhibitory effects of Korean medicinal plants and their main compounds on the 1,1-diphenyl-2-picrylhydrazyl radical. *Phytomedicine* 10, no. 6–7 (2003): 544–51.

Choi, J. Y., J. A. Lee, J. B. Lee, et al. Anti-inflammatory activity of Houttuynia cordata against lipoteichoic acid-induced inflammation in human dermal fibroblasts. *Chonnam Medical Journal* 46, no. 3 (2010): 140–47.

Chou, S.-C., C.-R. Su, Y.-C. Ku, et al. The constituents and their bioactivities of Houttuynia cordata. *Chemical & Pharmaceutical Bulletin* 57, no. 11 (2009): 1227–30.

Cui, X. H., L. Wang, and L. Cheng. Analysis of adverse events caused by irrational application of houttuynia injection. *Zhongguo Zhong Xi Yi Jie He Za Zhi* 31, no. 3 (2011): 407–12.

Deng, K., F. He, J. Shi, et al. Study on network compatibility of metabolisms in vivo rat for volatile oil in houttuynia herb and

2-undecanone. *Zhongguo Zhong Yao Za Zhi* 36, no. 15 (2011): 2076–83.

Dong, Y., Y. Zhang, L. Yi, et al. Transformation of antimicrobial peptide fusion gene of cecropin B and rabbit NP-1 to Houttuynia cordata. *Zhongguo Zhong Yao Za Zhi* 35, no. 13 (2010): 1660–65.

Duan, X., D. Zhong, and X. Chen. Derivatization of beta-dicarbonyl compound with 2,4-dinitrophenylhydrazine to enhance mass spectrometric detection: Application to quantitative analysis of houttuynin in human plasma. *Journal of Mass Spectrometry* 43, no. 6 (2008): 814–24.

Ground Cover – Pest Plants. Pest Plant Fact Sheet no. 15 from the Environment Bay of Plenty Regional Council (Whakatane, New Zealand), 2003.

Han, E. H., J. H. Park, J. Y. Kim, et al. Houttuynia cordata water extract suppresses anaphylactic reaction and IgE-mediated allergic response by inhibiting multiple steps of FcepsilonRI signaling in mast cells. *Food and Chemical Toxicology* 47, no. 7 (2009): 1659–66.

Hayashi, K., M. Kamiya, and T. Hayashi. Virucidal effects of the steam distillate from Houttuynia cordata and its components on HSV-1, influenza virus, and HIV. *Planta Medica* 61, no. 3 (1995): 237–41.

Ho, J.-C. The bioactivities of the essential oil and crude extracts from Houttuynia cordata. *Ta Hwa Institute of Technology* 1 (2007): 496–500.

Hou, Y., and X. Zhang. Antiphlogistic action of Houttuynia cordata injection in vitro and in mice. *Zhongguo Zhong Yao Za Zhi* 15, no. 4 (1990): 221–22, 255.

Houttuynia cordata 'Chameleon'. Species profile on the Ohio State University Department of Horticulture and Crop Science website, www.hcs.ohio-state.edu/hcs/TMI/Plantlist/ ho_rdata.html, accessed April 5, 2012.

Houttuynia cordata (heart-shaped houttuynia). Species profile on the Kew Royal Botanic Gardens website, www.kew.org/plants-fungi/Houttuynia-cordata.htm, accessed April 17, 2012.

Hu, S. H., and A. F. Du. Treatment of bovine mastitis with houttuynin sodium bisulphate. *Zentralblatt für Veterinärmedizin. Reihe B* 44, no. 6 (1997): 365–70.

Inouye, S., M. Takahashi, and S. Abe. The inhibitory activity of hydrosols prepared from 18 Japanese herbs of weakly aromatic flavor against filamentous formation and growth of Candida albicans. *Medical Mycology Journal* 53, no. 1 (2012): 33–40.

Jang, S. Y., J. S. Bae, Y. H. Lee, et al. Caffeic acid and quercitrin purified from Houttuynia cordata inhibit DNA topoisomerase I activity. *Natural Product Research* 25, no. 3 (2011): 222–31.

Ji, K. M., M. Li, J. J. Chen, et al. Anaphylactic shock and lethal anaphylaxis caused by Houttuynia cordata injection, a herbal treatment in China. *Allergy* 64, no. 5 (2009): 816–17.

Ji, W., K. Bi, Q. Chen, et al. Simultaneous determination of eight activate components in Houttuynia cordata injection and its quality control in productive process. *Journal of Separation Science* 34, no. 21 (2011): 3053–60.

Jiang, X.-L., and H.-F. Cui. Different therapy for different types of ulcerative colitis in China. *World Journal of Gastroenterology* 10, no. 10 (2004): 1513–20.

Kar, A., and S. K. Borthakur. Medicinal plants used against dysentery, diarrhea and cholera by the tribes of erstwhile Kameng district of Arunachal Pradesh. *Natural Product Radiance* 7, no. 2 (2008): 176–181.

Katzer, Gernot. Chameleon plant (Houttuynia cordata) Thunb. Entry in Gernot Katzer's Spice Pages, http://gernot-katzers-spice-pages.com/engl/Hout_cor.html?redirect=1, accessed April 17, 2012.

Kim, G. S., D. H. Kim, J. J. Lim, et al. Biological and antibacterial activities of the natural herb Houttuynia cordata water extract against the intracellular bacterial pathogen salmonella within the RAW 264.7 macrophage. *Biological and Pharmaceutical Bulletin* 31, no. 11 (2008): 2012–17.

Kim, I. S., J. H. Kim, C. Y. Yun, et al. The inhibitory effect of Houttuynia cordata extract on stem cell factor-induced HMC-1 cell migration. *Journal of Ethnopharmacology* 112, no. 1 (2007): 90–95.

Kim, J., C. S. Park, Y. Lim, et al. Paeonia japonica, Houttuynia cordata, and Aster scaber water extracts induce nitric oxide and cytokine production by lipopolysaccharide-activated macrophages. *Journal of Medicinal Food* 12, no. 2 (2009): 365–73.

Kim, S. K., S. Y. Ryu, J. No, et al. Cytotoxic alkaloids from Houttuynia cordata. *Archives of Pharmacal Research* 24, no. 6 (2001): 518–21.

Klawikkan, N., V. Nukoolkarn, S. Jirakanjanakit, et al. Effect of Thai medicinal plant extracts against dengue virus in vitro. *Mahidol University Journal of Pharmaceutical Science* 38, no. 1–2 (2011): 13–18.

Kusirisin, W., S. Srichairatanakool, P. Lerttrakarnnon, et al. Antioxidative activity, polyphenolic content and anti-glycation effect of some Thai medicinal plants traditionally used in diabetic patients. *Journal of Medicinal Chemistry* 5, no. 2 (2009): 139–47.

Lai, K. C., Y. J. Chiu, Y. J. Tang, et al. Houttuynia cordata Thunb extract inhibits cell growth and induces apoptosis in human primary colorectal cancer cells. *Anticancer Research* 30, no. 9 (2010): 3549–56.

Lau, K. M., K. M. Lee, C. M. Koon, et al. Immunomodulatory and anti-SARS activities of Houttuynia cordata. *Journal of Ethnopharmacology* 118, no. 1 (2008): 79–85.

Leardkamolkarn, V., W. Sirigulpanit, C. Phurimsak, et al. The inhibitory actions of Houttuynia cordata aqueous extract on dengue virus and dengue-infected cells. *Journal of Food Biochemistry* 36, no. 1 (2012): 86–92.

Lee, J. S., I. S. Kim, J. H. Kim, et al. Suppressive effects of Houttuynia cordata Thunb (Saururaceae) extract on Th2 immune response. *Journal of Ethnopharmacology* 117, no. 1 (2008): 34–40.

Li, C., Y. Zhao, C. Liang, et al. Observations of the curative effect with various liquid for post operative irrigation of ESS of treating chronic sinusitis and nasal polyps. *Lin Chuang Er Bi Yan Hou Ke Za Zhi* 15, no. 2 (2001): 53–54.

Li, G. Z., O. H. Chai, M. S. Lee, et al. Inhibitory effects of Houttuynia cordata water extracts on anaphylactic reaction and mast cell activation. *Biological and Pharmaceutical Bulletin* 28, no. 10 (2005): 1864–68.

Li, S., R. Wang, Y. Zhang, et al. Symptom combinations associated with outcome and therapeutic effects in a cohort of cases with SARS. *American Journal of Chinese Medicine* 34, no. 6 (2006): 937–47.

Li, W., P. Zhou, Y. Zhang, et al. Houttuynia cordata, a novel and selective COX-2 inhibitor with anti-inflammatory activity. *Journal of Ethnopharmacology* 133, no. 2 (2011): 922–27.

Liang, K. L., Y. C. Su, C. C. Tsai, et al. Postoperative care with Chinese herbal medicine or amoxicillin after functional endoscopic sinus surgery: A randomized, double-blind, placebo-controlled study. *American Journal of Rhinology & Allergy* 25, no. 3 (2011): 170–75.

Lin, T. Y., Y. C. Liu, J. R. Jheng, et al. Anti-enterovirus 71 activity screening of Chinese herbs with anti-infection and inflammation activities. *American Journal of Chinese Medicine* 37, no. 1 (2009): 143–58.

Liu, F. Z., H. Shi, Y. J. Shi, et al. Pharmacodynamic experiment of the antivirus effect of Houttuynia cordata injection on influenza virus in mice. *Yao Xue Xue Bao* 45, no. 3 (2010): 399–402.

Liu, G., H. Xiang, X. Tang, et al. Transcriptional and functional analysis shows sodium houttuyfonate-mediated inhibition of autolysis in Staphylococcus aureus. *Molecules* 16, no. 10 (2011): 8848–65.

Liu, L., W. Wu, Z. Fu, et al. Comparison of volatile oils of cultivated Houttaynia cordata populations with wild. *Zhongguo Zhong Yao Za Zhi* 35, no. 7 (2010): 876–81.

Lu, H., X. Wu, Y. Liang, et al. Variation in chemical composition and antibacterial activities of essential oils from two species of Houttuynia Thunb. *Chemical & Pharmaceutical Bulletin* 54, no. 7 (2006): 936–40.

Lu, H. M., Y. Z. Liang, L. Z. Yi, et al. Anti-inflammatory effect of Houttuynia cordata injection. *Journal of Ethnopharmacology* 104, no. 1–2 (2006): 245–49.

Lu, Y., X. Wang, D. Chen, et al. Polystyrene/graphene composite electrode fabricated by in situ polymerization for capillary electrophoretic determination of bioactive constituents in herba houttuyiae. *Electrophoresis* 32, no. 14 (2011): 1906–12.

Marsh, C. Houttuynia cordata — Thunb. Entry in the Plants for a Future database, www.pfaf.org/user/plant.aspx?latinname=Houttuynia+cordata, accessed April 29, 2012.

Meng, J., X. P. Dong, Z. H. Jiang, et al. Study on chemical constituents of flavonoids in fresh herb of Houttuynia cordata. *Zhongguo Zhong Yao Za Zhi* 31, no. 16 (2006): 1335–37.

Meng, J., X. P. Dong, Y. S. Zhou, et al. Studies on chemical constituents of phenols in fresh Houttuynia cordata. *Zhongguo Zhong Yao Za Zhi* 32, no. 10 (2007): 929–31.

Meng, J., K. S. Leung, X. P. Dong, et al. Simultaneous quantification of eight bioactive components of Houttuynia cordata and related Saururaceae medicinal plants by on-line high performance liquid chromatography-diode array detector-electrospray mass spectrometry. *Fitoterapia* 80, no. 8 (2009): 468–74.

Miyata, M., T. Koyama, and K. Yazawa. Water extract of Houttuynia cordata Thunb. leaves exerts anti-obesity effects by inhibiting fatty acid and glycerol absorption. *Journal of Nutritional Science and Vitaminology* 56 (2010): 150–56.

Ng, L. T., F. L. Yen, C. W. Liao, et al. Protective effect of Houttuynia cordata extract on bleomycin-induced pulmonary fibrosis in rats. *American Journal of Chinese Medicine* 35, no. 3 (2007): 465–75.

Nguyen, T. H., M. Sakakibara, S. Sano, et al. Uptake of metals and metalloids by plants growing in a lead-zinc mine area, northern Vietnam. *Journal of Hazardous Materials* 186, no. 2–3 (2011): 1384–91.

Pan, P., Y. J. Wang, L. Han, et al. Effects of sodium houttuyfonate on expression of NF-κB and MCP-1 in membranous glomerulonephritis. *Journal of Ethnopharmacology* 131, no. 1 (2010): 203–9.

Park, H., and M. S. Oh. Houttuyniae herba protects rat primary cortical cells from Aβ25-35-induced neurotoxicity via regulation of calcium influx and mitochondria-mediated apoptosis. *Human & Experimental Toxicology* 1 (2012): 1.

Puttawong, S., and S. Wongroung. Plucao (Houttuynia cordata) Thunb. and sabsua (Eupatorium odoratum L.) extracts suppress Colletotrichum capsici and Fusarium oxysporum. *Journal of Agricultural & Food Industrial Organization* 1, special issue (2009): S381–386.

Ren, X., X. Sui, and J. Yin. The effect of Houttuynia cordata injection on pseudorabies herpesvirus (PrV) infection in vitro. *Pharmaceutical Biology* 49, no. 2 (2011): 161–66.

Sarker, M. S. K., and C. J. Yang. Eosungcho (Houttuynia cordata) with multi strain probiotics as alternative to antibiotic for broiler production. *Journal of Medicinal Plants Research* 5, no. 18 (2011): 4411–17.

Shim, S. Y., Y. K. Seo, and J. R. Park. Down-regulation of FcepsilonRI expression by

Houttuynia cordata Thunb extract in human basophilic KU812F cells. *Journal of Medicinal Food* 12, no. 2 (2009): 383–88.

Shin, S., S. S. Joo, J. H. Jeon, et al. Anti-inflammatory effects of a Houttuynia cordata supercritical extract. *Journal of Veterinary Science* 11, no. 3 (2009): 273–75.

Su, Cory. Comments in the "Plant at a Time: Houttuynia" forum hosted on Susun Weed's Wise Woman Forum, June 22, 2007 (4:53 p.m.), www.healingwiseforum.com/viewtopic.php?t=17315.

Sun, W. W., Y. K. Li, and J. Y. Zhang. Anaphylactoid reactions inducing effect of polysorbate 80 and polysorbate 80 contained Houttuynia cordata injection on beagle. *Zhongguo Zhong Xi Yi Jie He Za Zhi* 31, no. 1 (2011): 90–93.

Tang, Y. J., J. S. Yang, C. F. Lin, et al. Houttuynia cordata Thunb extract induces apoptosis through mitochondrial-dependent pathway in HT-29 human colon adenocarcinoma cells. *Oncology Reports* 22, no. 5 (2009): 1051–56.

Toda, S. Antioxidative effects of polyphenols in leaves of Houttuynia cordata on protein fragmentation by copper-hydrogen peroxide in vitro. *Journal of Medicinal Food* 8, no. 2 (2005): 266–68.

Wang, F., F. Lu, and L. Xu. Effects of Houttuynia cordata Thunb on expression of BMP-7 and TGF-beta1 in the renal tissues of diabetic rats. *Journal of Traditional Chinese Medicine* 27, no. 3 (2007): 220–25.

Wang, F., P. Ouyang, Q. Zuo, et al. Effects of a new houttuyfonate derivative on proliferation of NIH3T3 cell and expression of syndecan-4 induced by tumor necrosis factor alpha. *Zhong Yao Cai* 33, no. 1 (2010): 92–96.

Wang, H. Y. and J. L. Bao. Effect of Houttuynia cordata aetherolea on adiponectin and connective tissue growth factor in a rat model of diabetes mellitus. *Journal of Traditional Chinese Medicine* 1 (2012): 1–2.

Wang, L., X. Cui, L. Cheng, et al. Adverse events to houttuynia injection: A systematic review. *Journal of Evidence-Based Medicine* 3, no. 3 (2010): 168–76.

Wu, L., J. Si, H. Zhou, et al. Study on chemical diversity of volatile oils in Houttuynia cordata and their genetic basis. *Zhongguo Zhong Yao Za Zhi* 34, no. 1 (2009): 64–67.

Wu, W., Y. L. Zheng, Y. Ma, et al. Analysis on yield and quality of different Houttuynia cordata. *Zhongguo Zhong Yao Za Zhi* 28, no. 8 (2003): 718–20, 771.

Xu, C. J., Y. Z. Liang, and F. T. Chau. Identification of essential components of Houttuynia cordata by gas chromatography/mass spectrometry and the integrated chemometric approach. *Talanta* 68, no. 1 (2005): 108–15.

Xu, X., H. Ye, W. Wang, et al. Determination of flavonoids in Houttuynia cordata Thunb. and Saururus chinensis (Lour.) Bail. by capillary electrophoresis with electrochemical detection. *Talanta* 68, no. 3 (2006): 759–64.

Yadav, A. K. Anticestodal activity of Houttuynia cordata leaf extract against Hymenolepis diminuta in experimentally infected rats. *Journal of Parasitic Diseases* 35, no. 2 (2011): 190–94.

Yang, Z., S. Luo, Z. Yu, et al. GC-MS analysis of the volatile compositions of Houttuynia cordata Thunb obtained by headspace solid-phase micro extraction (HS-SPME). *Modern Pharmaceutical Research* 2, no. 5 (2009): 90–96.

Yang, Z.-N., Q.-C. Peng, S.-Q. Luo, et al. Central properties of the metabolites of Houttuynia cordata Thunb. populations from different altitudes in Guizhou. *Journal of the Chinese Medical Association* 31, no. 16 (2010): 261–69.

Yin, J., G. Li, J. Li, et al. In vitro and in vivo effects of Houttuynia cordata on infectious bronchitis virus. *Avian Pathology* 40, no. 5 (2011): 491–98.

Yu-eui, R., Z. Yangyang, L. Wenjuan, et al. Research on the effect of Houttuynia cordata Thunb nutrient liquid for increase of white blood cells. *Preventive Medicine Tribune* 1999-01, CNKI.

Zhang, T. T., Y. Wu, and T. J. Hang. Study on HPLC fingerprint of flavonoids from Houttuynia cordata by comparing with fingerprint reference. *Zhong Yao Cai* 32, no. 5 (2009): 687–90.

Isatis (*Isatis tinctoria*)

Ahmad, I., et al. Butyrylcholinesterase, lipoxygenase inhibiting and antifungal alkaloids from Isatis tinctoria. *Journal of Enzyme Inhibition and Medicinal Chemistry* 23, no. 3 (2008): 313–16.

Ahmad, I., et al. Urease and serine protease inhibitory alkaloids from Isatis tinctoria. *Journal of Enzyme Inhibition and Medicinal Chemistry* 23, no. 6 (2008): 918–21.

Ahmad, I., et al. Xanthine oxidase/tyrosinase inhibiting, antioxidant, and antifungal oxindole alkaloids from Isatis costata. *Pharmaceutical Biology* 48, no. 6 (2010): 716–21.

An, Y. Q., et al. Content determination of epigoitrin in radix isatidis and its preparation by RP-HPLC. *Zhongguo Zhong Yao Za Zhi* 33, no. 18 (2008): 2074–76.

Angelini, L. G., et al. Response of woad (Isatis tinctoria L.) to different irrigation levels to optimise leaf and indigo production. In *Irrigation in Mediterranean Agriculture: Challenges and Innovation for the Next Decades*, ed. A. Santini, N. Lamaddalena, G. Severino, and M. Palladino, series A, no. 4 in *Options Méditerranéennes*. Bari, Italy: CIHEAM-IAMB, 2008.

Anonymous. Dyer's woad [Isatis tinctoria L.]. Plant profile on the website of the California Department of Food and Agriculture, www.cdfa.ca.gov/phpps/ipc/weedinfo/isatis.htm, accessed February 4, 2011.

Anonymous. Isatis L. woad. Entry in the U.S. Department of Agriculture Natural Resources Conservation Service PLANTS Database, http://plants.usda.gov/java/profile?symbol=ISTI, accessed February 4, 2011.

Anonymous. Heat Clearing Herbs to Clear Heat and Toxics: Isatis Root. Plant profile on ENaturalHealthCenter.com, www.e2121.com/herb_db/viewherb.php3?viewid=121&setlang=1, accessed February 5, 2011.

Anonymous. Isatis. Monograph on the Adam Herbs website, http://adamherbs.com/herbs/istatis.html, accessed February 5, 2011.

Anonymous. Isatis tinctoria. Monograph, *Alternative Medicine Review* 7, no. 6 (2002): 523–24.

Anonymous. Isatis tinctoria. Entry in *Wikipedia*, http://en.wikipedia.org/wiki/Isatis_tinctoria, accessed February 4, 2011.

Anonymous. Pharmacological research on banlangen. Free Papers Download Center, March 9, 2009, http://eng.hi138.com/?i133492.

Anonymous. Weed of the week: Dyer's woad. U.S. Department of Agriculture Forest Service, Forest Health Staff, Newtown Square, Penn., August 30, 2006, www. na.fs.fed.us/fhp/invasive_plants/weeds/dyers_woad.pdf.

Bagci, E., et al. Fatty acid and tocochromanol patterns of some Isatis L. (Brassicaceae) species from Turkey. *Pakistan Journal of Botany* 41, no. 2 (2009): 639–46.

Bogdana, K., et al. Inhibition of Toxoplasma gondii by indirubin and tryptanthrin analogs. *Antimicrobial Agents and Chemotherapy* 52, no. 12 (2008): 4466–69.

Brattström, A., et al. The plant extract Isatis tinctoria L. extract (ITE) inhibits allergen-induced airway inflammation and hyperactivity in mice. *Phytomedicine* 17, no. 8–9 (2010): 551–56.

Chen, L., et al. Immune responses to foot-and-mouth disease DNA vaccines can be enhanced by coinjection with the Isatis indigotica extract. *Intervirology* 48, no. 4 (2005): 207–12.

Chen, Z. W., et al. Mechanism study of anti-influenza effects of radix isatidis water extract by red blood cells capillary electrophoresis. *Zhongguo Zhong Yao Za Zhi* 31, no. 20 (2006): 1715–19.

Condurso, C., et al. The leaf volatile constituents of Isatis tinctoria by solid-phase microextraction and gas chromatography/mass spectrometry. *Planta Medica* 72, no. 10 (2006): 924–28.

Crouch, H. J. Somerset Rare Plant Register species account: Isatis tinctoria. Somerset Rare Plants Group, www.somersetrareplantsgroup.org.uk, accessed February 1, 2013.

Deng, X., et al. Qualitative and quantitative analysis of flavonoids in the leaves of Isatis indigatica Fort. by ultra-performance liquid chromatography with PDA and electrospray ionization tandem mass spectrometry detection. *Journal of Pharmaceutical and Biomedical Analysis* 48, no. 3 (2008): 562–67.

Dong, J., et al. Effective constituents contents in indigowood roots and leaves from different regions. *Ying Yong Sheng Tai Xue Bao* 17, no. 9 (2006): 1613–18.

Elliott, M. C., et al. Distribution and variation of indole glucosinolates in woad (Isatis tinctoria L.). *Plant Physiology* 48 (1971): 498–503.

Emam, S. S., et al. Primary metabolites and flavonoid constituents of Isatis microcarpa J. Gay ex Boiss. *IJournal of Natural Products* (online) 3 (2010): 12–26, www.journalofnaturalproducts.com/Volume3/3_Res_paper-2.pdf.

Fang, J., et al. Influence of radix isatidis on the endotoxin-induced release of TNF-alpha and IL-8 from HL-60 cells. *Journal of Huazhong University of Science and Technology. Medical Sciences* 25, no. 5 (2005): 546–48.

Fang, J. G., et al. The anti-endotoxic effect of o-aminobenzoic acid from radix isatidis. *Acta Pharmacologica Sinica* 26, no. 5 (2005): 593–97.

Fang, J. G., et al. Antiviral effect of folium isatidis on herpes simplex virus type I. *Zhongguo Zhong Yao Za Zhi* 30, no. 17 (2005): 1343–46.

Fatima, I., et al. Isatones A and B, new antifungal oxindole alkaloids from Isatis costata. *Molecules* 12, no. 2 (2007): 155–62.

Gilbert, K. G., et al. A high degree of genetic diversity is revealed in Isatis spp. (dyer's woad) by amplified fragment length polymorphism (AFLP). *Theoretical and Applied Genetics* 104 (2002): 1150–56.

Gilbert, K. G., et al. Quantitative analysis of indigo and indigo precursors in leaves of Isatis spp. and Polygonum tinctorium. *Biotechnology Progress* 20, no. 4 (2004): 1289–92.

Hamburger, M. Isatis tinctoria — from the rediscovery of an ancient medicinal plant towards a novel anti-inflammatory phytopharmaceutical. *Phytochemistry Review* 1, no. 3 (2002): 333–34.

Hamburger, M. New approaches in analyzing the pharmacological properties of herbal extracts. *Proceedings of the Western Pharmacology Society* 50 (2007): 156–61.

He, C. M. Experimental study on antivirus activity of traditional Chinese medicine. *Zhongguo Zhong Yao Za Zhi* 29, no. 5 (2004): 452–55.

He, L. W., et al. Chemical constituents from water extract of radix isatidis. *Yao Xue Xue Bao* 41, no. 12 (2006): 1193–96.

He, Y., et al. Clinical and experimental study on effects of huanglan granule in inhibiting rubella virus. *Zhongguo Zhong Xi Yi Jie He Za Zhi* 28, no. 4 (2008): 322–25.

Heinemann, C., et al. Prevention of experimentally induced irritant contact dermatitis by extract of Isatis tinctoria compared to pure tryptanthrin and its impact on UVB-induced erythema. *Planta Medica* 70, no. 5 (2004): 385–90.

Ho, Y. L., et al. Studies on the antinociceptive, anti-inflammatory and antipyretic effects of Isatis indigotica root. *Phytomedicine* 9, no. 5 (2002): 419–24.

Hsuan, S. L., et al. The cytotoxicity to leukemia cells and antiviral effects of Isatis indigotica extracts on pseudorabies virus. *Journal of Ethnopharmacology* 123, no. 1 (2009): 61–67.

Huang, C., et al. Affect of moroxydine and banlangen to rat with positive hepatitis. *Journal of Southwest Nationalities College*, 1997-02, CNKI.

Itrat, Fatima. A new alkaloid from Isatis costata. *Turkish Journal of Chemistry* 31 (2007): 443–47.

Jacobs, Jim, and Monica Pokorny. *Ecology and management of dyer's woad* (Isatis tinctoria L.). Invasive Species Technical Note MT-10. U.S. Department of Agriculture Natural Resources Conservation Service, March 2007. ftp://ftp-fc.sc.egov.usda.gov/MT/www/technical/invasive/Invasive_Species_Tech_Note_MT10.pdf.

Jiang, Z., et al. Effection of six Chinese medicinal herbs on activity of Newcastle disease virus. *Progress in Veterinary Medicine*, 2005-02, CNKI.

Kang, X., et al. Isatis tinctoria L. combined with co-stimulatory molecules blockade prolongs survival of cardiac allografts in alloantigen-primed mice. *Transplant Immunology* 23, no. 1–2 (2010): 34–39.

Kong, X., et al. Effects of Chinese herbal medicinal ingredients on peripheral lymphocyte proliferation and serum antibody titer after vaccination in chicken. *International Immunopharmacology* 4, no. 7 (2004): 975–82.

Kong, X. F., et al. Chinese herbal ingredients are effective immune stimulators for chickens infected with the Newcastle disease virus. *Poultry Science* 85, no. 12 (2006): 2169–75.

Lai, P., et al. Bifunctional modulating effects of an indigo dimer (bisindigotin) to CYP1A1 induction in H4IIE cells. *Toxicology* 226, no. 2–3 (2006): 188–96.

Li, A., et al. Anti-virus effect of traditional Chinese medicine yi-fu-qing granule on acute respiratory tract infections. *Bioscience Trends* 3, no. 4 (2009): 119–23.

Li, H. B., et al. Biological evaluation of radix isatidis based on neuraminidase activity assay. *Yao Xue Xue Bao* 44, no. 2 (2009): 162–66.

Li, H. B., et al. Establishment of bioassay method for antivirus potency of radix isatidis based on chemical fluorometric determination. *Guang Pu Xue Yu Guang Pu Fen Xi* 29, no. 4 (2009): 908–12.

Li, J., et al. Effect of radix isatidis on the expression of moesin mRNA induced by LPS in the tissues of mice. *Journal of Huazhong University of Science and Technology. Medical Sciences* 27, no. 2 (2007): 135–37.

Li, W., et al. Experiment studies on viricidal effects of radix isatis against HFRSV. *Practical Preventative Medicine*, 2006-06, CNKI.

Li, X., et al. New sphingolipids from the root of Isatis indigotica and their cytotoxic activity. *Fitoterapia* 78, no. 7–8 (2007): 490–95.

Lin, A. H., et al. Studies on anti-endotoxin activity of F022 from radix isatidis. *Zhongguo Zhong Yao Za Zhi* 27, no. 6 (2002): 439–42.

Lin, C. W., et al. Anti-SARS coronavirus 3C-like protease effects of Isatis indigotica root and plant-derived phenolic compounds. *Antiviral Research* 68, no. 1 (2005): 36–42.

Lingmin, Z., et al. Antiviral activity of the four monomers of isatis tinctoria L against Coxsackievirus B_3 in vitro. *Journal of Hubei Medical University*, 2005-01, CNKI.

Liu, J. F., et al. Isatisine A, a novel alkaloid with an unprecedented skeleton from leaves of Isatis indigotica. *Organic Letters* 9, no. 21 (2007): 4127–29.

Liu, J. F., et al. Studies on chemical constituents from leaves of Isatis indigotica. *Zhong Yao Za Zhi* 31, no. 23 (2006): 1961–65.

Liu, R., et al. Identification of 5 constituents of the aqueous extract of Isatis indigotica by HPLC-MS2. *Zhong Yao Cai* 28, no. 9 (2005): 772–74.

Liu, Y., et al. Anti-endotoxic effects of syringeic acid of radix isatidis. *Journal of Huazhong University of Science and Technology. Medical Sciences* 23, no. 2 (2003): 206–8.

Ma, L., et al. Determination of total organic acids and salicylic acid in extract of radix isatidis. *Zhongguo Zhong Yao Za Zhi* 31, no. 10 (2006): 804–6.

Mak, N. K., et al. Inhibition of RANTES expression by indirubin in influenza virus-infected human bronchial epithelial cells. *Biochemical Pharmacology* 67, no. 1 (2004): 167–74.

Moazzeni, H., et al. Isatis L. (Brassicaceae) in Iran: A new record and a new synonym. *Turkish Journal of Botany* 32 (2008): 243–47.

Moazzeni, H., et al. On the circumscription of Isatis tinctoria L. (Brassicaceae) in Iran. *Turkish Journal of Botany* 30 (2006): 455–58.

Mohn, Tobias. A comprehensive metabolite profiling of Isatis tinctoria leaf extracts. Ph.D. diss., University of Basel, 2009, http://edoc.unibas.ch/953/1/Dissertation_Tobias_Mohn.pdf.

Mohn, T., et al. A comprehensive metabolite profiling of Isatis tinctoria leaf extracts. *Phytochemistry* 70, no. 7 (2009): 924–34.

Mohn, T., et al. Quantification of active principles and pigments in leaf extracts of Isatis tinctoria by HPLC/UV/MS. *Planta Medica* 73, no. 2 (2007): 151–56.

Ni, Sein. Case report on virus hepatitis B treated with banlangen leading to seroconversion from positive to negative. *Myanmar Medical Journal*, 1995, conference issue: 97–99.

Oberthür, C., et al. The content of indigo precursors in Isatis tinctoria leaves — a comparative study of selected accessions and post-harvest treatments. *Phytochemistry* 65, no. 24 (2004): 3261–68.

Oberthür, C., et al. The elusive indigo precursors in woad (Isatis tinctoria L.) — identification of the major indigo precursor, isatan A, and a structure revision of isatan B. *Chemistry & Biodiversity* 1, no. 1 (2004): 174–82.

Oberthür, C., et al. Tryptanthrin content in Isatis tinctoria leaves — a comparative study of selected strains and post-harvest treatment. *Planta Medica* 70, no. 7 (2004): 642–45.

Pokorny, M., et al. Evaluating Montana's dyer's woad (Isatis tinctoria) cooperative eradication project. *Weed Technology* 21 (2007): 262–69.

Qi, C. X., et al. Clinical research of isatis root eyedrops on the acute bacterial conjunctivitis. *Zhong Yao Cai* 30, no. 1 (2007): 120–22.

Qui, Y., et al. Immunopotentiating effects of four Chinese herbal polysaccharides administered at vaccination in chickens. *Poultry Science* 86, no. 12 (2007): 2530–35.

Recio, M. C., et al. Anti-arthritic activity of a lipophilic woad (Isatis tinctoria) extract. *Planta Medica* 72, no. 8 (2006): 715–20.

Recio, M. C., et al. Anti-inflammatory and antiallergenic activity in vivo of lipophilic Isatis tinctoria extracts and tryptanthrin. *Planta Medica* 72, no. 6 (2006): 539–46.

Roxas, M., et al. Colds and influenza: A review of diagnosis and conventional, botanical and nutritional considerations. *Alternative Medicine Review* 12, no. 1 (2007): 25–48.

Ruan, J. L., et al. Studies on chemical constituents in leaf of Isatis indigotica. *Zhongguo Zhong Yao Za Zhi* 30, no. 19 (2005): 1525–26.

Rüster, G. U., et al. Inhibitory activity of indolin-2-one derivatives on compound 48/80-induced histamine release from mast cells. *Pharmazie* 59, no. 3 (2004): 236–37.

Smith, S. E. What is isatis? Plant profile on WiseGeek website, www.wisegeek.com/what-is-isatis.htm, accessed February 4, 2011.

Song, Z., et al. Effects of Chinese medicinal herbs on a rat model of chronic Pseudomonas aeruginosa lung function. *APMIS* 104, no. 5 (1996): 350–54.

Spataro, G., et al. Analysis of molecular variation in Isatis tinctoria L. populations from Europe and central Asia. Poster abstract H.21 in *Proceedings of the XLVIII Italian Society of Agricultural Genetics—SIFV-SIGA Joint Meeting, Lecce, Italy, 15/18 September, 2004*, www.siga.unina.it/SIGA2004/H_21.pdf.

Spencer, Neal R., ed. Prospects and progress in biological control of cruciferous weeds. In *Proceedings of the X International Symposium on Biological Control of Weeds, July 4–14, 1999*. Bozeman: Montana State University, 2000. www. invasive.org/publications/ xsymposium/proceed/submeet.pdf.

Süleyman, K. Morphological and agronomical characteristics of some wild and cultivated Isatis species. *Journal of Central European Agriculture* 7, no. 3 (2006): 479–84.

Verhille, B. Tinctorial plants, their therapeutic applications in ancient times. The particular case of isatis. *Histoire des Sciences Médicales* 43, no. 4 (2009): 357–67.

Yang, Z., et al. In vitro inhibition of influenza virus infection by a crude extract of Isatis indigotica root resulting in the prevention of viral attachment. *Molecular Medicine Reports* 5, no. 3 (2012): 793–99.

Wang, W., et al. Screening of anti-endotoxin components from radix isatidis. *Journal of Huazhong University of Science and Technology. Medical Sciences* 26, no. 2 (2006): 261–64.

Wang, X., et al. Determination of salylic acid, syringic acid, benzoic acid and anthranilic acid in radix isatidis by HPCE. *Zhongguo Zhong Yao Za Zhi* 34, no. 2 (2009): 189–92.

Wang, Y., et al. Evaluation on antiendotoxic action and antiviral action in vitro of tetraploid Isatis indigotica. *Zhongguo Zhong Yao Za Zhi* 25, no. 6 (2000): 327–29.

Wang, Y., et al. Synergistic effects of Isatis tinctoria L. and tacrolimus in the prevention of acute heart rejection in mice. *Transplant Immunology* 22, no. 1–2 (2009): 5–11.

Wei, X. Y., et al. Bisindigotin, a TCDD antagonist from the Chinese medicinal herb Isatis indigotica. *Journal of Natural Products* 68, no. 3 (2005): 427–29.

Wu, Y., et al. Novel indole C-glycosides from Isatis indigotica and their potential cytotoxic activity. *Fitoterapia* 82, no. 2 (2011): 288–92. Published electronically ahead of print October 30, 2010.

Xiao, Z., et al. Indirubin and meisoindigo in the treatment of chronic myelogenous leukemia in China. *Leukemia & Lymphoma* 43, no. 9 (2002): 1763–68.

Xu, T., et al. Production and analysis of organic acids in hairy-root cultures of Isatis indigotica Fort. (indigo woad). *Biotechnology and Applied Biochemistry* 39, pt. 1 (2004): 123–28.

Xu, X., et al. Antivirus effects of IRPS against good parvovirus in goose embryo. *Chinese Journal of Veterinary Science*, 2008-11, CNKI.

Yang, Z. C., et al. The synergistic activity of antibiotics combined with eight traditional Chinese medicines against two different strains of Staphylococcus aureus. *Colloids and Surfaces. B. Biointerfaces* 41, no. 2–3 (2005): 79–81.

You, W. C., et al. Effects of extracts from indigowood root (Isatis indigotica Fort.) on immune responses in radiation-induced mucositis. *Journal of Alternative and Complementary Medicine* 15, no. 7 (2009): 771–78.

You, W. C., et al. Indigowood root extract protects hematopoietic cells, reduces tissue damage and modulates inflammatory cytokines after total-body irradiation: Does indirubin play a role in radioprotection? *Phytomedicine* 16, no. 12 (2009): 1105–11.

Youshun, H., et al. Experimental study on inhibitory effect of ganlu xiaodu dan on Coxsackie virus in vitro. *Zhongguo Zhong Xi Yi Jie He Za Zhi* 18, no. 12 (1998): 737–40.

Zech-Matterne, V., et al. New archaeobotanical finds of Isatis tinctoria L. (woad) from Iron Age Gaul and a discussion of the importance of woad in ancient time, *Vegetation History and Archaeobotany* 19, no. 2 (2010): 137–42.

Zeng, Q., et al. Anti-virus activity of three Chinese herbs against porcine reproductive and respiratory syndrome virus in vitro. *Journal of Hunan Agricultural University*, 2010-04, CNKI.

Zhao, Y. L., et al. Effects of different extracts from radix isatidis lymphocytes of mice by biothermodynamics. *Zhongguo Zhong Yao Za Zhi* 31, no. 7 (2006): 590–93.

Zhao, Y. L., et al. Thermodynamics study on antibacterial effect of different extracts from radix isatis. *Chinese Journal of Integrative Medicine* 12, no. 1 (2006): 42–45.

Zou, P., et al. Chemical fingerprinting of Isatis indigotica root by RP-HPLC and hierarchical clustering analysis. *Journal of Pharmaceutical and Biomedical Analysis* 38, no. 3 (2005): 514–20.

Zou, P., et al. Determination of indicant, isatin, indirubin and indigotin in Isatis indigotica by liquid chromatography/electrospray ionization tandem mass spectrometry. *Rapid Communications in Mass Spectrometry* 21, no. 7 (2007): 1239–46.

Zuo, L., et al. Studies on chemical constituents in root of Isatis indigotica. *Zhongguo Zhong Yao Za Zhi* 32, no. 8 (2007): 688–91.

Licorice (*Glycyrrhiza glabra*)

Acharya, S. K., et al. A preliminary open trial on interferon stimulator (SNMC) derived from Glycyrrhiza glabra in the treatment of subacute hepatic failure, *Indian Journal of Medical Research* 98 (1993): 69–74.

Adams, L. S., et al. Analysis of the interactions of botanical extract combinations against the viability of prostate cancer cell lines. *Evidence-Based Complementary and Alternative Medicine* 3, no. 1 (2006): 117–24.

Agarwal, A., et al. An evaluation of the efficacy of licorice gargle for attenuating postoperative sore throat: A prospective, randomized, single-blind study. *Anesthesia and Analgesia* 109, no. 1 (2009): 77–81.

Aiyegoro, O. A., et al. Use of bioactive plant products in combination with standard antibiotics: Implications in antimicrobial chemotherapy. *Journal of Medicinal Plants Research* 3, no. 13 (2009): 1147–52.

Aly, A. M. Licorice: A possible anti-inflammatory and anti-ulcer drug. *AAPS PharmSciTech* 6, no. 1 (2005): E74–82.

Ambawade, S. D., et al. Anticonvulsant activity of roots and rhizomes of Glycyrrhiza glabra. *Indian Journal of Pharmacology* 34 (2002): 251–55.

Anonymous. Glycyrrhiza. Entry in *Wikipedia*, http://en.wikipedia.org/wiki/Glycyrrhiza, accessed February 7, 2011.

Anonymous. Glycyrrhiza. Plant profile on Botany.com, www.botany.com/glycyrrhiza.html, accessed February 7, 2011.

Anonymous. Glycyrrhiza glabra. Monograph, *Alternative Medicine Review* 10, no. 3 (2005): 230–37.

Anonymous. Glycyrrhiza L. Entry in the U.S. Department of Agriculture Natural Resources Conservation Service PLANTS Database, http://plants.usda.gov/java/profile?symbol=GLYCY, accessed February 7, 2011.

Anonymous. Glycyrrhiza lepidota Pursh. Entry in the U.S. Department of Agriculture Natural Resources Conservation Service PLANTS Database, http://plants.usda.gov/java/profile?symbol=GLLE3, accessed February 1, 2013.

Anonymous. Glycyrrhiza uralensis. Entry in *Wikipedia*, http://en.wikipedia.org/wiki/Glycyrrhiza_uralensis, accessed February 7, 2011.

Anonymous. Liquorice. Entry in *Wikipedia*, http://en.wikipedia.org/wiki/Liquorice, accessed February 7, 2011.

Aoki, F., et al. Clinical safety of licorice flavonoid oil (LFO) and pharmacokinetics of glabridin in healthy humans. *Journal of the American College of Nutrition* 26, no. 3 (2007): 209–18.

Armanini, D., et al. Treatment of polycystic ovary syndrome with spironolactone plus licorice. *European Journal of Obstetrics, Gynecology and Reproductive Biology* 131, no. 1 (2007): 61–67.

Ashfaq, U., et al. Glycyrrhizin as antiviral agent against hepatitis C virus. *Journal of Translational Medicine* 9 (2011): 112.

Asl, M., et al. Review of pharmacological effects of Glycyrrhiza sp. and its bioactive compounds. *Phytotherapy Research* 22, no. 6 (2008): 709–24.

Badam, L. In vitro antiviral activity of indigenous glycyrrhizin, licorice and glycyrrhizic acid (Sigma) on Japanese encephalitis virus. *Journal of Communicable Diseases* 29, no. 2 (1997): 91–99.

Badam, L. In vitro studies on the effect of glycyrrhizin from Indian Glycyrrhiza glabra Linn on some RNA and DNA viruses. *Indian Journal of Pharmacology* 26, no. 3 (1994): 194–99.

Barthomeuf, C., et al. Conferone from Ferula schtschurowskiana enhances vinblastine cytotoxicity in MDCK-MDR1 cells by competitively inhibiting P-glycoprotein transport. *Planta Medica* 72, no. 7 (2006): 634–39.

Belofsky, G., et al. Metabolites of the "smoke tree," Dalea spinosa, potentiate antibiotic activity against multidrug-resistant Staphylococcus aureus. *Journal of Natural Products* 69, no. 2 (2006): 261–64.

Belofsky, G., et al. Phenolic metabolites of Dalea versicolor that enhance antibiotic activity against model pathogenic bacteria. *Journal of Natural Products* 67, no. 3 (2004): 481–84.

Betoni, J. E. C., et al. Synergism between plant extract and antimicrobial drugs used on Staphylococcus aureus diseases. *Memórias do Instituto Oswaldo Cruz* 101, no. 4 (2006): 387–90.

Biavatti, Maique W. Synergy: An old wisdom, a new paradigm for pharmacotherapy. *Brazilian*

Journal of Pharmaceutical Sciences 45, no. 3 (2009): 371–78.

Biradar, Y. Synergistic evaluation of antiplasmodial compounds *in vitro*. Chapter 7 in Evaluation of antimalarial activity of selected plants of Indian systems of medicine and study: The synergistic activity of the compounds present therein. Ph.D. diss., Nirma University (India), December 9, 2010, www.ietd.inflibnet.ac.in/bitstream/10603/1379/12/12_chapter7.pdf.

Bojian, B., et al. Glycyrrhiza Linnaeus. In *Flora of China* 10, 509–11. St. Louis: Missouri Botanical Garden Press; Beijing: Science Press, 2010.

Burgess, J. A. Review of over-the-counter treatments for aphthous ulceration and results from use of a dissolving oral patch containing glycyrrhiza complex herbal extract. *Journal of Contemporary Dental Practice* 9, no. 3 (2008): 88–98.

Cantelli-Forti, G., et al. Interaction of licorice on glycyrrhizin pharmacokinetics. *Environmental Health Perspectives* 102, suppl. 9 (1994): 65–68.

Chérigo, L., et al. Bacterial resistance modifying tetrasaccharide agents from Ipomoea murucoides. *Phytochemistry* 70, no. 2 (2009): 222–27.

Chérigo, L., et al. Inhibitors of bacterial multidrug efflux pumps from the resin glycosides of Ipomoea murucoides. *Journal of Natural Products* 71, no. 6 (2008): 1037–45.

Chérigo, L., et al. Resin glycosides from the flowers of Ipomoea murucoides. *Journal of Natural Products* 69, no. 4 (2006): 595–99.

Cho, H. J., et al. Hexane/ethanol extract of Glycyrrhiza uralensis licorice exerts potent anti-inflammatory effects in murine macrophages and in mouse skin. *Food Chemistry* 121 (2010): 959–66.

Cinatl, J., et al. Glycyrrhizin, an active component of liquorice roots, and replication of SARS-associated coronavirus. *Lancet* 361, no. 9374 (2003): 2045–46.

Cortés-Selva F., et al. Dihydro-beta-agarofuran sesquiterpenes: A new class of reversal agents of the multidrug resistance phenotype mediated by P-glycoprotein in the protozoan parasite Leishmania. *Current Pharmaceutical Design* 11, no. 24 (2005): 3125–39.

Crance, J., et al. Interferon, ribavirin, 6-azauridine and glycyrrhizin: Antiviral compounds active against flaviviruses. *Antiviral Research* 58, no. 1 (2003): 73–79.

Dao, T. T., et al. Chalcones as novel influenza A (H1N1) neuraminidase inhibitors from Glycyrrhiza inflata. *Bioorganic & Medicinal Chemistry Letters* 21, no. 1 (2011): 294–98. Published electronically ahead of print November 5, 2010.

Dong, Y., et al. The anti-respiratory syncytial virus (RSV) effect of radix glycyrrhizae in vitro. *Zhong Yao Cai* 27, no. 6 (2004): 425–27.

Efferth, T., et al. Complex interactions between phytochemicals: The multi-target therapeutic concept of phytotherapy. *Current Drug Targets* 12, no. 1 (2011): 122–32.

Elmadjian, F., et al. The action of mono-ammonium glycyrrhizinate on adrenalectomized subjects and its synergism with hydrocortisone. *Journal of Clinical Endocrinology and Metabolism* 16, no. 3 (1956): 338–49.

Feng, W., et al. Content variation of saponins and flavonoids from growing and harvesting time of Glycyrrhiza uralensis. *Zhong Yao Cai* 31, no. 2 (2008): 184–86.

Fiore, C., et al. Antiviral effects of Glycyrrhiza species. *Phytotherapy Research* 22, no. 2 (2008): 141–48.

Follett, J., et al. Growing licorice (Glycyrrhiza glabra L.). New Zealand Center for Crop & Food Research broadsheet no. 121 (2000).

Foster, Steven. Licorice — Glycyrrhiza. Monograph, Steven Foster Group, Inc., www.stevenfoster.com/education/monograph/licorice.html, accessed February 7, 2011.

Fuhrman, B., et al. Lycopene synergistically inhibits LDL oxidation in combination with vitamin E, glabridin, rosmarinic acid, carnosic acid, or garlic. *Antioxidants & Redox Signaling* 2, no. 3 (2000): 491–506.

Gao, Q., et al. Comparative pharmacokinetic behavior of glycyrrhetic acid after oral administration of glycyrrhizic acid and gancao-fuzi-tang. *Biological & Pharmaceutical Bulletin* 27, no. 2 (2004): 226–28.

Gao, X., et al. Review of pharmacological effects of glycyrrhiza radix and its bioactive compounds. *Zhongguo Zhong Yao Za Zhi* 34, no. 21 (2009): 2695–700.

Genovese, T., et al. Glycyrrhizin reduces secondary inflammatory process after spinal cord compression injury in mice. *Shock* 31, no. 4 (2009): 367–75.

Grankina, V. P., et al. Trace element composition of Ural licorice *Glycyrrhiza uralensis* Fisch. (Fabaceae family). *Contemporary Problems of Ecology* 2, no. 4 (2009): 396–99. Abstract, accessed online via www.maik.ru/abstract/proecol/9/proecol0396_abstract.pdf.

Grover, I. S., et al. Effect of liquorice [Glycyrrhiza glabra Linn.] as an adjuvant in newly diagnosed sputum smear-positive patients of pulmonary tuberculosis on directly observed treatment short course (DOTS) therapy. *Chest* 130, no. 4, suppl. (2006): 95S.

Hammouda, F. M., et al. Glycyrrhiza glabra L. In *A Guide to Medicinal Plants in North Africa*, 147–50. Malaga, Spain: IUCN Center for Mediterranean Cooperation, 2005, www.uicnmed.org/nabp/database/HTM/PDF/p94.pdf.

Harada, S. The broad anti-viral agent glycyrrhizin directly modulates the fluidity of plasma membrane and HIV-1 envelope. *Biochemical Journal* 392 (2005): 191–99.

Hayashi, H., et al. Distribution pattern of saponins in different organs of Glycyrrhiza glabra. *Planta Medica* 59, no. 4 (1993): 351–53.

Hayashi, H., et al. Field survey of Glycyrrhiza plants in central Asia (2). Characterization of phenolics and their variation in the leaves of Glycyrrhiza plants collected in Kazakhstan. *Chemical and Pharmaceutical Bulletin* (Tokyo) 51, no. 11 (2003): 1147–52.

Hayashi, H., et al. Seasonal variation of glycyrrhizin and isoliquiritigenin glycosides in the root of Glycyrrhiza glabra L. *Biological & Pharmaceutical Bulletin* 21, no. 9 (1998): 987–89.

He, J., et al. Antibacterial compounds from Glycyrrhiza uralensis. *Journal of Natural Products* 69 (2006): 121–24.

He, X., et al. Down-regulation of Treg cells and up-regulation of TH1/TH2 cytokine ration were induced by polysaccharide from radix glycyrrhizae in H22 hepatocarcinoma bearing mice. *Molecules* 16, no. 10 (2011): 8343–52.

Hennell, J., et al. The determination of glycyrrhizic acid in Glycyrrhiza uralensis Fisch ex DC (zhi gan cao) root and the dried aqueous extract by LC-DAD. *Journal of Pharmaceutical and Biomedical Analysis* 47, no. 3 (2008): 494–500.

Hirabayashi, K., et al. Antiviral activities of glycyrrhizin and its modified compounds against human immunodeficiency virus type 1 (HIV-1) and herpes simplex virus type 1 (HSV-1) in vitro. *Chemical and Pharmaceutical Bulletin* (Tokyo) 39, no. 1 (1991): 112–15.

Hoever, G., et al. Antiviral activity of glycyrrhizic acid derivatives against SARS-coronavirus. *Journal of Medicinal Chemistry* 48, no. 4 (2005): 1256–59.

Hou, Y., et al. Profound difference of metabolic pharmacokinetics between pure glycyrrhizin and glycyrrhizin in licorice decoction. *Life Sciences* 76, no. 10 (2005): 1167–76.

Huang, M., et al. Investigation on medicinal plant resources of Glycyrrhiza uralensis in China and chemical assessment of its underground part. *Zhongguo Zhong Yao Za Zhi* 35, no. 8 (2010): 947–52.

Irani, M., et al. Leaves antimicrobial activity of Glycyrrhiza glabra L. *Iranian Journal of Pharmaceutical Research* 9, no. 4 (2010): 425–28.

Izadi, M., et al. An evaluation of antibacterial activity of Glycyrrhiza glabra extract on the growth of *Salmonella, Shigella* and ETEC *E. coli. Journal of Biological Sciences* 7, no. 5 (2007): 827–29.

Janke, R. *Farming a few acres of herbs: Licorice.* Kansas State University, May 2004, www.ksre.ksu.edu/bookstore/pubs/MF2616.pdf.

Jatav, V., et al. Recent pharmacological trends of Glycyrrhiza glabra Linn. *International Journal of Pharmaceutical Frontier Research* 1, no. 1 (2011): 170–85.

Jiang, X., et al. The content dynamics of glycyrrhizic acid and soluble sugar in glycyrrhizae radix et rhizoma. *Zhong Yao Cai* 34, no. 9 (2011): 1321–23.

Jing, L., et al. Comparative analysis of glycyrrhizin diammonium and lithium chloride on infectious bronchitis virus infection in vitro. *Avian Pathology* 38, no. 3 (2009): 215–21.

Johns, C. Glycyrrhizic acid toxicity caused by consumption of licorice candy cigars. *CJEM* 11, no. 1 (2009): 94–96.

Kim, S., et al. Glycyrrhizic acid affords robust neuroprotection in the postischemic brain via antiinflammatory effect by inhibiting HMGB1 phosphorylation and secretion. *Neurobiology of Disease* 46, no. 1 (2012): 147–56.

Kim, S., et al. The use of stronger neo-minophagen C, a glycyrrhizin-containing preparation, in robust neuroprotection in the postischemic brain, *Anatomy & Cell Biology* 44, no. 4 (2011): 304–13.

Ko, H. C., et al. The effect of medicinal plants used in Chinese folk medicine on RANTES secretion by virus-infected human epithelial cells. *Journal of Ethnopharmacology* 107, no. 2 (2006): 205–10.

Kojoma, M., et al. Variation of glycyrrhizin and liquiritin contents within a population of 5-year-old licorice (Glycyrrhiza uralensis) plant cultivated under the same conditions. *Biological & Pharmaceutical Bulletin* 34, no. 8 (2011): 1334–37.

Kolbe, L., et al. Anti-inflammatory efficacy of licochalcone A: Correlation of clinical potency and in vitro effects. *Archives of Dermatological Research* 298, no. 1 (2006): 23–30.

Kondo, K., et al. Constituent properties of licorices derived from Glycyrrhiza uralensis G. glabra, or G. inflata identified by genetic information. *Biological & Pharmaceutical Bulletin* 30, no. 7 (2007): 1271–77.

Krahenbuhl, S., et al. Kinetics and dynamics of orally administered 18 beta-glycyrrhetinic acid in humans. *Journal of Clinical Endocrinology and Metabolism* 78, no. 3 (1994): 581–85.

Kuo, K., et al. Water extract of Glycyrrhiza uralensis inhibited enterovirus 71 in a human foreskin fibroblast cell line. *American Journal of Chinese Medicine* 37, no. 2 (2009): 383–94.

Kusano, E. How to diagnose and treat a licorice-induced syndrome with findings similar to that of primary hyperaldosteronism. Editorial, *Internal Medicine* (Tokyo) 43, no. 1 (2004): 5–6.

Kushiev, H., et al. Remediation of abandoned saline soils using Glycyrrhiza glabra: A study from the Hungry Steppes of Central Asia. *International Journal of Agricultural Sustainability* 3, no. 2 (2005): 102.

Kwon, H., et al. Blockade of cytokine-induced endothelial cell adhesion molecule expression by licorice isoliquiritigenin through NF-kB signal disruption. *Experimental Biology and Medicine* 232, no. 2 (2007): 235–45.

Lapi, F., et al. Myopathies associated with red yeast rice and liquorice: Spontaneous reports from the Italian Surveillance System of Natural Health Products. *British Journal of Clinical Pharmacology* 66, no. 4 (2008): 572–74.

Li, X. L., et al. Antioxidant status and immune activity of glycyrrhizin in allergic rhinitis mice. *International Journal of Molecular Sciences* 12 (2011): 905–16.

Li, Y. Toxicity attenuation and efficacy potentiation effect of liquorice on treatment of rheumatoid arthriris with Tripterygium wilfodii. *Zhongguo Zhong Xi Yi Jie He Za Zhi* 26, no. 12 (2006): 1117–19.

Li, Y., et al. The use of albendazole and diammonium glycyrrhizinate in the treatment of eosinophilic meningitis in mice infected with Angiostrongylus cantonensis. *Journal of Helminthology* 13 (2011): 1–11.

Lin, J. C. Mechanism of action of glycyrrhizic acid in inhibition of Epstein-Barr virus replication in vitro. *Antiviral Research* 59, no. 1 (2003): 41–47.

Liu, X. R., et al. Treatment of intestinal metaplasia and atypical hyperplasia of gastric mucosa with xiao wei yan powder. *Zhongguo Zhong Xi Yi Jie He Za Zhi* 12, no. 10 (1992): 602–3, 580.

Lu, S., et al. Survey of study on the extraction, purification and determination methods of glycyrrhizic acid in licorice. *Zhongguo Zhong Yao Za Zhi* 31, no. 5 (2006): 357–60.

Martin, M. D., et al. A controlled trial of a dissolving oral patch concerning glycyrrhiza (licorice) herbal extract for the treatment of aphthous ulcers. *General Dentistry* 56, no. 2 (2008): 206–10.

Michaelis, M., et al. Glycyrrhizin inhibits highly pathogenic H5N1 influenza A virus-induced pro-inflammatory cytokine and chemokine expression in human macrophages. *Medical Microbiology and Immunology* 199, no. 4 (2010): 291–97.

Miyamura, M., et al. Properties of glycyrrhizin in Kampo extracts including licorice root and changes in the blood concentration of glycyrrhetic acid after oral administration of Kampo extracts. *Yakugaku Zasshi* 116, no. 3 (1996): 209–16.

Moghadamnia, A. A. The efficacy of the bioadhesive patches containing licorice extract in the management of recurrent aphthous stomatitis. *Phytotherapy Research* 23, no. 2 (2009): 246–50.

Molnár, J., et al. Reversal of multidrug resistance by natural substances from plants. *Current Topics in Medicinal Chemistry* 10, no. 17 (2010): 1757–68.

Montoro, P., et al. Metabolic profiling of roots of licorice (Glycyrrhiza glabra) from different geographical areas by ESI/MS/MS and determination of major metabolites by LC-ESI/ME and LC-ESI/MS/MS. *Journal of Pharmaceutical and Biomedical Analysis* 54, no. 3 (2011): 535–44.

Morel, C., et al. Isoflavones as potentiators of antibacterial activity. *Journal of Agricultural and Food Chemistry* 51, no. 19 (2003): 5677–79.

Muralidharan, P., et al. Cerebroprotective effect of Glycyrrhiza glabra Linn. root extract on hypoxic rats. *Bangladesh Journal of Pharmacology* 4 (2009): 60–64.

Nomura, T., et al. Chemistry of phenolic compounds of licorice (Glycyrrhiza species) and their estrogenic and cytotoxic activities. *Pure and Applied Chemistry* 74, no. 7 (2002): 1199–206.

Ozaki, Y., et al. Studies on concentration of glycyrrhizin in plasma and its absorption after oral administration of licorice extract and glycyrrhizin. *Yakugaku Zasshi* 110, no. 1 (1990): 77–81.

Parsaeimehr, A., et al. Producing friable callus for suspension of culture in Glycyrrhiza glabra. *Advances in Environmental Biology* 3, no. 2 (2009): 125–28.

Pati, A. K. Licorice (Glycyrrhiza glabra, G. uralensis). Press release from Best Nutrition Products, Inc., Hayward, Calif., July 10, 2010. On the website of PR Log at http://prlog. org/10780323-licorice-glycyrrhiza-glabra-uralensis-dr-abhay-kumar-pati-best-nutrition-hayward-ca-usa.html.

Ploeger, B., et al. The pharmacokinetics of glycyrrhizic acid evaluated by physiologically based pharmacokinetic modeling. *Drug Metabolism Reviews* 33, no. 2 (2001): 125–47.

Plouzek, C. A., et al. Inhibition of P-glycoprotein activity and reversal of multidrug resistance in vitro by rosemary extract. *European Journal of Cancer* 35, no. 10 (1999): 1541–45.

Pompei, R., et al. Antiviral activity of glycyrrhizic acid. *Experientia* 36, no. 3 (1980): 304.

Pompei, R., et al. Glycyrrhizic acid inhibits virus growth and inactivates virus particles. *Nature* 281, no. 5733 (1979): 689–90.

Qiao'e, W., et al. Study on the optimal harvest time of semi-wild Glycyrrhiza uralensis at Liangwai, Inner Mongolia. *Zhong Yao Cai* 27, no. 4 (2004): 235–37.

Raggi, M., et al. Bioavailability of glycyrrhizin and licorice extract in rat and human plasma as detected by HPLC method. *Pharmazie* 49, no. 4 (1994): 269–72.

Räikkönen, K., et al. Maternal licorice consumption and detrimental cognitive and psychiatric outcomes in children. *American Journal of Epidemiology* 170, no. 9 (2009): 1137–46.

Renjie, L., et al. Protective effect of Glycyrrhiza glabra polysaccharides against carbon tetrachloride-induced liver injury in rats. *African Journal of Microbiology Research* 4, no. 16 (2010): 1784–87.

Saeedi, M., et al. The treatment of atopic dermatitis with licorice gel. *Journal of Dermatological Treatment* 14, no. 3 (2003): 153–57.

Saif, M. W., et al. Phase I study of the botanical formulation PHY906 with capecitabine in advanced pancreatic and other gastrointestinal malignancies. *Phytomedicine* 17, no. 3–4 (2010): 161–69.

Sancar, M., et al. Comparative effectiveness of Glycyrrhiza glabra vs. omeprazole and misoprostol for the treatment of aspirin-induced gastric ulcers. *African Journal of Pharmacy and Pharmacology* 3, no. 12 (2009): 615–20.

Sato, J., et al. Antifungal activity of plant extracts against Arthrinium sacchari and Chaetomium funicola. *Journal of Bioscience and Bioengineering* 90, no. 4 (2000): 442–46.

Sato, Y., et al. Isoliquiritigenin, one of the anti-spasmodic principles of Glycyrrhiza ularensis roots, acts in the lower part of intestine. *Biological & Pharmaceutical Bulletin* 30, no. 1 (2007): 145–49.

Schröfelbauer, B., et al. Glycyrrhizin, the main active compound in liquorice, attenuates pro-inflammatory responses by interfering with membrane-dependent receptor signaling. *Biochemical Journal* 421, no. 3 (2009): 473–82.

Sekizawa, T., et al. Glycyrrhizin increases sur-vival of mice with herpes simplex encephali-tis. *Acta Virologica* 45, no. 1 (2001): 51–54.

Shamsa, F., et al. The anti-inflammatory and anti-viral effects of an ethnic medicine: Glycyrrhizin. *Journal of Medicinal Plants* 9, suppl. 6 (2010): 1–28.

Shibata, S. A drug over the millennia: Pharmacognosy, chemistry, and pharmacol-ogy of licorice. *Yakugaku Zasshi* 120, no. 10 (2000): 849–62.

Simões, M., et al. Understanding antimicrobial activities of phytochemicals against multi-drug resistant bacteria and biofilms. *Journal of Natural Products* 26 (2009): 746–57.

Sofia, H. N., and T. M. Walter. Review of Glycyrrhiza glabra, Linn. Siddha Papers 02 (01) (LR), ISSN 0974-2522, January 12, 2009, http://openmed.nic.in/3195/01/Glycyrrhiza_final.pdf.

Stavri, M., et al. Bacterial efflux pump inhibitors from natural sources. *Journal of Antimicrobial Chemotherapy* 59 (2007): 1247–60.

Strandberg, T. E., et al. Birth outcome in relation to licorice consumption during pregnancy. *American Journal of Epidemiology* 153, no. 11 (2001): 1085–88.

Strandberg, T. E., et al. Preterm birth and licorice consumption during pregnancy. *American Journal of Epidemiology* 156, no. 9 (2002): 803–5.

Sui, X., et al. Antiviral effect of diammonium glycyrrhizinate and lithium chloride on cell infection by pseudorabies herpesvirus. *Antiviral Research* 85, no. 2 (2010): 346–53.

Sultana, S., et al. Antimicrobial, cytotoxic and antioxidant activity of methanolic extract of Glycyrrhiza glabra. *Agriculture and Biology Journal of North America* (2010). doi:10.5251/abjna.2010.1.5.957.960.

Tancevski, I., et al. Images in cardiovascular medicine: Malicious licorice. *Circulation* 117 (2008): e299.

Teelucksingh, S., et al. Potentiation of hydro-cortisone activity in skin by glycyrrhetinic. *Lancet* 335, no. 8697 (1990): 1060–63.

Uto, T., et al. Analysis of the synergistic effect of glycyrrhizin and other constituents in lico-rice extract on lipopolysaccharide-induced nitric oxide production using knock-out extract. *Biochemical and Biophysical Research Communications* 417, no. 2 (2012): 473–78.

Utsunomiya, T., et al. Glycyrrizin, an active component of licorice roots, reduces morbid-ity and mortality of mice infected with lethal doses of influenza virus. *Antimicrobial Agents and Chemotherapy* 41, no. 3 (1997): 551–56.

Vibha, J., et al. A study on the pharmacokinetics and therapeutic efficacy of Glycyrrhiza gla-bra: A miracle medical herb. *Botany Research International* 2, no. 3 (2009): 157–63.

Wagner, H., et al. Natural products chemistry and phytomedicine research in the new mil-lennium: New developments and challenges. *ARKIVOC* 7 (2004): 277–84.

Wang, X., et al. The anti-respiratory syncytial virus effect of active compound of Glycyrrhiza GD4 in vitro. *Zhong Yao Cai* 29, no. 7 (2006): 692–94.

Wang, Z., et al. Gastrointestinal absorption char-acteristics of glycyrrhizin from Glycyrrhiza extract. *Biological & Pharmaceutical Bulletin* 18, no. 9 (1995): 1238–41.

Williamson, E. M., et al. Synergy: Interactions within herbal medicines. *European Phytojournal* 8, no. 5 (2001): 401–9.

Wolkerstoerfer, A., et al. Glycyrrhizin inhib-its influenza A virus uptake into the cell. *Antiviral Research* 83, no. 2 (2009): 171–78.

Wu, T. H., et al. Hypouricemic effect and regulatory effects on autonomic function of shao-yao gan-cao tang, a Chinese herbal prescription, in asymptomatic hyperuricemic vegetarians. *Rheumatology International* 28, no. 1 (2007): 27–31.

Yamamoto, Y. Pharmaceutical evaluation of Glycyrrhiza uralensis roots cultivated in eastern Nei-Meng-Gu of China. *Biological & Pharmaceutical Bulletin* 26, no. 8 (2003): 1144–49.

Yamashiki, M., et al. Effects of the Japanese herbal medicine "sho-saiko-to" (TJ-9) on interleukin-12 production in patients with HCV-positive liver cirrhosis. *Developmental Immunology* 7, no. 1 (1999): 17–22.

Yasue H., et al. Severe hypokalemia, rhabdo-myolysis, muscle paralysis, and respiratory impairment in a hypertensive patient taking herbal medicines containing licorice. *Internal Medicine* 46, no. 9 (2007): 575–78.

Yim, S. B., et al. Protective effect of glycyr-rhizin on 1-methyl-4-phenylpyridinium-induced mitochondrial damage and cell death in differentiated PC12 cells. *Journal of Pharmacology and Experimental Therapeutics* 321, no. 2 (2007): 816.

Yuan, H. N., et al. A randomized, crossover com-parison of herbal medicine and bromocriptine against risperidone-induced hyperprolac-tinemia in patients with schizophrenia. *Journal of Clinical Psychopharmacology* 28, no. 3 (2008): 264–370.

Zhang, L., et al. Study on adscription of plasma effective constituents of rat after adminis-trated with Paeonia laclifora and Glycyrrhiza uralensis. *Zhongguo Zhong Yao Za Zhi* 32, no. 17 (2007): 1789–91.

Zhu, S., et al. Survey of glycyrrhizae radix sources in Mongolia: Chemical assessment of the underground part of Glycyrrhiza uralensis and comparison with Chinese glycyrrhiza radix. *Journal of Natural Medicine* 63, no. 2 (2009): 137–46.

Zore, G., et al. Chemoprofile and bioactivities of Taverniera cuneifolia (Roth) Arn: A wild relative and possible substitute of Glycyrrhiza glabra L. *Phytomedicine* 15, no. 4 (2008): 292–300.

Lomatium (*Lomatium dissectum*)

Anonymous. Bradshaw's desert parsley. Species fact sheet from the U.S. Fish and Wildlife Service Oregon Fish & Wildlife Office, updated September 22, 2008, www.fws.gov/oregonfwo/Species/Data/BradshawsLomatium/.

Anonymous. Lomatium extract. Product description for BrainChild Nutritionals, www.brainchildnutritionals.com/lomatium-extract-331.html, accessed February 1, 2013.

Anonymous. Lomatium Raf. Entry in the U.S. Department of Agriculture Natural Resources Conservation Service PLANTS Database, http://plants.usda.gov/java/profile?symbol=LOMAT, accessed January 31, 2011.

Anonymous. Lomatium sandbergii Coult. & Rose. In *Field Guide to Selected Rare Vascular Plants of Washington.* Washington Natural Heritage Program and USDI Bureau of Land Management, 2005, www1.dnr.wa.gov/nhp/refdesk/fguide/pdf/lomsan.pdf.

Anonymous. Lomatium tuberosum Hoover. In *Field Guide to Selected Rare Vascular Plants of Washington.* Washington Natural Heritage Program and USDI Bureau of Land Management, 2005, www1.dnr.wa.gov/nhp/refdesk/fguide/pdf/lotu.pdf.

Anonymous. What is Lomatium dissectum? Brief monograph on the website Lomatium.com, www.lomatium.com/botany.htm, accessed November 25, 2010.

Asuming, W., et al. Essential oil composition of four *Lomatium* Raf. species and their chemotaxonomy. *Biochemical Systematics and Ecology* 33, no. 1 (2005): 17–26.

Atwood, D., and A. DeBolt. Packard's lomatium. In *Field Guide to the Special Status Plants of the Bureau of Land Management Lower Snake River District.* Boise, Id.: USDI Bureau of Land Management Lower Snake River District, April 2000, www.blm.gov/pgdata/etc/medialib/blm/id/publications/field_guide_to_the.Par.68503.File.dat/plomatium.pdf.

Bairamian, S., et al. California lomatiums part III. Composition of the hydrodistilled oils from two varieties of Lomatium dissectum. Isolation of a new hydrocarbon. *Journal of Essential Oil Research* 16, no. 5 (2004): 461–68. doi:10.1080/10412905.2004.9698772.

Barneby, R. C., et al. A new species of Lomatium (Apiaceae) from Utah. *Brittonia* 31, no. 1 (1979): 96–100.

Beauchamp, P. S., et al. California Lomatiums part IV(a). Composition of the essential oils of Lomatium rigidum (M.E. Jones) Jepson. Structures of two new funebrene epimers and a tridecatriene. *Journal of Essential Oil Research* 16, no. 6 (2004): 571–78.

Beauchamp, P. S., et al. Essential oil composition of six Lomatium species attractive to Indra swallowtail butterfly (Papilio indra): Principal component analysis against essential oil composition of Lomatium dissectum var. multifidum. *Journal of Essential Oil Research* 21 (2009): 535–42.

Bergner, Paul. Antiviral botanicals in herbal medicine. *Medical Herbalism* 14, no. 3 (2005): 1–12.

Carlson, H. J., et al. Antibiotic agents separated from the root of lace-leaved Leptotaenia. *Journal of Bacteriology* 55, no. 5 (1948): 615–21.

Chou, S. C., et al. Antibacterial activity of components from Lomatium californicum. *Phytotherapy Research* 20, no. 2 (2006): 153–56.

Curini, M., et al. Chemistry and biological activity of natural and synthetic prenyloxycoumarins. *Current Medicinal Chemistry* 13, no. 2 (2006): 199–222.

Dev, V., et al. Lomatium grayi and Indra swallowtail butterfly. Composition of the essential oils of three varieties of Lomatium grayi (J.M. Coult et Rose) J.M. Coult et Rose. *Journal of Essential Oil Research* 19, no. 3 (2007): 244–48. doi: 10.1080/10412905.2007.9699270.

Drum, Ryan. Three herbs: Yarrow, Indian consumption plant, coral root. Presentation at the Southwest Conference on Botanical Medicine, Tempe, Ariz., 2006. Available on the website of Island Herbs at http://ryandrum.com/threeherbs2.htm.

Garry Oak Ecosystems Recovery Team. Lomatium dissectum var. dissectum. In *Species at Risk in Garry Oak & Associated Ecosystems in British Columbia.* Victoria, B.C.: Garry Oak Ecosystems Recovery Team, 2003, www.goert.ca/documents/inserts/Lomatium_dissectum_Insert_Sheet.pdf.

Garry Oak Ecosystems Recovery Team. Lomatium grayi. In *Species at Risk in Garry Oak & Associated Ecosystems in British Columbia.* Victoria, B.C.: Garry Oak Ecosystems Recovery Team, 2003, www.goert.ca/documents/PARFS_lomagray.pdf.

Gupta, P. K., et al. Coumarins. 3. Identification of the lactone of Leptotaenia multifida. *Journal of Pharmaceutical Sciences* 53 (1964): 1543–44.

Henry, C. and J. D. Lomatium dissectum. *The Provisionary* (a newsletter of Therapeutic Environments, Albuquerque, N.M.) 5, no. 2 (2009): 1–4.

Keville, Kathi. Herb profile *Lomatium. American Herb Association Quarterly Newsletter* 19, no. 2 (2003): 3.

Lee, C. L., et al. Influenza A (H(1)N(1)) antiviral and cytotoxic agents from Ferula assa-foetida. *Journal of Natural Products* 72, no. 9 (2009): 1568–72.

Lee, K. H., et al. Coumarins. VII. The coumarins of Lomatium nuttallii. *Journal of Pharmaceutical Sciences* 57, no. 5 (1968): 865–68.

Lee, T. T., et al. Suksdorfin: An anti-HIV principle from Lomatium suksdorfii, its structure-activity correlation with related coumarins, and synergistic effects with anti-AIDS nucleosides. *Bioorganic & Medicinal Chemistry* 2, no. 10 (1994): 1051–56.

Matson, G. A., et al. Antibiotic studies on an extract from Leptotaenia multifeda. *Journal of Clinical Investigation* 28, no. 5, pt. 1 (1949): 903–8.

McCutcheon, A. R., et al. Antibiotic screening of medicinal plants of the British Columbian native peoples. *Journal of Ethnopharmacology* 37, no. 3 (1992): 213–23.

McCutcheon, A. R., et al. Anti-mycobacterial screening of British Columbian medicinal plants. *Pharmaceutical Biology* 35, no. 2 (1997): 77–83.

McCutcheon, A. R., et al. Antiviral screening of British Columbian medicinal plants. *Journal of Ethnopharmacology* 49 (1995): 101–10.

Meepagala, K. M., et al. Phytotoxic and antifungal compounds from two Apiaceae species, Lomatium californicum and Ligusticum hultenii, rich sources of Z-ligustilide and apiol, respectively. *Journal of Chemical Ecology* 31, no. 7 (2005): 1567–78.

Pendergrass, K. Introduction to Bradshaw's lomatium, a federally listed endangered species, and a key and photo guide to the *Lomatium* species that occur within its range. U.S. Department of Agriculture Natural Resources Conservation Service Technical Note 40b (2010): 1–21.

Pettinato, F. A., et al. An analysis of the volatile oil of *Lomatium suksdorfii*. *Journal of the American Pharmaceutica Association* 49, no. 1 (1960): 45–48.

Pettinato, F. A., et al. A note on the preliminary phytochemical and biological study of Lomatium suksdorfii. *Journal of the American Pharmaceutical Association* 48, no. 7 (1959): 423.

Pettinato, F. A., et al. A note on the volatile oil from the fruits of Lomatium grayi. *Journal of the American Pharmaceutical Association* 48, no. 5 (1959): 302.

Scholten, M., et al. Environmental regulation of dormancy loss in seeds of Lomatium dissectum (Apiaceae). *Annals of Botany* 103 (2009): 1091–100.

Starlord. Ancient Amerindian medicine kills the H1N1 virus. Post on the ConspiracyCafé. net website, October 20, 2009 (8:47 p.m.), www.conspiracycafe.net/forum/index.php?/topic/24684-ancient-amerindian-medicine-kills-the-h1n1-virus/.

Steck, Warren. Coumarins and chromones from 'Lomatium macrocarpum.' Prepared for the National Research Council of Canada Saskatoon (Saskatchewan) Prairie Regional Lab, March 19, 1973. Accessed online via the Open Archives Initiative at http://oai.dtic. mil/oai/oai?verb=getRecord&metadataPrefix =html&identifier=AD0769141.

VanWagenen, B. C., et al. Native American food and medicinal plants, 7. Antimicrobial tetronic acids from Lomatium dissectum. *Tetrahedron* 42 (1986): 1117.

VanWagenen, B. C., et al. Native American food and medicinal plants, 8. Water-soluble constituents of Lomatium dissectum. *Journal of Natural Products* 51, no. 1 (1988): 136–41.

Yates, Gene. Final report: Lomatium erythrocarpum survey. U.S. Department of Agriculture Forest Service, October 2005, http://fs.fed. us/r6/sfpnw/issssp/.../inv-rpt-va-loer-waw-surveys-2005-10.pdf.

Zakay-Rones, Z. N., et al. Lomatium dissectum: An herbal virucide? *Complementary Medicine* 2, no. 5 (1987): 32–34.

Red Root (*Ceanothus* spp.)

Alakurtti, S., et al. Pharmacological properties of the ubiquitous natural product betulin. *European Journal of Pharmaceutical Sciences* 1 (2006): 1–13.

Berry, A. M., et al. Bacteriohopanetetrol: Abundant lipid in *Frankia* cells and in nitrogen-fixing nodule tissue. *Plant Physiology* 95, no. 1 (1991): 111–15.

Bishop, J. G., et al. The effect of ceanothyn on blood coagulation time. *Journal of the American Pharmaceutical Association* 46, no. 7 (1957): 396–98.

Cichewicz, R. H. Chemistry, biological activity, and chemotherapeutic potential of betulinic acid for the prevention and treatment of cancer and HIV infection. *Medical Research Reviews* 24, no. 1 (2004): 90–114.

Cook, William. Ceanothus americanus. Entry in *The Physiomedical Dispensatory* (1869). Electronic version hosted on the website of *Medical Herbalism* journal, http://medherb. com/cook/home.htm.

de Sá, M. S., et al. Antimalarial activity of betulinic acid and derivatives in vitro against Plasmodium falciparum and in vivo in P. berghei-infected mice. *Parasitology Research* 105, no. 1 (2009): 275–79.

Delwiche, C. C., et al. Nitrogren fixation by Ceanothus. *Plant Physiology* 40, no. 6 (1965): 1045–47.

Eichenmüller, M., et al. Betulinic acid induces apoptosis and inhibits hedgehog signaling in rhabdomyosarcoma. *British Journal of Cancer* 103, no. 1 (2010): 43–51.

Emile, A., et al. Bioassay-guided isolation of antifungal alkaloids from Melochia odorata. *Phytotherapy Research* 21, no. 4 (2007): 398–400.

Fisher, J. B., et al. What the towers don't see at night: Nocturnal sap flow in trees and shrubs at two AmeriFlux sites in California. *Tree Physiology* 27, no. 4 (2007): 597–610.

Fu, J. Y. Betulinic acid ameliorates impairment of endothelium-dependent relaxation induced by oxidative stress in rat aorta. *Zhejiang Da Xue Xue Bao Yi Xue Ban* 39, no. 5 (2010): 523–29.

Giordano, A. A. S., et al. Ceanothus americanus: Its effect on the coagulation time of the blood. *Archives of Otolaryngology* 7, no. 6 (1928): 618–22.

Groot, J. T., et al. The pharmacology of Ceanothus americanus I. Preliminary studies: Hemodynamics and the effects on coagulation, *Journal of Pharmacology and Experimental Therapeutics* 30, no. 4 (1926): 275–91.

Klein, F. K., et al. Ceanothus alkaloids. Americine. *Journal of the American Chemical Society* 90, no. 9 (1968): 2398–404.

Kommera, H., et al. Synthesis and anticancer activity of novel betulinic acid and betulin derivatives. *Archiv der Pharmazie* (Weinheim, Germany) 343, no. 8 (2010): 449–57.

Laferriere, J. E., et al. Mineral composition of some traditional Mexican teas. *Plant Foods for Human Nutrition* 41 (1991): 277–82.

Lan, P., et al. Understanding the structure-activity relationship of betulinic acid derivatives as anti-HIV-1 agents by using 3D-QSAR and docking. *Journal of Molecular Modeling* 17, no. 7 (2011): 1643–59. Published electronically ahead of print October 27, 2010.

Laszczyk, M. N. Pentacytic triterpenes of the lupane, oleanane and ursane group as tools in cancer therapy. *Planta Medica* 75, no. 15 (2009): 1549–60.

Leal, I. C., et al. Ceanothane and lupane type triterpenes from Ziziphus joazeiro — an anti-staphylococcal evaluation. *Planta Medica* 76, no. 1 (2010): 47–52.

Lee, S. M., et al. Anti-complementary activity of triterpenoides from fruit of Zizyphus jujuba. *Biological & Pharmaceutical Bulletin* 27, no. 11 (2004): 1883–86.

Lee, S. S., et al. Preparation and cytotoxic effect of ceanothic acid derivatives. *Journal of Natural Products* 61, no. 11 (1998): 1343–47.

Li, X. C., et al. Antimicrobial compounds from Ceanothus americanus against oral pathogens. *Phytochemistry* 46, no. 1 (1997): 97–102.

Li, Y., et al. Betulin induces mitochondrial cytochrome c release associated apoptosis in human cancer cells. *Molecular Carcinogenesis* 49, no. 7 (2010): 630–40.

Lo, Y. C. Betulinic acid stimulates the differentiation and mineralization of osteoblastic MC3T3-E1 cells: Involvement of BMP/Runx2 and beta-catenin signals. *Journal of Agricultural and Food Chemistry* 58, no. 11 (2010): 6643–49.

Lucas, Joy. Ceanothus — a nice cup of tea & a piece of ague cake. On the Homeopathic Materia Medica website, updated August 30, 2003, www.web.mac.com/joylucas/iWeb/Site/Materia%20Medica%20(2)_files/Ceanothus.pdf.

Lucero, M. E., et al. Composition of *Ceanothus gregii* oil as determined by stream distillation and solid-phase microextraction. *Journal of Essential Oil Research* 22 (2010): 104–42.

Lynch, T. A., et al. An investigation of the blood coagulation principles from Ceanothus americanus. *Journal of the American Pharmaceutical Association* 47, no. 11 (1958): 816–19.

McCutcheon, A. R., et al. Antifungal screening of medicinal plants of British Columbian native peoples. *Journal of Ethnopharmacology* 44, no. 3 (1994): 157–69.

McCutcheon, A. R. et al. Antiviral screening of British Columbian medicinal plants. *Journal of Ethnopharmacology* 49, no. 2 (1995): 101–10.

Moore, M. Ceanothus: Red root. Folio on the website of the Southwest School of Botanical Medicine, www.swsbm.com/FOLIOS/RedRtFol.pdf, accessed July 12, 2011.

Rooney, R. F., et al. A case of poisoning from Ceanothus velutinus, resembling Rhus poisoning. *California State Journal of Medicine* 3, no. 9 (1905): 290–91.

Roscoe, C. W., et al. A preliminary study of the alkaloidal principles of Ceanothus americanus and Ceanothus velutinus. *Journal of the American Pharmaceutical Association* 49, no. 2 (1960): 108–12.

Saaby, L., et al. Isolation of immunomodulatory triterpene acids from a standardized rose hip powder (Rosa canina L.). *Phytotherapy Research* 25, no. 2 (2011): 195–201. Published electronically ahead of print, 2010.

Salazar-Aranda, R., et al. Antimicrobial and antioxidant activities of plants from northeast of Mexico. *Evidence-Based Complementary and Alternative Medicine* (2011). doi: 10.1093/ecam/nep127.

Servis, Robert, et al. Ceanothus alkaloids. II. Peptide alkaloids from Ceanothus americanus. *Journal of the American Chemical Society* 91, no. 20 (1969): 5619–24.

Spjut, Richard W. *Ceanothus* Rhamnacea. On the website of World Botanical Associates, www.worldbotanical.com/ceanothus.htm, accessed December 9, 2010.

Steele, J. C., et al. In vitro and in vivo evaluation of betulinic acid as an antimalarial. *Phytotherapy Research* 13, no. 2 (1999): 115–19.

Suksamram, S., et al. Ceanothane- and lupane-type triterpenes with antiplasmodial and antimycobacterial activities from Ziziphus cambodiana. *Chemical and Pharmaceutical Bulletin* (Tokyo) 54, no. 4 (2006): 535–37.

Takada, Y., et al. Betulinic acid suppresses carcinogen-induced NF-kappa B activation through inhibition of I kappa B alpha kinase and p65 phosphorylation: Abrogation of cyclooxygenase-2 and matrix metalloprotease-9. *Journal of Immunology* 171, no. 6 (2003): 3278–86.

Theraldsen, C. E., et al. Notes on blood reactions of the alkaloids of Ceanothus americanus. *American Journal of Physiology* 79, no. 3 (1926): 545–52.

Tortoriello, J., et al. Spasmolytic activity of medicinal plants used to treat gastrointestinal diseases in the Highland of Chiapas. *Phytomedicine* 2, no. 1 (1995): 57–66.

Tschesche, R., et al. Alkaloids from Rhamnaceae. IV. Integerrin, an additional peptide alkaloid from Ceanothus integgerrimus Hock and Arn. *Tetrahedron Letters* 11 (1968): 1311–15.

Tschesche, R., et al. Integerressin and integerrenin, two peptide alkaloids from Ceanothus integerrimus Hook. and Arn. *Chemische Berichte* 100, no. 12 (1967): 3924–36.

Vijayan, V., et al. Betulinic acid inhibits endotoxin stimulated phosphorylation cascade and pro-inflammatory prostaglandin E(2) production in human peripheral blood mononuclear cells. *British Journal of Pharmacology* 162, no. 6 (2011):1291–303. Published electronically ahead of print, 2010.

Wastle, H. Influence of tea leaves from Ceanothus americanus on blood pressure of hypertensive rats. *Federation Proceedings* 7, no. 1, pt. 1 (1948): 131.

Wollenweber, E., et al. Exudate flavonoids of eight species of Ceanothus (Rhamnaceae). *Zeitschrift für Naturforschung C* 59, no. 7–8 (2004): 459–62.

Yi, J. E., Immunomodulatory effects of betulic acid from the bark of white birch on mice. *Journal of Veterinary Science* 11, no. 4 (2010): 305–13.

Yogeeswari, P., et al. Betulinic acid and its derivatives: A review on their biological properties. *Current Medicinal Chemistry* 12, no. 6 (2005): 657–66.

Yoon, J. J., et al. Betulinic acid inhibits high glucose-induced vascular smooth muscle cells proliferation and migration. *Journal of Cellular Biochemistry* 111, no. 6 (2010): 1501–11.

Yun, Y., et al. Immunomodulatory activity of betulinic acid by producing pro-inflammatory cytokines and activation of macrophages. *Archives of Pharmacal Research* 26, no. 12 (2003): 1087–95.

Rhodiola (*Rhodiola* spp.)

Abidov, M., et al. Effect of extracts from Rhodiola rosea and Rhodiola crenulata (Crassulaceae) roots on ATP content in mitochondria of skeletal muscles. *Bulletin of Experimental Biology and Medicine* 136, no. 6 (2003): 585–87.

Abidov, M., et al. Extract of Rhodiola rosea radix reduces the level of C-reactive protein and creatinine kinase in the blood. *Bulletin of Experimental Biology and Medicine* 138, no. 1 (2004): 63–64.

Abidoff, M., and Z. Ramazanov. Rhodiola rosea: The herbal heavyweight from Russia. *Muscle Development*, January 2003, www.pdfking.

com/images/large/9862-rhodiola-muscle-development.gif.

Akgul, Y., et al. Lotaustralin from Rhodiola rosea roots. *Fitoterapia* 75, no. 6 (2004): 612–14.

An, F., et al. Determination of salidroside in eight Rhodiola species by TLC-UV spectrometry. *Zhongguo Zhong Yao Za Zhi* 23, no. 1 (1998): 43–44, 64.

Anonymous. Queen's crown: Rhodiola rhodantha. Plant profile from Natural Medicinal Herbs, www.naturalmedicinalherbs.net/herbs/r/rhodiola-rhodantha=queen's-crown. php, accessed December 10, 2010. (Profile drawn from the database of Plants for a Future, www.pfaf.org.)

Anonymous. Rhodiola. Plant profile from Paradise Herbs, www.paradiseherbs.com/media/uploads/research/Rhodiola.pdf, accessed February 1, 2013.

Anonymous. Rhodiola integrifolia Raf. Entry in the U.S. Department of Agriculture Natural Resources Conservation Service PLANTS Database, http://plants.usda.gov/java/profile?symbol=RHINI, accessed December 10, 2010.

Anonymous. Rhodiola rhodantha (A. Gray) H. Jacobsen. Entry in the U.S. Department of Agriculture Natural Resources Conservation Service PLANTS Database, http://plants.usda.gov/java/profile?symbol=RHRH4, accessed December 10, 2010.

Anonymous. Rhodiola rosea. Entry in *Wikipedia*, http://en.Wikipedia.org/wiki/Rhodiola_rosea, accessed February 12, 2011.

Anonymous. Rhodiola rosea. Monograph, *Alternative Medicine Review* 7, no. 5 (2002): 421–23.

Anonymous. Rhodiola rosea L. Entry in the Global Biodiversity Information Facility database, http://data.gbif.org/search/taxa/Rhodiola%20rosea, accessed December 10, 2010.

Anonymous. *Rhodiola rosea* L. Entry in the U.S. Department of Agriculture Natural Resources Conservation Service PLANTS Database, http://plants.usda.gov/java/profile?symbol=RHRO3, accessed December 10, 2010.

Anonymous. Study on the chemical constituents from Rhodiola bupleuroldes. Master's thesis, abstract, available via the website of China Papers, http://mt.china-papers.com/2/?p=48858, posted September 8, 2010..

Arora, R., et al. Evaluation of radioprotective activities Rhodiola imbricata Edgew — a high altitude plant. *Molecular and Cellular Biochemistry* 273, no. 1–2 (2005): 209–23.

Aslanyan, G., et al. Double-blind, placebo-controlled, randomized study of single dose effects of ADAPT-232 on cognitive functions. *Phytomedicine* 17, no. 7 (2010): 494–99.

Battistelli, M., et al. Rhodiola rosea as antioxidant in red blood cells: Ultrastructural and hemolytic behaviour. *European Journal of Histochemistry* 49, no. 3 (2005): 243–54.

Bocharova, O. A., et al. The effect of a Rhodiola rosea extract on the incidence of recurrences of a superficial bladder cancer (experimental clinical research). *Urologiia i nefrologiia* (Moscow) 2 (1995): 46–47.

Brown, R. P., et al. Rhodiola rosea: A phytomedicinal overview. *HerbalGram* 56 (2002): 40–52.

Bystritsky, A., et al. A pilot study of Rhodiola rosea (Rhodax) for generalized anxiety disorder (GAD). *Journal of Alternative and Complementary Medicine* 14, no. 2 (2008): 175–80.

Calcabrini, C., et al. Rhodiola rosea ability to enrich cellular antioxidant defences of cultured human keratinocytes. *Archives of Dermatological Research* 302, no. 3 (2010): 191–200.

Cao, L. L., et al. The effect of salidroside on cell damage induced by glutamate and intracellular free calcium in PC12 cells. *Journal of Asian Natural Products Research* 8, no. 1–2 (2006): 159–65.

Chem, X., et al. Hypoglycemic effect of Rhodiola sachalinensis A. Bor. polysaccharides: Comparison of administration in different ways. *Zhongguo Zhong Yao Za Zhi* 21, no. 11 (1996): 685–87.

Chen, C. H., et al. Antioxidant activity of some plant extracts towards xanthine oxidase, lipoxygenase and tyrosinase. *Molecules* 14, no. 8 (2009): 2947–58.

Chen, Q. G., et al. The effects of Rhodiola rosea extract on 5-HT level, cell proliferation and quantity of neurons at cerebral hippocampus of depressive rats. *Phytomedicine* 16, no. 9 (2009): 830–38.

Chen, T. S., et al. Antioxidant evaluation of three adaptogen extracts. *American Journal of Chinese Medicine* 36, no. 6 (2008): 1209–17.

Chen, X., et al. Protective effect of salidroside against H2O2-induced cell apoptosis in primary culture of rat hippocampal neurons. *Molecular and Cellular Biochemistry* 332, no. 1–2 (2009): 85–93.

Cui, S., et al. Determination of p-tyrosol and salidroside in three samples of Rhodiola crenulata and one of Rhodiola kirilowii by capillary zone electrophoresis. *Analytical and Bioanalytical Chemistry* 377, no. 2 (2003): 370–74.

Darbinyan, V., et al. Clinical trial of Rhodiola rosea L. extract SHR-5 in the treatment of mild to moderate depression. *Nordic Journal of Psychiatry* 61, no. 5 (2007): 343–48.

Darbinyan, V., et al. *Rhodiola rosea* in stress induced fatigue — a double blind cross-over study of a standardized extract SHR-5 with a repeated low-dose regimen on the mental performance of healthy physicians during night duty. *Phytomedicine* 7, no. 5 (2000): 365–71.

De Bock, K., et al. Acute Rhodiola rosea intake can improve endurance exercise performance. *International Journal of Sport Nutrition and Exercise Metabolism* 14, no. 3 (2004): 298–307.

De Sanctis, R., et al. In vitro protective effect of Rhodiola rosea extract against hypochlorous acid-induced oxidative damage in human erythrocytes. *Biofactors* 20, no. 3 (2004): 147–59.

Dieamant, G. C., et al. Neuroimmunomodulatory compound for sensitive skin care: In vitro and clinical assessment. *Journal of Cosmetic Dermatology* 7, no. 2 (2008): 112–19.

Evdokimov, V. G., et al. Effect of cryopowder Rhodiola rosea L. on cardiorespiratory parameters and physical performance of humans. *Aviakosmicheskaia i Ekologicheskaia Meditsina* 43, no. 6 (2009): 52–56.

Evstatieva, L., et al. Chemical composition of the essential oils of Rhodiola rosea L. of three different origins. *Pharmacognosy Magazine* 6, no. 24 (2010): 256–58.

Fan, W., et al. Prolyl endopeptidase inhibitors from the underground part of Rhodiola sachalinensis. *Chemical and Pharmaceutical Bulletin* (Tokyo) 49, no. 4 (2001): 396–401.

Fintelmann, V., et al. Efficacy and tolerability of a Rhodiola rosea extract in adults with physical and cognitive deficiencies. *Advances in Therapy* 24, no. 4 (2007): 929–39.

Galambosi, B. Demand and availability of *Rhodiola rosea* L. raw material. Chapter 16 in *Medicinal and Aromatic Plants*, ed. R. J. Bogers et al., 223–36. Wageningen UR Frontis series, vol. 17. Springer, 2006.

Gao, D., et al. Antidiabetic potential of Rhodiola sachalinensis root extract in streptozotocin-induced diabetic rats. *Methods and Findings in Experimental and Clinical Pharmacology* 31, no. 6 (2009): 375–81.

Gauger, K. J., et al. Rhodiola crenulata inhibits the tumorigenic properties of invasive mammary epithelial cells with stem cell characteristics. *Journal of Medicinal Plants Research* 4, no. 6 (2010): 446–54.

Goel, H. C., et al. Radioprotection by Rhodiola imbricata in mice against whole-body lethal irradiation. *Journal of Medicinal Food* 9, no. 2 (2006): 154–60.

Grace, M. H., et al. Phytochemical characterization of an adaptogenic preparation from Rhodiola heterodonta. *Natural Products Communications* 4, no. 8 (2009): 1053–58.

Guest, Heidi. Molecular phylogeography of Rhodiola integrifolia (Crassulaceae) and its postglacial recolonization of north-western North America. Poster presented at the Botany 2006 conference at California State University at Chico, July 28–August 2, 2006, http://2006.botanyconference.org/engine/search/index.php?func=detail&aid=668.

Guest, Heidi. Systematic and phylogeographic implications of molecular variation in the western North American roseroot, Rhodiola integrifolia (Crassulaceae). Master's thesis, University of Victoria (British Columbia), 2001, http://hdl.handle.net/1828/2812.

Guo, Yibing. Synthesis, biological activity of salidroside and its analogues. *Chemical and*

Pharmaceutical Bulletin (Tokyo) 58, no. 12 (2010): 1627–29.

Gupta, A., et al. Effects of Rhodiola imbricata on dermal wound healing. *Planta Medica* 73, no. 8 (2007): 774–77.

Gupta, V., et al. Anti-oxidative effect of Rhodiola imbricata root extract in rats during cold, hypoxia and restraint (C-H-R) exposure and post-stress recovery. *Food and Chemical Toxicology* 48, no. 4 (2010): 1019–25.

Gupta, V., et al. A dose dependent adaptogenic and safety evaluation of Rhodiola imbricata Edgew, a high altitude rhizome. *Food and Chemical Toxicology* 46, no. 5 (2008): 1645–52.

Gupta, V., et al. Mechanism of action of Rhodiola imbricata Edgew during exposure to cold, hypoxia and restraint (C-H-R) stress induced hypothermia and post stress recovery in rats. *Food and Chemical Toxicology* 47, no. 6 (2009): 1239–45.

Ha, Z., et al. The effect of rhodiola and acetazolamide on the sleep architecture and blood oxygen saturation in men living at high altitude. *Zhonghua Jie He He Hu Xi Za Zhi* 25, no. 9 (2002): 527–30.

Hellum, B. H., et al. Potent in vitro inhibition of CYP3A4 and P-glycoprotein by Rhodiola rosea. *Planta Medica* 76, no. 4 (2010): 331–38.

Huang, S. C., et al. Attenuation of long-term Rhodiola rosea supplementation on exhaustive swimming-evoked oxidative stress in the rat. *Chinese Journal of Physiology* 52, no. 5 (2009): 316–24.

Hung, S. K., et al. The effectiveness and efficacy of Rhodiola rosea L.: A systematic review of randomized clinical trials. *Phytomedicine* 18, no. 4 (2011): 235–44. Published electronically ahead of print October 30, 2010.

Ip, Siu-Po, et al. Association of free radicals and the tissue renin-angiotensin system: Prospective effects of Rhodiola, a genus of Chinese herb, on hypoxia-induced pancreatic injury. *Journal of the Pancreas* 2, no. 1 (2001): 16–25.

Jafari, M., et al. *Rhodiola*: A promising anti-aging Chinese herb. *Rejuvenation Research* 10, no. 4 (2007): 587–602.

Jang, S. L. Salidroside from Rhodiola sachalinensis protects neuronal PC12 cells against cytotoxicity induced by amyloid-beta. *Immunopharmacology and Immunotoxicology* 25, no. 3 (2003): 295–304.

Jeong, H. J., et al. Neuraminidase inhibitory activities of flavonoids isolated from Rhodiola rosea roots and their in vitro anti-influenza viral activities. *Bioorganic & Medicinal Chemistry* 17, no. 19 (2009): 6816–23.

Kang, S., et al. Comparative study of the constituents from 10 Rhodiola plants. *Zhong Yao Cai* 20, no. 12 (1997): 616–18.

Kanupriya, et al. Cytoprotective and antioxidant activity of Rhodiola imbricata against tert-butyl hydroperoxide induced oxidative injury in U-937 human macrophages. *Molecular and Cellular Biochemistry* 275, no. 1–2 (2005): 1–6.

Kelly, G. S. *Rhodiola rosea*: A possible plant adaptogen. *Alternative Medicine Review* 6, no. 3 (2001): 293–302.

Khanum, F., et al. *Rhodiola rosea*: A versatile adaptogen. *Comprehensive Reviews in Food Science and Food Safety* 4 (2005): 55–62.

Kobayashi, K., et al. Constituents of Rhodiola rosea showing inhibitory effect on lipase activity in mouse plasma and alimentary canal. *Planta Medica* 74, no. 14 (2008): 1716–19.

Kormosh, N., et al. Effect of a combination of extract from several plants on cell-mediated and humoral immunity of patients with advanced ovarian cancer. *Phytotherapy Research* 20, no. 5 (2006): 424–25.

Kucinskaite, A., et al. Evaluation of biologically active compounds in roots and rhizomes of Rhodiola rosea L. cultivated in Lithuania. *Medicina* (Kaunas, Lithuania) 43, no. 6 (2007): 487–94.

Kucinskaite, A., et al. Experimental analysis of therapeutic properties of Rhodiola rosea L. and its possible application in medicine. *Medicina* (Kaunas, Lithuania) 40, no. 7 (2004): 614–19.

Kwon, Y. I., et al. Evaluation of Rhodiola crenulata and Rhodiola rosea for management of type II diabetes and hypertension. *Asia Pacific Journal of Clinical Nutrition* 15, no. 3 (2006): 425–32.

Laremiĭ, I. N., et al. Hepatoprotective properties of liquid extract of Rhodiola rosea. *Eksperimental'naia i Klinicheskaia Farmakologiia* 65, no. 6 (2002): 57–59.

Lee, F. T., et al. Chronic Rhodiola rosea extract supplementation enforces exhaustive swimming tolerance. *American Journal of Chinese Medicine* 37, no. 3 (2009): 557–72.

Lee, M. W., et al. Antioxidative phenolic compounds from the roots of Rhodiola sachalinensis A. Bor. *Archives of Pharmacal Research* 23, no. 5 (2000): 455–58.

Lei, Y., et al. Chemical composition of the essential oils of two Rhodiola species from Tibet. *Zeitschrift für Naturforschung C* 58, no. 3 (2003): 161–64.

Li, C., et al. Study on the extraction process for salidroside and p-tyrosol in Rhodiola crenulata. *Zhong Yao Cai* 29, no. 11 (2006): 1239–41.

Li, H. B., et al. Salidroside stimulated glucose uptake in skeletal muscle cells by activating AMP-activated protein kinase. *European Journal of Pharmacology* 588, no. 2–3 (2008): 165–69.

Li, H. X., et al. Production of Th1- and Th2-dependent cytokines induced by the Chinese medicine herb, Rhodiola algida, on human peripheral blood monocytes. *Journal of Ethnopharmacology* 123, no. 2 (2009): 257–66.

Li, J., et al. Effect of rhodiola on expressions of Flt-1, KDR and Tie-2 in rats with ischemic myocardium. *Zhongguo Zhong Xi Yi Jie He Za Zhi* 25, no. 5 (2005): 445–48.

Li, T., et al. Identification and comparative determination of rhodionin in traditional Tibetan medicinal plants of fourteen *Rhodiola* species by high-performance liquid chromatography-photodiode array detection and electrospray ionization-mass spectrometry. *Chemical and Pharmaceutical Bulletin* (Tokyo) 56, no. 6 (2008): 807–14.

Li, T., et al. Pharmacological studies on the sedative and hypnotic effect of salidroside from the Chinese medicinal plant Rhodiola sachalinensis. *Phytomedicine* 14, no 9 (2007): 601–4.

Li, X., et al. Bioactive constituents from Chinese natural medicines. XXIX. Monoterpene and monoterpene glycosides from the roots of Rhodiola sachalinensis. *Chemical and Pharmaceutical Bulletin* (Tokyo) 56, no. 4 (2008): 612–15.

Liu, Q., et al. Phenolic components from Rhodiola dumulosa. *Zhongguo Zhong Yao Za Zhi* 33, no. 4 (2008): 411–13.

Lovieno, N., et al. Second-tier natural antidepressants: Review and critique. *Journal of Affective Disorders* 130, no. 3 (2011): 343–57. Published electronically ahead of print June 26, 2010.

Luo, D., et al. Studies on the chemical constituents from Rhodiola dumulosa (I). *Zhong Yao Cai* 28, no. 2 (2005): 98–99.

Ma, G., et al. Rhodiolosides A-E, monoterpene glycosides from Rhodiola rosea. *Chemical and Pharmaceutical Bulletin* (Tokyo) 54, no. 8 (2006): 1229–33.

Majewska, A., et al. Antiproliferative and antimitotic effect, S phase accumulation and induction of apoptosis and necrosis after treatment of extract from Rhodiola rosea rhizomes on HL-60 cells. *Journal of Ethnopharmacology* 103, no. 1 (2006): 43–52.

Maslov, L. N., et al. Antiarrhythmic activity of phytoadaptogens in short-term ischemia-reperfusion of the heart and postinfarction cardiosclerosis. *Bulletin of Experimental Biology and Medicine* 147, no. 3 (2009): 331–34.

Maslova, L. V., et al. The cardioprotective and antiadrenergic activity of an extract of Rhodiola rosea in stress. *Eksperimental'naia i Klinicheskaia Farmakologiia* 57, no. 6 (1994): 61–63.

Mattioli, L., et al. Effects of Rhodiola rosea L. extract on behavioural and physiological alterations induced by chronic mild stress in female rats. *Journal of Psychopharmacology* 23, no. 2 (2009): 130–42. Abstract, online at http://jop.sagepub.com/content/23/2/130. abstract.

Mattioli, L., et al. Rhodiola rosea L. extract reduces stress- and CRF-induced anorexia in rats. *Journal of Psychopharmacology* 21, no. 7 (2007): 742–50.

Meng, L. Q., et al. Effection of observation Xinnaoxin capsules in treatment of chronic cerebral circulatory insufficiency. *Zhongguo Zhong Yao Za Zhi* 32, no. 17 (2007): 1798–800.

Ming, D. S., et al. Bioactive compounds from Rhodiola rosea (Crassulaceae). *Phytotherapy Research* 19, no. 9 (2005): 740–43.

Mishra, K. P., et al. Adjuvant effect of aqueous extract of Rhodiola imbricata rhizome on the immune responses to tetanus toxoid and ovalbumin in rats. *Immunopharmacology and Immunotoxicology* 32, no. 1 (2010): 141–46.

Mishra, K. P., et al. Aqueous extract of Rhodiola imbricata rhizome inhibits proliferation of an erythroleukemic cell line K-562 by inducing apoptosis and cell cycle arrest at G2/M phase. *Immunobiology* 213, no. 2 (2008): 125–31.

Mishra, K. P., et al. Aqueous extract of Rhodiola imbricata rhizome stimulates proinflammatory mediators via phosphorylated IkappaB and transcription factor nuclear factor-kappaB. *Immunopharmacology and Immunotoxicology* 28, no. 2 (2006): 201–12.

Mishra, K. P., et al. Aqueous extract of Rhodiola imbricata rhizome stimulates Toll-like receptor 4, granzyme-B and Th1 cytokines in vitro. *Immunobiology* 214, no. 1 (2009): 27–31.

Mook-Jung, I., et al. Neuroprotective effects of constituents of the Oriental crude drugs, Rhodiola sacra, R. sachalinensis and tokaku-joki-to, against beta-amyloid toxicity, oxidative stress and apoptosis. *Biological & Pharmaceutical Bulletin* 25, no. 8 (2002): 1101–4.

Moran, R. V. Rhodiola integrifolia. In *Flora of North America* 8, ed. Flora of North America Steering Committee, 164–66. New York and Oxford, 2009. www.efloras.org/florataxon. aspx?flora_id=1&taxon_id=250092043.

Morgan, M., and K. Bone. *Rhodiola rosea—Rhodiola. MediHerb Newsletter* 47 (2005): 1-4.

Nakamura, S., et al. Bioactive constituents from Chinese natural medicines. XXXVI. Chemical structures and hepatoprotective effects of constituents from roots of Rhodiola sachalinensis. *Chemical and Pharmaceutical Bulletin* (Tokyo) 55, no. 10 (2007): 1505–11.

Nakamura, S., et al. Bioactive constituents from Chinese natural medicines. XXXVIII. Chemical structures of acyclic glycosides from the roots of Rhodiola crenulata. *Chemical and Pharmaceutical Bulletin* (Tokyo) 56, no. 4 (2008): 536–40.

Narimanian, M., et al. Impact of Chisan (ADAPT-232) on the quality-of-life and its efficacy as an adjuvant in the treatment of acute non-specific pneumonia. *Phytomedicine* 12, no. 10 (2005): 723–29.

Olsson, E. M., et al. A randomized, double-blind, placebo-controlled, parallel-group study of the standardized extract shr-5 of the roots of Rhodiola rosea in the treatment of subjects with stress-related fatigue. *Planta Medica* 75, no. 2 (2009): 105–12.

Pae, H. O., et al. Rhodiola sachalinesis induces the expression of inducible nitric oxide synthase gene by murine fetal hepatocytes (BNL CL.2). *Immunopharmacology and Immunotoxicology* 23, no. 1 (2001): 25–33.

Panossian, A., et al. Comparative study of Rhodiola preparations on behavioral despair of rats. *Phytomedicine* 15, no. 1–2 (2008): 84–91.

Panossian, A., et al. Evidence-based efficacy of adaptogens in fatigue, and molecular mechanisms related to their stress-protective activity. *Current Clinical Pharmacology* 4, no. 3 (2009): 198–219.

Panossian, A., et al. Rosenroot (Rhodiola rosea): Traditional use, chemical composition, pharmacology and clinical efficacy. *Phytomedicine* 17, no. 7 (2010): 481–93.

Parisi, A., et al. Effects of chronic Rhodiola rosea supplementation on sport performance and antioxidant capacity in trained male: Preliminary results. *Journal of Sports Medicine and Physical Fitness* 50, no. 1 (2010): 57–63.

Pashkevich, I. A., et al. Comparative evaluation of effects of p-tyrosol and Rhodiola rosea extract on bone marrow cells in vivo. *Eksperimental'naia i Klinicheskaia Farmakologiia* 66, no. 4 (2003): 50–52.

Peng, J. N., et al. Chemical constituents of Rhodiola kirilowii (Regel) Regel. *Zhongguo Zhong Yao Za Zhi* 19, no. 11 (1994): 676–77, 702.

Peng, J. N., et al. Studies on the chemical constituents of Rhodiola fastigita. *Yao Xue Xue Bao* 31, no. 10 (1996): 798–800.

Pererva, T. P., et al. Interaction of Ungernia victoris, Rhodiola rosea and Polyscias filicifolia plant extracts with bacterial cells. *Tsitologiia i Genetika* 44, no. 4 (2010): 34–40.

Perfumi, M., et al. Adaptogenic and central nervous sytem effects of single doses of 3% rosavin and 1% salidroside Rhodiola rosea L. extract in mice. *Phytotherapy Research* 21, no. 1 (2007): 37–43.

Pickut, W. The uses of the Rhodiola integrifolia herb. LIVESTRONG.com, July 13, 2010, www.livestrong.com/article/173782-the-uses-of-the-rhodiola-integrifolia-herb/.

Platikanov, S., et al. Introduction of wild golden root (Rhodiola rosea L.) as a potential economic crop in Bulgaria. *Economic Botany* 20, no. 10 (2008): 1–7.

Pooja, et al. Anti-inflammatory activity of Rhodiola rosea — "a second-generation adaptogen." *Phytotherapy Research* 23, no. 8 (2009): 1099–102.

Qin, Y. J., et al. Effects of Rhodiola rosea on level of 5-hydroxytryptamine, cell proliferation and differentiation, and number of neuron in cerebral hippocampus of rats with depression induced by chronic mild stress. *Zhongguo Zhong Yao Za Zhi* 33, no. 23 (2008): 2842–46.

Qu, Z. Q., et al. Pretreatment with Rhodiola rosea extract reduces cognitive impairment induced by intracerebroventricular streptozotocin in rats: Implications of anti-oxidative and neuroprotective effects. *Biomedical and Environmental Sciences* 22, no. 4 (2009): 318–26.

Rohloff, J., et al. Volatiles from rhizomes of Rhodiola rosea L. *Phytochemistry* 59, no. 6 (2002): 655–61.

Ruan, X., et al. Analysis on the trace element and amino acid content in xinjiang 6 series Rhodiola L. plant. *Guang Pu Xue Yu Guang Pu Fen Xi* 21, no. 4 (2001): 542–44.

Schittko, U., et al. Rhodiola integrifolia: Hybrid origin and medicinal ancestry. *Proceedings of the North Dakota Academy of Science*, April 1, 2008.

Schriner, S. E., et al. Decreased mitochondrial superoxide levels and enhanced protection against paraquat in Drosophila melanogaster supplemented with Rhodiola rosea. *Free Radical Research* 43, no. 9 (2009): 836–43.

Schriner, S. E., et al. Protection of human cultured cells against oxidative stress by Rhodiola rosea without activation of antioxidant defenses. *Free Radic Biology & Medicine* 47, no. 5 (2009): 577–84.

Schutgens, F. W., et al. The influence of adaptogens on ultraweak biophoton emission: A pilot-experiment. *Phytotherapy Research* 23, no. 8 (2009): 1103–8.

Seikou, N., et al. Bioactive constituents from Chinese natural medicines. XXVI. Chemical structures and hepatoprotective effects of constituents from roots of *Rhodiola sachalinensis*. *Chemical and Pharmaceutical Bulletin* (Tokyo) 55, no. 10 (2007): 1505–11.

Seo, W. G., et al. The aqueous extract of Rhodiola sachalinensis root enhances the expression of inducible nitric oxide synthase gene in RAW264.7 macrophages. *Journal of Ethnopharmacology* 76, no. 1 (2001): 119–23.

Shen, W., et al. Effects of rhodiola on expression of vascular endothelial cell growth factor and angiogenesis in aortic atherosclerotic plaque of rabbits. *Zhongguo Zhong XI Yi Jie He Za Zhi* 28, no. 11 (2008): 1022–25.

Shevtsov, V. A., et al. A randomized trial of two different doses of a SHR-5 Rhodiola rosea extract versus placebo and control of capacity for mental work. *Phytomedicine* 19, no. 2–3 (2003): 95–105.

Shi, C. D., et al. Automatic nervous system mediates the cardiovascular effects of Rhodiola sacra radix in rats. *Journal of Ethnopharmacology* 119, no. 2 (2008): 284–90.

Shim, C., et al. Isolation and identification of antimicrobial active substances from Rhodiola sachlinensis. *Korean Journal of Food Preservation* 11, no. 1 (2004): 63–70.

Skopinska-Rózewska, E., et al. The effect of Rhodiola quadrifida extracts on cellular immunity in mice and rats. *Polish Journal of Veterinary Sciences* 11, no. 2 (2008): 105–11.

Skopinska-Rózewska, E., et al. The influence of Rhodiola quadrifida 50% hydro-alcoholic extract and salidroside on tumor-induced angiogenesis in mice. *Polish Journal of Veterinary Sciences* 11, no. 2 (2008): 97–104.

Smith, H. I. Materia medica of the Bella Coola and neighboring tribes of British Columbia. In *Annual Report for 1927*, bulletin no. 56 of the Canada Department of Mines National Museum of Canada Bulletin, 47–68. Ottawa: F. A. Acland, 1929. Reproduced online at http://wolf.mind.net/swsbm/Ethnobotany/Bella_Coola_Materia_Medica.pdf.

Spasov, A. A., et al. A double-blind, placebo-controlled pilot study of the stimulating and adaptogenic effect of Rhodiola rosea SHR-5 extract on the fatigue of students caused by stress during an examination period with a repeated low-dose regimen. *Phytomedicine* 7, no. 2 (2000): 85–89.

Spasov, A. A., et al. The effect of the preparation rodakson on the psychophysiological and physical adaptation of students to an academic load. *Eksperimental'naia i Klinicheskaia Farmakologiia* 63, no. 1 (2000): 76–78.

Tan, C. B., et al. Protective effect of salidroside on endothelial cell apoptosis induced by cobalt chloride. *Biological & Pharmaceutical Bulletin* 32, no. 8 (2009): 1359–63.

Tolonen, A., et al. Phenylpropanoid glycosides from Rhodiola rosea. *Chemical and Pharmaceutical Bulletin* (Tokyo) 51, no. 4 (2003): 467–70.

Tu, Y., et al. Rhodiola crenulata induces death and inhibits growth of breast cancer cell lines. *Journal of Medicinal Food* 11, no. 3 (2008): 413–23.

van Diermen, D., et al. Monoamine oxidase inhibition by Rhodiola rosea L. roots. *Journal of Ethnopharmacology* 122, no. 2 (2009): 397–401.

Walker, T. B., et al. Does Rhodiola rosea possess ergogenic properties? *International Journal of Sport Nutrition and Exercise Metabolism* 16, no. 3 (2006): 305–15.

Wang, H., et al. The in vitro and in vivo antiviral effects of salidroside from Rhodiola rosea L. against Coxsackievirus B3. *Phytomedicine* 16, no. 2–3 (2009): 146–55.

Wang, Q., et al. Salidroside protects the hypothalamic-pituitary-gonad axis of male rats undergoing negative psychological stress in experimental navigation and intensive exercise. *Zhonghua Nan Ke Xue* 15, no. 4 (2009): 331–36.

Wiedenfeld, H., et al. Phytochemical and analytical studies of extracts from *Rhodiola rosea* and *Rhodiola quadrifida*. *Pharmazie* 62, no. 4 (2007): 308–11.

Wójcik, R., et al. The effect of Chinese medicinal herb Rhodiola kirilowii extracts on cellular immunity in mice and rats. *Polish Journal of Veterinary Sciences* 12, no. 3 (2009): 399–405.

Wong, Y. C., et al. Chemical constituents and anti-tuberculosis activity of root of Rhodiola kirilowii. *Zhongguo Zhong Yao Za Zhi* 33, no. 13 (2008): 1561–65.

Wu, T., et al. Cardioprotection of salidroside from ischemia/reperfusion injury by increasing N-acetylglucosamine linkage to cellular proteins. *European Journal of Pharmacology* 613, no. 1–3 (2009): 93–99.

Wu, Y. L., et al. Hepatoprotective effects of salidroside on fulminant hepatic failure induced by D-galactosamine and lipopolysaccharide in mice. *Journal of Pharmacy and Pharmacology* 61, no. 10 (2009): 1375–82.

Xu, K. J., et al. Preventive and treatment effect of composite Rhodiolae on acute lung injury in patients with severe pulmonary hypertension during extracorporeal circulation. *Zhongguo Zhong Xi Yi Jie He Za Zhi* 23, no. 9 (2003): 648–50.

Yan, X., et al. Seasonal variations in biomass and salidroside content in roots of Rhodiola sachalinensis as affected by gauze and red film shading. *Ying Yong Sheng Tai Xue Bao* 15, no. 3 (2004): 382–86.

Yang, Y., et al. Lignans from the root of Rhodiola crenulata. *Journal of Agricultural and Food Chemistry* 60, no. 4 (2012): 964–72.

Yoshikawa, M., et al. Bioactive constituents of Chinese natural medicines. II. Rhodiolae radix. (1). Chemical structures and antiallergic activity of rhodiocyanosides A and B from the underground part of Rhodiola quadrifida (Pall.) Fisch. et May. (Crassulaceae). *Chemical and Pharmaceutical Bulletin* (Tokyo) 44, no. 11 (1996): 2086–91.

Yoshikawa, M., et al. Bioactive constituents of Chinese natural medicines. IV. Rhodiolae radix. (2). On the histamine release inhibitors from the underground part of Rhodiola sacra (Prain ex Hamet) S. H. Fu (Crassulaceae): Chemical structures of rhodiocyanoside D and sacranosides A and B. *Chemical and Pharmaceutical Bulletin* (Tokyo) 45, no. 9 (1997): 1498–503.

Yoshikawa, M., et al. Rhodiocyanosides A and B, new antiallergic cyanoglycosides from Chinese natural medicine "si lie hong jing tain," the underground part of Rhodiola quadrifida (Pall.) Fisch. et Mey. *Chemical and Pharmaceutical Bulletin* (Tokyo) 43, no. 7 (1995): 1245–47.

Yousef, G. G., et al. Comparative phytochemical characterization of three *Rhodiola* species. *Phytochemistry* 67 (2006): 2380–91.

Yu, S., et al. Involvement of ERK1/2 pathway in neuroprotection by salidroside against hydrogen peroxide-induced apoptotic cell death. *Journal of Molecular Neuroscience* 40, no. 3 (2010): 321–31.

Yu, S., et al. Neuroprotective effects of salidroside in the PC12 cell model exposed to hypoglycemia and serum limitation. *Cellular and Molecular Neurobiology* 28, no. 8 (2008): 1067–78.

Zhang, J., et al. Salidroside protects cardiomyocyte against hypoxia-induced death: A HIF-1alpha-activated and VEGF-mediated pathway. *European Journal of Pharmacology* 607, no. 1–3 (2009): 6–14.

Zhang, L., et al. Neuroprotective effects of salidroside against beta-amyloid-induced oxidative stress in SH-SY5Y human neuroblastoma cells. *Neurochemistry International* 57, no. 5 (2010): 547–55.

Zhang, L., et al. Protective effects of salidroside on hydrogen peroxide-induced apoptosis in SH-SY5Y human neuroblastoma cells. *European Journal of Pharmacology* 564, no. 1–3 (2007): 18–25.

Zhang, S., et al. Early use of Chinese drug rhodiola compound for patients with post-trauma amd inflammation in prevention of ALI/ARDS. *Zhonghua Wai Ke Za Zhi* 37, no. 4 (1999): 238–40.

Zhang, S., et al. Extraction of flavonoids from Rhodiola sachalinesis A. Bor by UPE and the antioxidant activity of its extract. *Natural Product Research* 22, no. 2 (2008): 178–87.

Zhang, W. S., et al. Protective effects of salidro-side on injury induced by hypoxia/hypoglyce-mia in cultured neurons. *Zhongguo Zhong Yao Za Zhi* 29, no. 5 (2004): 459–62.

Zhang, Z., et al. The effect of Rhodiola capsules on oxygen consumption of myocardium and coronary artery blood flow in dogs. *Zhongguo Zhong Yao Za Zhi* 23, no. 2 (1998): 104–6.

Zhao, H. W., et al. Rhodiola sacra aqueous extract (RSAE) improves biochemical and sperm characteristics in cryopreserved boar semen. *Theriogenology* 71, no. 5 (2009): 849–57.

Zhou, X., et al. Rhodiola sachalinensis sup-presses T241 fibrosarcoma tumor cells prolif-eration in vitro and growth in vivo. *Zhong Yao Cai* 31, no. 9 (2008): 1377–80.

Zhou, X., et al. Salidroside production by hairy roots of Rhodiola sachalinensis obtained after transformation with Agrobacterium rhizogenes. *Biological & Pharmaceutical Bulletin* 30, no. 3 (2007): 439–42.

Zhu, B. W., et al. Reduction of noise-stress-induced physiological damage by radices of Astragali and Rhodiolae: Glycogen, lactic acid and cholesterol contents in liver of the rat. *Bioscience, Biotechnology, and Biochemistry* 67, no. 9 (2003): 1930–36.

Zhu, B. W., et al. Resistance imparted by tradi-tional Chinese medicines to the acute change of glutamic pyruvic transaminase, alkaline phosphatase and creatine kinase activi-ties in rat blood caused by noise. *Bioscience, Biotechnology, and Biochemistry* 68, no. 5 (2004): 1160–63.

Zhu, L., et al. Prevention of rhodiola-astragalus membranaceus compounds against simulated plateau hypoxia brain injury in rat. *Space Medicine and Medical Engineering* (Beijing) 18, no. 4 (2005): 303–5.

Zhuravlev, Y. N., et al. Medicinal plants of the Kurile Islands. *Botanical News from the Russian Far East* 2 (2005): 1–2.

Zubeldia, J. M., et al. Exploring new applications for Rhodiola rosea: Can we improve the qual-ity of life of patients with short-term hypo-thyroidism induced by hormone withdrawal? *Journal of Medicinal Food* 13, no. 6 (2010): 1287–92.

Zuo, G., et al. Activity of compounds from Chinese herbal medicine Rhodiola kirilowii (Regel) Maxim against HCV NS3 serine protease. *Antiviral Research* 76, no. 1 (2007): 86–92.

INDEX

Other Storey Titles
You Will Enjoy

ADHD Alternatives by Aviva and Tracy Romm

A guide to parents and educators to taking a more holistic, natural, and effective approach to the problems of attention, impulsivity, and hyperactivity.
160 pages. Paper. ISBN 978-1-58017-248-6.

Healthy Bones & Joints by David Hoffmann

An introduction to a natural approach to treating arthritis, osteoporosis, and other diseases of the bones and joints.
128 pages. Paper. ISBN 978-1-58017-253-0.

Herbs for Hepatitis C and the Liver by Stephen Harrod Buhner

Important information and practical guidance for protecting the liver and strengthening the immune system.
160 pages. Paper. ISBN 978-1-58017-255-4.

Homegrown Herbs by Tammi Hartung

A complete guide to growing, using, and enjoying more than 100 herbs.
256 pages. Paper. ISBN 978-1-60432-703-6.

Rosemary Gladstar's Medicinal Herbs: A Beginner's Guide

How to grow, harvest, prepare, and use 33 of the most common and versatile healing plants.
408 pages. Paper. ISBN 978-1-60342-078-5.

Rosemary Gladstar's Herbal Recipes for Vibrant Health

A practical compendium of herbal lore and know-how for wellness, longevity, and boundless energy.
224 pages. Paper. ISBN 978-1-61212-005-8.

By the Same Author

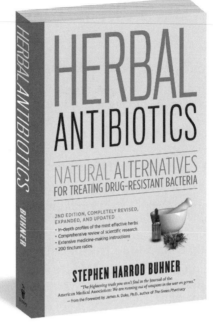

480 pages. Paper. ISBN 978-1-60342-987-0.

Praise for Stephen Harrod Buhner's *Herbal Antibiotics*

"In this timely book, Buhner reveals that plants are people's medicine, possessing attributes that pharmaceuticals never will."

— Taste for Life *magazine*

"A comprehensive introduction worthy to be on the shelf of any holistic practitioner, herbalist, farmer or parent. The book . . . shows an appreciation for the melding of traditional practices, tools, and wisdom with modern research and insight."

— Wise Traditions in Food, Farming, and the Healing Arts, the quarterly magazine of the Weston A. Price Foundation

"Buhner correlates the latest research and identifies the plant sources that are most effective in combating virulent new strains of antibiotic-resistant bacteria."

— American Free Press